Nutritional Value of Meat and Meat Products and Their Role in Human Health

Nutritional Value of Meat and Meat Products and Their Role in Human Health

Editor

Joanna Stadnik

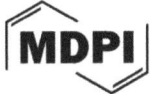

Basel • Beijing • Wuhan • Barcelona • Belgrade • Novi Sad • Cluj • Manchester

Editor
Joanna Stadnik
Department of Animal Food
Technology, Faculty of Food
Science and Biotechnology,
University of Life Sciences in
Lublin
Lublin
Poland

Editorial Office
MDPI AG
Grosspeteranlage 5
4052 Basel, Switzerland

This is a reprint of articles from the Special Issue published online in the open access journal *Nutrients* (ISSN 2072-6643) (available at: https://www.mdpi.com/journal/nutrients/special_issues/Nutritional_Value_Meat_Human_Health).

For citation purposes, cite each article independently as indicated on the article page online and as indicated below:

Lastname, A.A.; Lastname, B.B. Article Title. *Journal Name* **Year**, *Volume Number*, Page Range.

ISBN 978-3-7258-1755-9 (Hbk)
ISBN 978-3-7258-1756-6 (PDF)
doi.org/10.3390/books978-3-7258-1756-6

© 2024 by the authors. Articles in this book are Open Access and distributed under the Creative Commons Attribution (CC BY) license. The book as a whole is distributed by MDPI under the terms and conditions of the Creative Commons Attribution-NonCommercial-NoDerivs (CC BY-NC-ND) license.

Contents

About the Editor vii

Joanna Stadnik
Nutritional Value of Meat and Meat Products and Their Role in Human Health
Reprinted from: *Nutrients* **2024**, *16*, 1446, doi:10.3390/nu16101446 1

Gavin Connolly and Wayne W. Campbell
Poultry Consumption and Human Cardiometabolic Health-Related Outcomes: A Narrative Review
Reprinted from: *Nutrients* **2023**, *15*, 3550, doi:10.3390/nu15163550 5

Paulina Kęska, Joanna Stadnik, Aleksandra Łupawka and Agata Michalska
Novel α-Glucosidase Inhibitory Peptides Identified In Silico from Dry-Cured Pork Loins with Probiotics through Peptidomic and Molecular Docking Analysis
Reprinted from: *Nutrients* **2023**, *15*, 3539, doi:10.3390/nu15163539 29

Andrea Turnes, Paula Pereira, Helena Cid and Ana Valente
Meat Consumption and Availability for Its Reduction by Health and Environmental Concerns: A Pilot Study
Reprinted from: *Nutrients* **2023**, *15*, 3080, doi:10.3390/nu15143080 46

Clara S. Lau, Victor L. Fulgoni III, Mary E. Van Elswyk and Shalene H. McNeill
Trends in Beef Intake in the United States: Analysis of the National Health and Nutrition Examination Survey, 2001–2018
Reprinted from: *Nutrients* **2023**, *15*, 2475, doi:10.3390/nu15112475 59

Sanjiv Agarwal and Victor L. Fulgoni III
Association of Pork (All Pork, Fresh Pork and Processed Pork) Consumption with Nutrient Intakes and Adequacy in US Children (Age 2–18 Years) and Adults (Age 19+ Years): NHANES 2011–2018 Analysis
Reprinted from: *Nutrients* **2023**, *15*, 2293, doi:10.3390/nu15102293 76

Jean-Pierre Chouraqui
Risk Assessment of Micronutrients Deficiency in Vegetarian or Vegan Children: Not So Obvious
Reprinted from: *Nutrients* **2023**, *15*, 2129, doi:10.3390/nu15092129 88

Sanjiv Agarwal, Kathryn R. McCullough and Victor L. Fulgoni III
Nutritional Effects of Removing a Serving of Meat or Poultry from Healthy Dietary Patterns—A Dietary Modeling Study
Reprinted from: *Nutrients* **2023**, *15*, 1717, doi:10.3390/nu15071717 103

Kellie E. Mayfield, Julie Plasencia, Morgan Ellithorpe, Raeda K. Anderson and Nicole C. Wright
The Consumption of Animal and Plant Foods in Areas of High Prevalence of Stroke and Colorectal Cancer
Reprinted from: *Nutrients* **2023**, *15*, 993, doi:10.3390/nu15040993 117

Hikaru Takeuchi and Ryuta Kawashima
Nutrients and Dementia: Prospective Study
Reprinted from: *Nutrients* **2023**, *15*, 842, doi:10.3390/nu15040842 128

Victoria C. Wilk, Michelle K. McGuire and Annie J. Roe
Early Life Beef Consumption Patterns Are Related to Cognitive Outcomes at 1–5 Years of Age: An Exploratory Study
Reprinted from: *Nutrients* **2022**, *14*, 4497, doi:10.3390/nu14214497 . . . . **146**

Alessandro Dal Bosco, Alice Cartoni Mancinelli, Gaetano Vaudo, Massimiliano Cavallo, Cesare Castellini and Simona Mattioli
Indexing of Fatty Acids in Poultry Meat for Its Characterization in Healthy Human Nutrition: A Comprehensive Application of the Scientific Literature and New Proposals
Reprinted from: *Nutrients* **2022**, *14*, 3110, doi:10.3390/nu14153110 . . . . **160**

About the Editor

Joanna Stadnik

Prof. dr hab. Joanna Stadnik has been employed at the Faculty of Food Science and Biotechnology, University of Life Sciences in Lublin (ULSL), since 2004. She has worked as a full professor at the Department of Meat Technology and Food Quality since 2019. She also servs as the President of the Polish Food Technologists' Society. Her scientific interests focuses mainly on the use of probiotic bacteria in the production of dry cured meats, and in particular on their impact on proteolytic transformations and the formation of biogenic amines in the products. She also conducted research on the peptidegenic potential of muscle proteins in silico and in vitro, in which the potential of proteins (sarcoplasmic and myofibrillar) of dry cured meats as precursors of biologically active peptides under conditions of simulated digestion and absorption in the gastrointestinal tract was determined. She is the author and co-author of more than 150 scientific publications. She managed the project funded by the National Science Centre (Decarboxylating activity of selected strains of lactic acid bacteria in model systems) and Ministry of Science and Higher Education (Food production and packaging systems ensuring the preservation of its bioactive compounds important in the prevention of lifestyle diseases) under the program Regional Initiative of Excellence. In 2010, she was awarded "IUFoST's Young Scientist Presentation Award" granted by The International Union of Food Science and Technology. Polish Academy of Sciences granted her award for a young active researcher (2012).

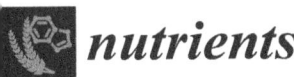 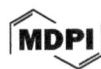

Editorial

Nutritional Value of Meat and Meat Products and Their Role in Human Health

Joanna Stadnik

Department of Animal Food Technology, Faculty of Food Science and Biotechnology, University of Life Sciences in Lublin, Skromna 8, 20-704 Lublin, Poland; joanna.stadnik@up.lublin.pl

Meat and meat products are among the most nutrient-dense food sources in the human diet. They fulfill most of our bodily requirements, acting as important sources of energy and a variety of essential nutrients, such as high-quality protein, several micronutrients (such as readily bioavailable iron, zinc, and selenium), vitamins (B6, B12, and folic acid), and bioactive compounds (taurine, carnitine, carnosine, ubiquinone, glutathione, and creatine) which are needed for a whole series of metabolic functions. Meat and meat products played a vital role in human evolution and are important components of a healthy and well-balanced diet [1–3]. The nutritional composition of meat and meat products differs depending on the cut, leanness, and processing level of the meat. Meat and meat products may also have other nutritive and non-nutritive components, such as sodium, saturated fat, nitrites, heterocyclic aromatic amines, and polycyclic aromatic hydrocarbons, which are associated with negative health-related outcomes. For this reason, frequent and excessive meat consumption, especially of red and processed meat (e.g., meat that is grilled, cured, or smoked), is currently a topic of scientific controversy, and there is a great deal of confusion as to the relationship between such consumption and adverse health outcomes, such as increased risk of cardiovascular diseases and multiple types of cancers, particularly colorectal cancer [4–8]. Moreover, concerns have also been raised regarding the environmental and climate-related effects of animal-sourced food production [9,10]. However, recommendations to limit or eliminate meat from our diets to minimize its environmental impacts present a broad spectrum of nutritional consequences, which vary by nutrient status, population, life course phase, and replacement food [3].

These matters are addressed in the Special Issue "Nutritional Value of Meat and Meat Products and Their Role in Human Health", which aims to present recent developments in the field of the nutritional value and health effects of meat and meat products.

Twenty-four manuscripts were submitted for consideration for this Special Issue of Nutrients, and all of them were subjected to the journal's rigorous peer-review process. In total, thirteen papers (nine research papers, two reviews, and two other papers) were accepted for publication and inclusion in this Special Issue. The contributions are listed below:

Contribution 1 evaluated alpha-glucosidase-inhibiting peptides obtained from dry-cured pork loins inoculated with probiotic/potentially probiotic strains of LAB. The most promising sequences (VATPPPPPPK, DIPPPPM, TPPPPPG, and TPPPPPPK) showed potential as antidiabetic agents.

Contribution 2 conducted a cross-sectional analytical study to assess the frequency of meat intake and willingness to reduce consumption on health and environmental grounds in residents of the Lisbon metropolitan region. The findings revealed that less frequent meat consumers were more amenable to reducing their meat consumption for environmental and health reasons than those who consumed meat more frequently.

Contribution 3 characterizes the consumption levels of total beef (i.e., any beef type) and individual beef types (fresh lean beef, ground beef, and processed beef) in Americans aged 2 years and older over an 18-year period using NHANES 2001–2018 data. The findings

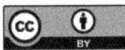

Citation: Stadnik, J. Nutritional Value of Meat and Meat Products and Their Role in Human Health. *Nutrients* **2024**, *16*, 1446. https://doi.org/10.3390/nu16101446

Received: 9 April 2024
Accepted: 22 April 2024
Published: 11 May 2024

Copyright: © 2024 by the author. Licensee MDPI, Basel, Switzerland. This article is an open access article distributed under the terms and conditions of the Creative Commons Attribution (CC BY) license (https://creativecommons.org/licenses/by/4.0/).

of the study indicate that beef consumption in children, adolescents, and adults declined, while consumption remained consistent in older adults. To date, no studies have evaluated beef-specific usual intake data on both a per capita and consumer basis.

The findings of this study were also mentioned in Contribution 13, in which the Authors emphasized the environmental effects of producing and consuming beef, and subsequent recommendations among expert bodies encouraged populations to reduce their red meat intake to support human and planetary health.

Contribution 4 investigated the relationship between pork intake (including fresh pork and processed pork) and overall nutrient intake, as well as the ability to meet nutrient recommendations in US children and adults, using the National Health and Nutrition Examination Survey (NHANES) 2011–2018. The research showed that pork intake was associated with higher intake and adequate amounts of certain key nutrients in children (age 2–18 years) and in adults (age 19+ years).

Contribution 5 assessed the potential unintended consequences of limiting meat and poultry by modeling the effect of removing a serving of meat/poultry on nutrient profiles of the Healthy Dietary Patterns (HDPs) identified in the Dietary Guidelines for Americans, 2020–2025, and assessed whether the modeled changes led to meaningful differences in intake. The results of this dietary modeling analysis show that removing a serving of meat or poultry could lead to decreases (10% or more from baseline) in protein and several key nutrients (iron, phosphorus, potassium, zinc, selenium, thiamine, riboflavin, niacin, vitamin B_6, vitamin B_{12}, and choline) as well as cholesterol and sodium in the HDPs.

Contribution 6 examined the association between Stroke Belt (eight southern U.S. states) residence and colorectal cancer incidence in relation to food consumption. This cross-sectional study found that Stroke Belt residency was associated with consuming greater quantities of meat, particularly red meat. The same associations were not observed for colorectal cancer quartiles and meat consumption, nor were there any associations between state residency and healthy food consumption.

Contribution 7 aimed to reveal the association between the intake of 23 nutrients and the risk of dementia in a large cohort after adjusting for a wide range of confounding factors. A greater risk of dementia was associated with no alcohol intake (compared with moderate to higher intake), higher intake of total sugars and carbohydrates (compared with lower intake), the highest or lowest fat intake (compared with moderate intake), quintiles of highest or lowest magnesium intake (compared with the quintile of the second highest intake), and the highest protein intake (compared with moderate intake).

Contribution 8 explored early feeding practices related to the introduction of beef in the rural US west (Idaho); parental perceptions of beef as a first food; and associations between early dietary beef, protein, iron, zinc, and choline intake and child cognition at 1–5 years of age. The findings of the study indicate that higher intake of beef, zinc, and choline at 6–12 months was associated with better attention and inhibitory control at 3–5 years of age. The results of this study show that early-life beef consumption patterns are related to cognitive outcomes.

Contribution 9 defined the state of the art of lipid nutritional indexing in poultry meat and, on this basis, conceived three progressive indexes (QuantiN-3 Index; Healthy Fatty Indexes 1 and 2) that more effectively explore potential uses in the determination of nutritional properties by comparing two divergent poultry genotypes with different growth rates and meat traits.

In Contribution 10, the authors conducted a narrative literature analysis on poultry consumption and human cardiometabolic health-related outcomes. Nutritional profiles of commonly consumed poultry products, consumption trends, and dietary recommendations in the United States were described. The associations between (and effects of) poultry consumption on body composition and body weight, type II diabetes mellitus, and cardiovascular disease were discussed.

Contribution 11 narratively reviewed the most recent literature on the relevance of micronutrient deficiency risk in vegetarian or vegan children based on the available data. It primarily focused on their intake of iron, zinc, iodine, and vitamins B12 and D. The findings revealed a lack of well-designed studies to assert the risk of micronutrient deficiency in vegetarian children. The results of the study indicate a need for education, regular medical/dietic supervision, and individually assessed supplementation.

Contribution 12 responds to Contribution 13, stating that sustainability was outside the scope of Contribution 3. This research endeavored to provide objective data on beef intake trends using a publicly available database (i.e., National Health and Nutrition Examination Survey (NHANES)) in the context of the example patterns from the 2020–2025 Dietary Guidelines for Americans (DGA).

Overall, this Special Issue, "Nutritional Value of Meat and Meat Products and Their Role in Human Health", identifies several potential research opportunities and future directions:

- Comprehensive analysis of intake of individual meat types across all life stages is needed to evaluate the relationships between red and processed meat intake and disease risk and to support the development of evidence-based dietary advice.
- Public health interventions aimed at reducing diet-related health disparities should consider the confluence of location and meat consumption in the development of lifestyle behavior change strategies and targeting practices.
- Models are needed to help define what foods would need to be consumed in greater quantities to replace nutrients previously gained from consuming meat if it was removed from the diet.
- More data on the relationship between residing in a high stroke area, colorectal cancer incidence levels, and red meat and processed meat consumption are needed.
- The ways in which access to preventative medical care and healthcare professionals confounds poor dietary choices associated with chronic diseases should also be explored further.

In light of the success of this Special Issue, we are pleased to announce a second Special Issue on this topic, entitled "Nutritional Value of Meat and Meat Products and Their Role in Human Health-2nd Edition". We are seeking original research papers and reviews on the nutritional value and health effects of meat and meat products. We believe that this Special Issue will broaden the horizons of our knowledge on the role of meat and meat products in human health.

Acknowledgments: Thanks to all the authors and peer reviewers for their valuable contributions to this Special Issue "Nutritional Value of Meat and Meat Products and Their Role in Human Health". We would also like to express our gratitude to the Editorial Office involved in this Special Issue. Finally, we give special thanks to the special issue Editor.

Conflicts of Interest: The authors declare no conflict of interest.

List of Contributions:

1. Kęska, P.; Stadnik, J.; Łupawka, A.; Michalska, A. Novel α-Glucosidase Inhibitory Peptides Identified In Silico from Dry-Cured Pork Loins with Probiotics through Peptidomic and Molecular Docking Analysis. *Nutrients* **2023**, *15*, 3539. https://doi.org/10.3390/nu15163539.
2. Turnes, A.; Pereira, P.; Cid, H.; Valente, A. Meat Consumption and Availability for Its Reduction by Health and Environmental Concerns: A Pilot Study. *Nutrients* **2023**, *15*, 3080. https://doi.org/10.3390/nu15143080.
3. Lau, C.S.; Fulgoni, V.L., III; Van Elswyk, M.E.; McNeill, S.H. Trends in Beef Intake in the United States: Analysis of the National Health and Nutrition Examination Survey, 2001–2018. *Nutrients* **2023**, *15*, 2475. https://doi.org/10.3390/nu15112475.
4. Agarwal, S.; Fulgoni, V.L., III. Association of Pork (All Pork, Fresh Pork and Processed Pork) Consumption with Nutrient Intakes and Adequacy in US Children (Age 2–18 Years) and Adults (Age 19+ Years): NHANES 2011–2018 Analysis. *Nutrients* **2023**, *15*, 2293. https://doi.org/10.3390/nu15102293.

5. Agarwal, S.; McCullough, K.R.; Fulgoni, V.L., III. Nutritional Effects of Removing a Serving of Meat or Poultry from Healthy Dietary Patterns—A Dietary Modeling Study. *Nutrients* **2023**, *15*, 1717. https://doi.org/10.3390/nu15071717.
6. Mayfield, K.E.; Plasencia, J.; Ellithorpe, M.; Anderson, R.K.; Wright, N.C. The Consumption of Animal and Plant Foods in Areas of High Prevalence of Stroke and Colorectal Cancer. *Nutrients* **2023**, *15*, 993. https://doi.org/10.3390/nu15040993.
7. Takeuchi, H.; Kawashima, R. Nutrients and Dementia: Prospective Study. *Nutrients* **2023**, *15*, 842. https://doi.org/10.3390/nu15040842.
8. Wilk, V.C.; McGuire, M.K.; Roe, A.J. Early Life Beef Consumption Patterns Are Related to Cognitive Outcomes at 1–5 Years of Age: An Exploratory Study. *Nutrients* **2022**, *14*, 4497. https://doi.org/10.3390/nu14214497.
9. Dal Bosco, A.; Cartoni Mancinelli, A.; Vaudo, G.; Cavallo, M.; Castellini, C.; Mattioli, S. Indexing of Fatty Acids in Poultry Meat for Its Characterization in Healthy Human Nutrition: A Comprehensive Application of the Scientific Literature and New Proposals. *Nutrients* **2022**, *14*, 3110. https://doi.org/10.3390/nu14153110.
10. Connolly, G.; Campbell, W.W. Poultry Consumption and Human Cardiometabolic Health-Related Outcomes: A Narrative Review. *Nutrients* **2023**, *15*, 3550. https://doi.org/10.3390/nu15163550.
11. Chouraqui, J.-P. Risk Assessment of Micronutrients Deficiency in Vegetarian or Vegan Children: Not So Obvious. *Nutrients* **2023**, *15*, 2129. https://doi.org/10.3390/nu15092129.
12. Lau, C.S.; Fulgoni, V.L., III; Van Elswyk, M.E.; McNeill, S.H. Reply to Consavage Stanley, K.; Kraak, V.I. Comment on "Lau et al. Trends in Beef Intake in the United States: Analysis of the National Health and Nutrition Examination Survey, 2001–2018. *Nutrients* **2023**, *15*, 2475". *Nutrients* **2023**, *15*, 3936. https://doi.org/10.3390/nu15183936.
13. Consavage Stanley, K.; Kraak, V.I. Comment on Lau et al. Trends in Beef Intake in the United States: Analysis of the National Health and Nutrition Examination Survey, 2001–2018. *Nutrients* **2023**, *15*, 2475. *Nutrients* **2023**, *15*, 3935. https://doi.org/10.3390/nu15183935.

References

1. Klurfeld, D.M. Research gaps in evaluating the relationship of meat and health. *Meat Sci.* **2015**, *109*, 86–95. [CrossRef] [PubMed]
2. Pereira, P.M.; Vicente, A.F. Meat nutritional composition and nutritive role in the human diet. *Meat Sci.* **2013**, *93*, 586–592. [CrossRef]
3. Leroy, F.; Smith, N.W.; Adesogan, A.T.; Beal, T.; Iannotti, L.; Moughan, P.J.; Mann, N. The role of meat in the human diet: Evolutionary aspects and nutritional value. *Anim. Front.* **2023**, *13*, 11–18. [CrossRef]
4. Papier, K.; Fensom, G.K.; Knuppel, A.; Appleby, P.N.; Tong, T.Y.N.; Schmidt, J.A.; Travis, R.C.; Key, T.J.; Perez-Cornago, A. Meat consumption and risk of 25 common conditions: Outcome-wide analyses in 475,000 men and women in the UK Biobank study. *BMC Med.* **2021**, *19*, 53. [CrossRef] [PubMed]
5. Giromini, C.; Givens, D.I. Benefits and Risks Associated with Meat Consumption during Key Life Processes and in Relation to the Risk of Chronic Diseases. *Foods* **2022**, *11*, 2063. [CrossRef] [PubMed]
6. González, N.; Marquès, M.; Nadal, M.; Domingo, J.L. Meat consumption: Which are the current global risks? A review of recent (2010–2020) evidences. *Food Res. Int.* **2020**, *137*, 109341. [CrossRef] [PubMed]
7. Salter, A.M. The effects of meat consumption on global health. *Rev. Sci. Tech.* **2018**, *37*, 47–55. [CrossRef] [PubMed]
8. Zhao, Z.; Feng, Q.; Yin, Z.; Shuang, J.; Bai, Z.; Yu, P.; Guo, M.; Zhao, Q. Red and processed meat consumption and colorectal cancer risk: A systematic review and meta-analysis. *Oncotarget* **2017**, *8*, 83306. [CrossRef]
9. Gerber, P.J.; Steinfeld, H.; Henderson, B.; Mottet, A.; Opio, C.; Dijkman, J.; Falcucci, A.; Tempio, G. *Tackling Climate Change through Livestock: A Global Assessment of Emissions and Mitigation Opportunities*; Food and Agriculture Organization of the United Nations (FAO): Rome, Italy, 2013.
10. Herrero, M.; Gerber, P.; Vellinga, T.; Garnett, T.; Leip, A.; Opio, C.; Westhoek, H.J.; Thornton, P.K.; Olesen, J.; Hutchings, N.; et al. Livestock and greenhouse gas emissions: The importance of getting the numbers right. *Anim. Feed Sci. Technol.* **2011**, *166*, 779–782. [CrossRef]

Disclaimer/Publisher's Note: The statements, opinions and data contained in all publications are solely those of the individual author(s) and contributor(s) and not of MDPI and/or the editor(s). MDPI and/or the editor(s) disclaim responsibility for any injury to people or property resulting from any ideas, methods, instructions or products referred to in the content.

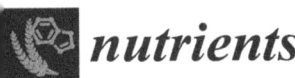

Review

Poultry Consumption and Human Cardiometabolic Health-Related Outcomes: A Narrative Review

Gavin Connolly and Wayne W. Campbell *

Department of Nutrition Science, Purdue University, West Lafayette, IN 47907, USA; connolg@purdue.edu
* Correspondence: campbeww@purdue.edu; Tel.: +1-(765)-494-8236

Abstract: Poultry meats, in particular chicken, have high rates of consumption globally. Poultry is the most consumed type of meat in the United States (US), with chicken being the most common type of poultry consumed. The amounts of chicken and total poultry consumed in the US have more than tripled over the last six decades. This narrative review describes nutritional profiles of commonly consumed chicken/poultry products, consumption trends, and dietary recommendations in the US. Overviews of the scientific literature pertaining to associations between, and effects of consuming chicken/poultry on, body weight and body composition, cardiovascular disease (CVD), and type II diabetes mellitus (T2DM) are provided. Limited evidence from randomized controlled trials indicates the consumption of lean unprocessed chicken as a primary dietary protein source has either beneficial or neutral effects on body weight and body composition and risk factors for CVD and T2DM. Apparently, zero randomized controlled feeding trials have specifically assessed the effects of consuming processed chicken/poultry on these health outcomes. Evidence from observational studies is less consistent, likely due to confounding factors such as a lack of a description of and distinctions among types of chicken/poultry products, amounts consumed, and cooking and preservation methods. New experimental and observational research on the impacts of consuming chicken/poultry, especially processed versions, on cardiometabolic health is sorely needed.

Keywords: chicken; turkey; protein; animal-based; animal protein; cardiovascular; type 2 diabetes mellitus; metabolic disease

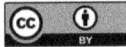

1. Introduction

Poultry meats, with chicken being the predominant type of poultry consumed, is the most consumed type of meat in the United States (US) [1]. Central to providing high-quality protein and other nutrients, poultry meats are generally considered as healthy [2]. Poultry meats, in particular chicken, are relatively affordable and easily accessible resulting in high rates of consumption globally [3] and in the US [1].

In 2022, we published a systematically searched scoping review pertinent to poultry intake and all facets of human health [4]. Among 13,141 articles identified, 525 met inclusion criteria. Among these 525 articles, 41 were on cardiovascular disease (CVD) morbidity and mortality; 52 on CVD risk factors; 32 on type II diabetes mellitus (T2DM) morbidity and mortality; 33 on T2DM risk factors; and 42 on body weight and body composition [4]. This scoping review did not present results described in the articles. The findings and articles included from the scoping review, along with more recently published articles, were used as a foundation for this narrative review on poultry consumption and human cardiometabolic health-related outcomes. Overviews of the scientific literature pertaining to associations between, and effects of consuming varying amounts and types of poultry on body weight and body composition, CVD, and T2DM are provided.

2. Nutritional Content of Chicken/Poultry

Chicken and other poultry meats provide macronutrients and micronutrients considered essential for human health and physiological functioning [5,6]. Essential nutrients are compounds the human body cannot make or cannot make in sufficient quantities and must be obtained via dietary sources. Chicken and other poultry-based proteins, like all other animal-based proteins such as other meats, milk, and eggs, as well as plant-based soy protein, are considered high-quality complete protein sources [5]. These foods provide a full complement of all 20 amino acids and adequate quantities of the nine essential amino acids.

Chicken and other poultry products have varying energetic and nutrient profiles and do not naturally contain carbohydrates (Table 1). Chicken contains 23–31 g of protein per 100 g or 3.5 oz, depending on the cut of chicken. The total fat content can vary from 3.6–2.1 g per 100 g, or 3.5 oz, in the leanest cuts such as cooked skinless chicken breast and cooked skinless turkey breast, respectively, to 16.9 g per 100 g/3.5 oz in cooked chicken wings with the skin. For example, cooked skinless chicken and turkey breast have 19% and 13%, respectively, of total energy content from fat, while cooked chicken wings with skin have 60%. The proportion of total fat from saturated fat is consistently about 27–29% (1–5 g per 100 g serving) for various cuts of chicken. Monounsaturated and polyunsaturated fats are about 32–46% and 20–23% (1.2–7.7 g and 0.8–3.6 g per 100 g serving), respectively, of the total fat content for different cuts of chicken [7].

Chicken and other poultry products also provide essential nutrients that are commonly under-consumed, including the minerals magnesium, phosphorous, potassium, selenium, and iron, and the B-group vitamins including thiamin (B1), riboflavin (B2), niacin (B3), pantothenic acid (B5), pyridoxal (B6), cobalamin (B12), and choline [6]. Unprocessed chicken and other poultry products are naturally low in salt. Chicken and other poultry products can be purchased as fresh unprocessed cuts (no preservation techniques other than refrigeration or freezing) or as processed items preserved by smoking, curing, salting, and/or the addition of chemical preservatives [6,8]. As sodium is a common preservative added to chicken and other poultry products to prolong shelf life and/or as a flavor enhancer, processed chicken and other poultry products may contain high or very high amounts of sodium [5]. As such, the sodium content of unprocessed and processed chicken and other poultry products can vary from <100 mg per 100 g serving in fresh, cooked, cuts of chicken to >2000 mg per 100 g serving in turkey bacon. The process of curing meats utilizes both NaCl and a synthetic nitrate or nitrite salt to preserve meat by inhibiting bacterial growth [9]. Many processed poultry deli meats contain either synthetic nitrate or nitrite salts, or nitrates from natural sources such as celery root powder. The addition of these preservatives can catalyze the formation of carcinogens, notably nitrosyl heme, when added to meat products that contain heme iron [9].

Table 1. Nutrient contents of selected poultry products [Source: United States Department of Agriculture FoodData Central [7]].

Nutrient	Unprocessed Poultry Products								Values per 100 g Cooked Product				Processed Poultry Products			
	Chicken Breast, Skinless, Boneless, Roasted	Dark Chicken Meat, Skinless, Boneless, Roasted	Chicken Drumstick, Skinless, Boneless, Roasted	Chicken Drumstick, Skin-on	Chicken Thigh, Skinless	Chicken Thigh, Skin-on, Roasted	Chicken Wing, Skinless	Chicken Wing, Skin-on, Roasted	Ground Turkey, 93% Lean, 7% Fat, Pan-Broiled	Turkey Patty, 93%, 7% Fat, Broiled	Turkey patty, 85%, 15% fat, broiled		Chicken Nuggets, White Meat, Breaded, Precooked, Frozen	Chicken Tenders, Breaded, Precooked, Frozen	Chicken, Luncheon Meat	Turkey, Luncheon Meat
Calories (kcal)	165	205	155	191	179	232	203	254	213	207	249		261	240	98	106
Protein (g)	31.0	27.4	24.2	23.4	24.8	23.3	30.5	23.8	27.1	25.9	25.9		14.4	14.6	17.4	14.8
Total fat (g)	3.6	9.7	5.7	10.2	8.2	14.7	8.1	16.9	11.6	11.4	16.2		15.4	13.6	1.9	3.8
Saturated fat (g)	1.0	2.7	2.1	2.7	2.3	4.1	2.3	5.0	3.0	3.0	4.1		3.4	2.4	0.6	0.9
Monounsaturated fat (g)	1.2	3.6	3.1	4.2	3.4	6.3	2.6	7.7	3.8	3.9	5.5		4.7	4.1	0.7	1.1
Polyunsaturated fat (g)	0.8	2.3	1.6	2.1	1.7	3.0	1.8	3.6	3.5	3.5	4.2		6.2	6.2	0.5	1.0
Carbohydrates (g)	0.0	0.0	0.0	0.0	0.0	0.0	0.0	0.0	0.0	0.0	0.0		16.2	14.9	0.0	0.0
Cholesterol (mg)	85	93	128	130	133	133	85	141	104	106	105		34	36	51	49
Sodium (mg)	74	93	128	123	106	102	92	98	90	91	81		538	527	1032	898
Vitamin D (µg)	0.1	0.1	0.1	0.1	0.2	0.2	0.1	0.2	0.2	0.2	0.2		0.1	0.1	0.1	0.2
Calcium (mg)	15	15	11	11	9	9	16	18	31	29	48		38	39	11	14
Iron (mg)	1.0	1.3	1.1	1.1	1.1	1.1	1.2	0.8	1.6	1.7	2.0		1.4	0.8	0.4	0.4
Potassium (mg)	256	240	256	247	269	253	210	212	304	247	242		281	281	360	371
Vitamin B2 [riboflavin] (mg)	0.1	0.2	0.2	0.2	0.2	0.2	0.1	0.2	0.3	0.2	0		0.1	0.1	0.1	0.1
Vitamin B3 [niacin] (mg)	13.7	6.5	5.6	5.4	6.2	5.8	7.3	6.3	8.1	6.6	7		6.7	5.9	9.1	7.2
Vitamin B5 [pantothenic acid] (mg)	1.0	1.2	1.1	1.1	1.3	1.2	1.0	0.9	1.4	1.3	1		0.9	0.9	1.0	0.6
Vitamin B6 (mg)	0.6	0.4	0.4	0.4	0.5	0.4	0.6	0.6	0.5	0.5	0.4		0.3	0.3	0.4	0.4
Vitamin B12 (µg)	0.3	0.3	0.4	0.4	0.4	0.4	0.3	0.4	1.9	1.8	1.4		0.2	0.2	0.1	0.4
Phosphorus (mg)	228	179	205	200	230	216	166	147	259	210	235		213	200	257	249
Magnesium (mg)	29	23	24	22	24	22	21	19	29	25	25		35	29	26	19
Zinc (mg)	1.0	2.8	2.6	2.4	1.9	1.7	2.1	1.6	3.8	3.7	3.3		0.8	0.6	0.5	0.9
Selenium (µg)	27.6	18.0	25.2	28.1	27.1	25.3	24.7	25.5	28.4	27.5	35.1		17.0	19.3	13.2	13.0
Choline (mg)	85.3	74.0	63.4	67.8	71.8	67.6	79.6	111.3	78.7	77.7	79.1		45.5	46.1	44.2	30.1

3. Chicken and Poultry Consumption in the US

Chicken meat is the most consumed meat in the US per capita [1]. The US has the largest broiler chicken industry in the world and more chicken is consumed in the US than in any other country. In 2022, annual consumption of chicken and turkey in the US per capita was estimated to be 100.6 pounds (lb) and 14.7 lb, respectively, for a total of 115.3 lb of poultry. In comparison, annual consumption of beef and pork was 59.4 lb and 51.4 lb per capita, respectively, for a total of 111.3 lb of red meat. Total consumption of commercial fish and shellfish was 16.1 lb per capita (last reported in 2018) [1]. From 1960 to 2022, chicken and total poultry consumption steadily increased and more than tripled. In contrast, pork consumption remained stable and beef and total red meat intakes have decreased (Figure 1).

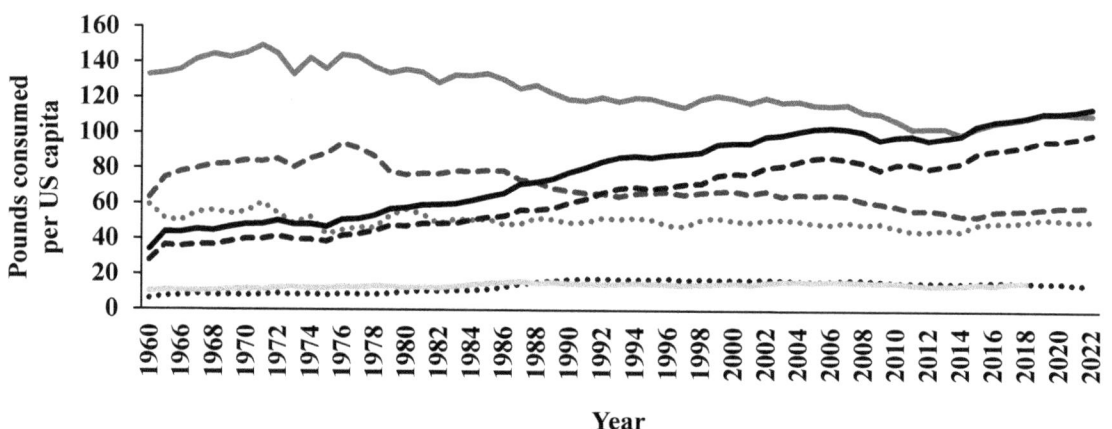

Figure 1. Pounds consumed per US capita for meats, fish, and shellfish from 1960 to 2022. Source: This figure was created using United States Department of Agriculture open-source data presented in tabular form by the National Chicken Council [1].

In the US, the National Health and Nutrition Examination Survey (NHANES) is a nationally representative sample of 5000 individuals per data collection period which assesses the health and nutritional status of adults and children. Based on NHANES data, protein intake is estimated to be 97 g/d and 67 g/d for males and females, respectively [10], which for both sexes equate to about 16% of total energy intake [11]. Animal-derived protein sources account for about two-thirds of total protein intake [10,12]. Based on an overall average intake of 83 g protein/d, poultry intake is estimated to be 12.5 g/d or 0.44 oz/d.

Although poultry was the top source of total dietary protein intake (10%), it ranked 6th for total dietary energy intake (<4%) [13]. More specifically, data from 2007 to 2010 indicate chicken whole pieces were the number one source of animal protein, accounting for 13.9% of total animal protein intake, 7.2% of total protein intake, and 2.8% of total energy intake. Turkey, duck, and other poultry ranked 17th, accounting for 1.9% of total animal protein intake, 0.9% of total protein intake, and 0.3% of total energy intake [10].

4. Dietary Guidance in the United States

The estimated average requirement (EAR) for total protein is 0.66 g/kg/d for men and women 19+ years of age The EAR is assumed to meet the protein requirement of 50% of the healthy adult population. The recommended dietary allowance (RDA) for total protein is 0.8 g/kg/d, which is two standard deviations above the EAR. The RDA is assumed to meet the protein needs of 97.5% of healthy adults 19+ years of age.

The Dietary Guidelines for Americans (DGA), updated and re-published every 5 years since 1980, serves as the evidence-based foundation for nutrition education by the US Federal Government to inform the development of food, nutrition, and health policies and programs. The intended audiences for the DGA are policymakers and health professionals. A primary focus of the DGA is disease prevention [6]. The 2020–2025 DGA states that "common characteristics of dietary patterns associated with positive health outcomes include relatively higher intakes of vegetables, fruits, legumes, whole grains, low- or non-fat dairy, lean meats and poultry, seafood, nuts, and unsaturated vegetable oils, and relatively lower consumption of red and processed meats, sugar-sweetened foods and beverages, and refined grains" [6].

The 2020–2025 DGA provides examples of three healthy dietary patterns. The three dietary patterns are the Healthy US-Style Dietary Pattern, the Healthy Mediterranean-Style Dietary Pattern, and the Healthy Vegetarian Dietary Pattern. In 2011, the DGA released the MyPlate icon to support the recommendations and translation of healthy dietary patterns. The MyPlate icon is a visual representation of a plate sectioned into the major food groups to aid individuals in choosing recommended amounts and types of healthy foods at mealtimes. The major food groups represented on the plate are vegetables, fruits, grains, and protein, accompanied by another circle for dairy.

Regarding the Protein Foods Group, the DGA provides guidance on protein foods from animal and plant sources in nutrient-dense forms, based on quantities measured in ounce-equivalents as defined by the United States Department of Agriculture [6,14]. The recommendation for protein foods in the Healthy US-Style Dietary Pattern at the 2000 kcal/d energy level is 5.5 ounce-equivalents of protein foods per day. The Protein Foods Group consists of meat (red), poultry, seafood, eggs, nuts and seeds (including nut and seed butters), legumes (beans and peas), and soy products (excluding calcium added soy milk assigned to the Dairy Group, and raw, green soybean assigned to the Vegetables Food Group) [6,14].

The Meat and Poultry components are further subdivided into Meat, Poultry, Organ Meat, and Cured Meat. The Meat component includes red meats such as beef, goat, lamb, pork (includes fresh or uncured ham), veal, and game meat (e.g., bear, bison, moose, opossum, rabbit, raccoon, squirrel, venison). The Poultry component includes chicken, Cornish hens, dove, duck, game birds (e.g., ostrich, pheasant, quail), goose, and turkey. The Cured Meat component includes cured or smoked meat products such as frankfurters, sausages, and luncheon meats, and cured meat made from beef, chicken, pork, and turkey. The Organ Meat component includes brain, chitterlings, giblets, gizzard, heart, kidney, stomach, sweetbreads, thymus, tongue, and tripe [14].

Supporting the 2020–2025 key health recommendations, individuals who consume omnivorous dietary patterns are encouraged to choose lean meats and animal products (<10 g of total fats and ≤4.5 g of saturated fats). Since processed meats and poultry (e.g., luncheon meats, bacon, sausages, beef jerky) are generally high sodium foods, limiting their intake will help meet the 2300 mg/d sodium intake recommendation [6]. Poultry (excluding deli and mixed dishes) contributes an estimated 4% of total saturated fat and 5% of sodium intakes in the US [6]. It is postulated that limiting red meat and poultry products high in saturated fat and sodium will be beneficial in limiting total energy, saturated fat, and sodium intakes. Currently, most of the US population consume these dietary components in excess [6]. The incorporation of lean, unprocessed chicken and other poultry products will provide individuals with high-quality sources of dietary protein and important nutrients, including heme-iron, selenium, and niacin, when consumed within energy requirements [6].

5. Experimental Approaches and Considerations When Studying the Influence of Poultry Intake on Human Health

5.1. Experimental Approaches

Both observational and experimental human trials provide valuable information regarding dietary choices and human health. However, findings from these studies do not always result in the same conclusions. Observational studies provide associations between a variable of interest and an outcome. These types of studies generally have large sample sizes, as they may be conducted at a population level, in highly diverse populations, and include long follow-up periods. While these observations can be insightful, potential confounding and uncontrolled variables preclude establishing a cause-and-effect relationship. Randomized controlled trials (RCTs) are generally considered the "gold standard" to assess a variable of interest and a specific outcome. In RCTs, participants are randomized to either an experimental intervention or a non-experimental or alternative intervention control group, and the outcome of interest is compared between groups. RCTs aim to keep as many variables—as is feasible—the same between groups, thereby reducing the risk of bias and the effects of confounding. Importantly, RCTs have relatively smaller sample sizes compared to observational studies. They also may lack generalizability and real-world application. Observational studies may assess endpoints, such as disease onset or death, whereas RCTs generally assess intermediary risk factors for disease [15]. For a more detailed description and comparison of these study designs, the reader may refer to articles addressing this topic by Hébert et al. [16], Booth and Tannock [17], Faraoni and Schaefer [18], and Barton [19].

Observational and experimental studies may be used to investigate the influences of individual nutrients, individual foods, or overall dietary patterns on human health [15]. Humans do not consume nutrients or foods in isolation, but within a dietary pattern dependent upon their available resources and/or personal preferences. This hierarchy of consumption—nutrients, foods, and patterns—will be applied in the following sections in addressing how chicken and/or other poultry consumption influence body weight and body composition, CVD, and T2DM. When limited evidence is available pertaining to chicken, we will supplement it with information pertaining to total poultry consumption. The definition of poultry included within this review is based on and consistent with the definition for the Poultry Food Group in the DGA 2020–2025; stating, "poultry includes chicken, Cornish hens, dove, duck, game birds (e.g., ostrich, pheasant, quail), goose, and turkey" [6].

5.2. Potential Explanatory Variables

Published research on poultry is complicated by the lack of a clear definition used among studies for poultry, a lack of reporting on whether the poultry products were unprocessed or processed, and cooking methods, all of which influence human health outcomes [20,21]. This is likely attributable to using food frequency questionnaires to assess dietary intake in observational studies [22] along with broad food categories [20,23].

5.2.1. Definitions

Poultry and health research is hampered by the lack of a clear definition used among studies. A 2020 systematic review and landscape analysis by O'Connor et al. [20], determined that of 52 identified studies assessing poultry consumption and health outcomes, only 63% provided a definition for poultry. In addition, poultry is often defined as "white meat", which may or may not also include fish and/or rabbit, or the definition of poultry includes rabbit. While "rabbit" should be considered a red meat, it is commonly included as poultry due to similarities in nutrition profiles [24,25]. These broad and inconsistent classifications make it problematic when trying to determine the influence of such foods on health outcomes. Classifying poultry, fatty fish, and lean fish, as "white meat" does not account for differences in nutritional profiles [23]. For example, fatty fish, which is higher in omega-3 fatty acids, have cardioprotective benefits [26]. The commonly used classification of "white meat" that includes fatty fish, lean fish, and poultry, may lead to the cardioprotective benefits of fatty fish being attributed to lean fish and poultry products. Adding to confusion, poultry contains both "white" and "dark" meat, which differ in macronutrient composition.

5.2.2. Processing

Processed meats, compared to unprocessed meats, contain high amounts of preservatives, such as sodium and nitrates. The sodium content of processed meats may be 400% higher than unprocessed meats, contributing to associations between processed meat intake and increased blood pressure [21,27]. Nitrates in processed meats may increase coagulation, inflammatory cytokines, and reactive oxygen species [28]. These indexes of endothelial cell dysfunction are involved in the process of atherosclerotic lesion manifestation and progression as well as increases in insulin resistance [29]. Heme-iron in meats increases oxidative stress and is associated with the atherosclerotic processes and cardiometabolic disease risk factors such as hypertension, hypercholesterolemia, endothelial dysfunction, insulin resistance, and T2DM [29–31]. Substituting white meats, especially unprocessed white meats, for red meats may reduce the risk of CVD [21] and all-cause mortality [32].

5.2.3. Cooking Methods

Varied cooking methods of poultry products introduce variability in the concentrations of non-nutritive compounds. Heterocyclic aromatic amines are formed in cooked meats through a reaction between amino acids, creatine, and sugars. Burned or charred meats have higher levels of heterocyclic aromatic amines and benzopyrene in comparison to meats cooked at a lower temperature or are not visibly blackened. Barbequed and grilled poultry products contain higher concentrations of heterocyclic aromatic amines than baked or boiled products. Polycyclic aromatic hydrocarbons are formed when cooking meat products at high temperatures, particularly during the process of smoking, grilling, roasting, and frying [10,11]. High-heat cooking methods, such as frying and grilling, produce higher amounts of advanced glycation end-products. Prior to and following cooking, these highly oxidant glycotoxins are found in greater amounts in animal-based meats compared to carbohydrate-based foods such as fruits, vegetables, and whole grains, and dairy products [12].

Advanced glycation end products are linked with increased insulin resistance and blood glucose concentrations [29]. These compounds can increase the risk of adverse cardiometabolic health-related outcomes, as they decrease the vascular endothelium response by a reduction in vasodilation and increased oxidative stress and inflammation [33,34]. The consumption of chicken cooked by open flame and/or high temperature has been associated with a 15% increased risk of T2DM [35]. Frying and the frequency of fried chicken consumption, has also been associated with increased CVD mortality in older-aged women in the WHI [36] and an increased incidence of T2DM in the Black Women's Health Study [37]. Along with advanced glycation end products, high-heat cooking methods, level of doneness, and processing of meats (which commonly use high-heat cooking methods) lead to the formation heterocyclic aromatic amines and polycyclic aromatic hydrocarbons, which are associated with an increased risk of CVD and T2DM [33].

6. Poultry Consumption and Body Weight and Body Composition

In the US, an estimated 73.6% of adults are classified as overweight (31.7%) or obese (41.9%) [38], while approximately 36% of children and adolescents aged 2–19 years are classified as overweight (16.6%) or obese (19.7%) [39]. Over a 20-year period (1999–2018) in the US, the prevalence of obesity and severe obesity have increased from 30.5% to 41.9%, and 4.7% to 9.2%, respectively [38]. Obesity may also lead to preventable and modifiable morbidities, such as CVD and T2DM, that are leading causes of premature death in the US and worldwide. Obesity comes with a large financial burden and obesity and obesity-related chronic diseases are a top priority for public health policy in the US. Obesity was estimated to cost the US at least $147 billion in direct medical costs in 2018 and another $4 billion in indirect costs, such as lost productivity. On an individual basis, people with obesity were estimated to have $1429 higher medical costs per year than people who were normal weight [40,41].

Diet and physical activity are two of the most effective ways to decrease the risk of or prevent overweight and obesity and related comorbidities [42–44]. Body weight and body composition are influenced by energy balance. Energy balance is determined by the relationship between energy intake via foods and beverages and energy expenditure via basal metabolic rate and the thermic effects of feeding and physical activity [42,45,46]. The relationship between energy intake and energy expenditure determines whether there is weight loss, weight maintenance, or weight gain [42,46]. Higher dietary protein intake, inclusive of chicken and/or other poultry products, may aid in weight control and favorable body composition changes, including decreased fat mass and/or increased lean body mass [47,48].

Evidence regarding weight management indicates the consumption of dietary protein and a higher protein diet can: (1) increase satiety; (2) increase thermogenesis; and (3) increase, maintain, or attenuate the loss of lean body mass [45,46,49,50]. The following sections document evidence from identified RCTs and observational studies specifically pertaining to chicken/poultry consumption on body mass and body composition.

6.1. RCTs

The available evidence from RCTs specific to chicken/poultry consumption and body weight or body composition, suggests chicken/poultry consumption has a neutral effect on body weight and body composition in the context of weight maintenance in adult men and women [51], and a favorable effect on body mass and body composition in the context of diet-induced weight loss in adult women classified as overweight [52] or with obesity [53]. Moreover, chicken protein in supplemental form in combination with resistance exercise training was beneficial for body composition changes in young adults [54].

A nine-month randomized cross-over trial by Murphy et al. [51] investigated the effects of regular consumption of pork, beef, or chicken on indices of adiposity via anthropometric and DEXA assessments. Forty-nine adults classified as overweight or obese were randomly assigned to consume five (for women) to seven (for men) 140–150 g per serving/week of pork, chicken, or lean beef by incorporating it into their habitual diets for the initial three-month period, followed by two more three-month periods consuming each of the alternative meats. There were no differences reported for energy or macronutrient intakes during each intervention period, indicating participants were substituting the meats in their diets without changing total energy or macronutrient intakes. The results showed no differences in body mass, BMI, any index of adiposity (% body fat, FM, abdominal fat, waist-to-hip ratio), or measures of lean mass among the pork, beef, or chicken diets. Consistent with the author's hypothesis, purposefully consuming known amounts of different meats (lean pork, chicken, or beef) did not influence body weight or body composition after each three-month intervention period [51].

In a 12-week RCT, 61 women characterized as obese, middle aged, and moderately physically active consumed individualized 500 kcal/d energy deficit diets with 20% of total energy intake primarily from lean beef versus lean chicken [53]. The diets were also designed to be equivalent in terms of total energy and percentage of energy from fat with the primary outcomes being bodyweight and body composition (assessed by hydrodensitometry). The beef and chicken groups each reduced body weight (-5.6 ± 0.6 kg and -6.0 ± 0.5 kg, respectively (mean $\pm$ standard error (SE)) and body fat ($-3.6 \pm 3.3\%$ and $-4.1 \pm 3.3\%$, respectively) from baseline to post-intervention, with no differences between groups [53].

Similarly, an RCT by Mahon et al. [52] investigated the effects of dietary protein intake on energy restriction-induced changes in body mass and body composition (assessed via DEXA) in 54 women classified as overweight and postmenopausal. For the nine-week intervention, three energy restricted groups consumed 1000 kcal/d of a lacto-ovo vegetarian base diet along with 250 kcal/d of either beef, chicken, or carbohydrate/fat foods; a non-interventional control group consumed their habitual diets. Energy intake was not different among the three energy restriction groups with total protein intake constituting 25% of total energy intake in the chicken and beef groups and 17% in the carbohydrate/fat group. Combined, the energy restricted groups decreased their body mass (-6.7 ± 2.4 kg; mean $\pm$ standard deviation (SD)), fat mass (-4.6 ± 1.9 kg, 13%), and fat-free mass (-2.1 ± 1.1 kg, 5%). There were no differences among the three energy restricted groups, except for body mass, as the chicken group lost more body mass than the carbohydrate/fat group: -7.9 ± 2.6 kg compared to -5.6 ± 1.8 kg, respectively [52].

The benefits of protein and higher protein intakes for body weight and body composition are well documented [45,46,49,50]. Dietary protein supplements are increasingly popular sources of protein [55]. Chicken and other forms of poultry can be produced as dietary protein supplements. Dairy- and plant-based proteins are typically used for research, often in combination with resistance exercise training [54]. Our literature search identified one double-blind, parallel, RCT with 41 young adult men ($n = 19$) and women ($n = 22$) investigating the effects (after eight weeks) of consuming beef protein isolate, hydrolyzed chicken, whey protein concentrate, and maltodextrin (as a control) consumption on resistance exercise training-induced changes in body composition [54]. Total energy intake and macronutrient intakes were not different among groups, with carbohydrate, fat, and protein intakes averaging 48%, 29%, and 23% of energy intake, respectively. This protein intake equates to 2.0–2.2 g/kg/d, with participants consuming a 46 g bolus of protein or control immediately post-exercise or at a similar time on non-training days [54].

There were no differences among groups for lean body mass and fat mass at baseline. The chicken, beef, and whey protein groups each increased lean body mass and decreased fat mass from baseline to post-intervention with no differences among groups. Interestingly, while total energy intake and total protein intake did not differ among the protein groups and control group, no changes in either lean body mass or fat mass were observed over time in the control group [54]. These findings indicate that consuming a higher protein diet, which may be obtained by the consumption of a supplemental form of chicken protein, aids in promoting increases in lean body mass and decreases in fat mass during resistance exercise training in young adults.

6.2. Observational Studies

Observational studies show that chicken/poultry consumption has either a positive or neutral association with body weight and BMI in adults or children and adolescents. An important consideration regarding observational studies is that inconsistencies in the findings may, in part, be explained by a lack of distinction and specific categorizations of chicken/poultry products (e.g., unprocessed vs. processed) and cooking methods, which influence the energy and nutrient profiles, and potentially, measures of body weight and body composition.

6.2.1. Observational Studies in Adults

A prospective observational study of 3902 men and women aged 55–69 years from the Netherlands Cohort Study found no association between total meat intake and changes in BMI over a 14-year follow-up period. Subgroup analysis of different types of meat indicated men and women in the highest quintile for chicken intake (>22.8 g/d) had a greater increase in BMI (men: +0.19 kg/m^2; women: +0.53 kg/m^2) compared to those in the lowest quintile who consumed no chicken [56]. A cross-sectional analysis in the US of 508 men (mean age of 53.7 years) and 1293 women (mean age of 49.5 years) classified as obese showed greater consumption of fried chicken was associated with higher BMI, in both sex groups [57]. A cross-sectional analysis of a community-based cohort of 204 African American/Black men indicated 90% ate their chicken fried. Consuming fried chicken with skin was associated with higher BMI [58]. A cross-sectional analysis of 287 individuals classified as obese and 1871 individuals classified as normal weight, aged 18–68 years, in India, found individuals classified as obese consumed greater amounts of fried/grilled chicken compared to individuals classified as normal weight [59].

In contrast, there is also evidence of neutral associations between poultry consumption and body weight and body composition. A prospective observational study in a cohort of 1638 men and women aged 18–60 years examined associations between unhealthy eating behaviors and weight gain over a 3.5-year follow-up period [60]. The investigators reported no association with never/almost never removing skin from chicken and weight gain, compared to those who removed skin from chicken. Additionally, cross-sectional data from 418 adults and older adults showed no associations between poultry intake and BMI or waist circumference [61].

6.2.2. Observational Studies in Children and Adolescents

Based on cross-sectional data from 1562 children aged 10 years from the Bogalusa Heart Study, no associations were observed between poultry consumption and overweight and obesity classifications [62]. Additionally, no associations were observed between poultry consumption and overweight and obesity classifications for ethnic−gender groups, namely, Euro-American males, Euro-American females, African-American males, and African-American females [62]. Harris et al. [63], using data from a prospective cohort study with adolescents, investigated associations between different types of meat with measures of body composition. They observed higher poultry intake in males at 10 years of age was positively associated with a higher fat mass index at 15 years of age. No associations were observed between poultry consumption and body composition changes in females [63].

The incongruence of these findings may be partially explained by lack of distinctions in the types and/or cooking methods of chicken/poultry consumed. More specific details on the type of poultry consumed were provided in the Avon Longitudinal Study of Parents and Children in the United Kingdom. Among the 4646 boys and girls aged 7–13 years of age, consuming greater amounts of coated (breaded or battered), but not uncoated poultry, was associated with excess weight gain [64]. The Harris et al. [63] study was done with all types of poultry products included, while the Dong et al. [64] study divided poultry products into coated and uncoated subcategories.

Cross-sectional analysis of data from 2525 freshmen university students in Turkey aged 18–22 years, revealed no association between chicken (excluding fried chicken) or burgers/fried chicken consumption and BMI [65]. In line with this finding, a cross-sectional analysis of data from 406 female students in Jordan, found consuming chicken more frequently (≥ 4 vs. <4 times/week) did not predict an increased likelihood of being classified as obese [66]. In contrast, cross-sectional data from 300 university students in Iran indicated consumption of fried chicken was associated with 40% increased odds of being classified as obese [67].

7. Poultry Consumption and CVD

Cardiovascular disease encompasses a group of heart and blood vessel disorders, including coronary heart disease (CHD), heart failure, cerebrovascular disease/stroke, and peripheral arterial disease [68,69]. CVD is the leading cause of diet-related deaths worldwide and deaths in the US, accounting for 9.5 million and greater than 877,500 deaths in 2017 [70] and 2020 [71,72], respectively. In the US, CVD accounts for approximately one third of all deaths and increases with age [71,73]. CVD comes with significant societal and economic burdens with direct medical costs for CVD estimated to be $216 billion, with an additional $147 billion in indirect costs, in 2020 [73,74]. As CVD is the leading cause of diet-related deaths worldwide, dietary components can differentially influence risk factors for CVD and the occurrence of CVD. The following sections will focus on evidence from RCTs and observational studies on the effects and associations of chicken/poultry consumption and CVD health-related outcomes.

7.1. RCTs

RCTs with lean chicken/poultry as the primary protein source in diets show neutral or beneficial effects on CVD risk factors.

A controlled-feeding RCT by Bergeron et al. [75] including 113 "generally healthy" adults (69 females, 34 males) investigated the effects of consuming a typical American diet with varying protein food sources and saturated fat intakes on blood lipids and lipoproteins. Protein sources were 12% of energy from lean poultry, lean red meat, or nonmeat sources and saturated fat intakes were 13% or 7% of energy intake. Participants were randomized to one of two parallel arms, either high- (n = 63) or low- (n = 52) saturated fat, and within each arm consumed either poultry, red meat, or nonmeat protein sources for four weeks in a three-period cross-over design, with a two-to-seven-week washout period between each intervention period. The higher-saturated fat intake was achieved primarily via the consumption of high-fat dairy products and butter.

Independent of saturated fat intake, consuming the nonmeat diet, but not the poultry or beef diet reduced total cholesterol, LDL cholesterol, non-HDL cholesterol, HDL cholesterol, apolipoprotein B, and apolipoprotein A1. Protein source did not influence triglycerides or total to HDL cholesterol ratio among the three diets. Independent of dietary protein source, higher-saturated fat intake resulted in increased total cholesterol, LDL cholesterol, and non-HDL cholesterol compared to lower-saturated fat intake [75]. These findings indicate that source of dietary protein and saturated fat intake each independently affect multiple CVD risk factors. The results also support the health promoting properties of consuming nonmeat protein foods compared to animal-based protein foods.

Two controlled-feeding RCTs have investigated the effects of lean chicken/poultry intake on blood lipids and lipoproteins in males with hypercholesterolemia [76,77]. In a randomized crossover design study by Beauchesne-Rondeau et al. [76] 17 white, weight-stable males classified as overweight and hypercholesterolemic (mean age ± SD of 50.1 ± 3.3 years) consumed an American Heart Association-style dietary pattern for 26-day periods. The pattern had a high polyunsaturated-to-saturated fatty acid ratio and a high fiber content as a base diet, as well as either lean poultry (skinless chicken and ground turkey), lean beef, or lean fish. Each experimental treatment period was separated by a six-week washout. The poultry, beef, and fish diets each reduced total cholesterol, LDL cholesterol, apolipoprotein B, total to HDL cholesterol ratio, and triglycerides from pre-to post-intervention, with no differences between interventions [76]. These findings suggest the health promoting properties of an American Heart Association-style diet may be achieved when the primary source of protein is lean poultry, beef, or fish.

Scott et al. [77] provide further support for these findings. In this RCT, 38 men with hypercholesterolemia consumed an American Heart Association-style diet with 85 g per 1000 kcal of lean chicken or lean beef for five weeks. Both diet groups reduced total and LDL cholesterol, with no differences between diets [77]. However, in contrast to Beauchesne-Rondeau et al. [76], Scott et al. [77] did not observe any changes in triglyceride concentrations or total to HDL cholesterol ratios for either diet. Taken together, the findings from these two RCTs indicate that when lean meats (chicken/poultry, red meat, or fish) are the primary protein food source consumed as part of this healthy dietary pattern, it can result in favorable changes in blood lipids and lipoproteins in males with hypercholesterolemia, most notably total and LDL cholesterol.

In the two RCTs previously described by Mahon et al. [52] and Melanson et al. [53], women classified as overweight and obese consumed energy restricted diets for 9–12 weeks, with chicken or beef as the primary protein source. Both diets decreased total and LDL cholesterol, with no differences between groups. Additionally, Mahon et al. [52] found no changes over time with the chicken or beef diet on triglycerides, HDL cholesterol, or C-reactive protein. Melanson et al. [53] also reported no differences in triglycerides from baseline to post-intervention for the chicken or beef groups and no differences between groups. Another randomized cross-over trial by Mateo-Gallego et al. [78] investigated the effects of consuming lean red meat (lean breed lamb) and lean chicken as part of an energy balanced diet, each for a period of five weeks, on lipid profiles in 36 older (mean age of 71 years) women classified as overweight and obese [78]. No differences were observed for total and LDL cholesterol, triglycerides, apolipoprotein B or lipoprotein (a) from baseline to post-intervention for the chicken or red meat diet, or between groups for any outcome [78].

7.2. Observational Studies

Evidence indicates chicken/poultry consumption has either neutral or beneficial associations with CVD morbidity and mortality, and neutral or adverse associations with blood pressure and hypertension.

7.2.1. CVD

A 2021 systematic review and meta-analysis of 10 prospective cohort studies by Papp et al. [2] found no association between the highest and lowest intakes of poultry and risk for CVD or CHD. Linear dose response meta-analyses found no association per 100 g/d increase in poultry intake for CVD or CHD based on nine and 10 studies, respectively. Non-linear meta-analysis showed evidence for an association between poultry consumption and CVD, but not CHD [2]. These findings should be interpreted with caution, due to the certainty of evidence being deemed weak for CVD and CHD using the GRADE approach. A meta-analysis of prospective cohort studies by Abete et al. [30] found no relationship between poultry intake and CVD or ischemic heart disease mortality between the highest and lowest intakes or in the dose–response meta-analysis [30]. A pooled analysis of eight prospective cohort studies conducted in Asia found no associations between poultry consumption and CVD [79].

In line with these findings, several prospective cohort studies have shown no associations between poultry consumption and CVD. Analyses of two large Chinese population-based prospective cohort studies, The Shanghai Women's Health Study (SWHS) and The Shanghai Men's Health Study (SMHS), as well as The Japan Collaborative Cohort (JACC), showed no associations between poultry consumption and CVD mortality [80,81]. The Pan-European EPIC cohort, The JACC, and the Atherosclerosis Risk in Communities (ARIC) Study, showed that poultry consumption was not associated with risk of ischemic heart disease [81–83]. Similarly, the ARIC Study showed no associations between poultry consumption and peripheral arterial disease [84].

There is also evidence from prospective cohort studies that higher intakes of chicken/poultry are associated with a decreased risk of CVD among men and women in a dose–response relationship [85] and CHD among women in the Nurses' Health Study (NHS) with a 26-year follow-up [86]. The Korean Genome and Epidemiology Study (KoGES) showed a dose–response association between intakes of unprocessed chicken and decreased CVD risk. Those in the highest quintile of chicken intake were 32% less likely to develop CVD compared to those in the lowest quintile (1.41 vs. 0 median servings/week) [85]. Moreover, in the NHS, when compared to one serving/d of red meat, one serving/d of poultry was associated with a 19% lower risk of CHD [86]. Additionally, the Costa Rica Heart Study, a population-based case-control study showed lower odds of myocardial infarction when substituting 50 g of chicken without skin and without fat for total red meat (25% reduction), unprocessed red meat (11% reduction), and processed red meat (41% reduction) [87].

In contrast, as part of the Lifetime Risk Pooling Project, data were pooled from six prospective US cohort studies comprising the ARIC Study, CARDIA (Coronary Artery Risk Development in Young Adults) Study, CHS (Cardiovascular Health Study), FHS (Framingham Heart Study), FOS (Framingham Offspring Study), and MESA (Multi-Ethnic Study of Atherosclerosis). Findings showed each additional two servings/week of poultry was associated with a 4% increase in incident CVD [88]. Additionally, evidence from 474,985 middle-aged men and women in the UK Biobank study showed that an increase of 30 g/d of poultry consumption was associated with an 8% increased risk for ischemic heart disease over an eight-year follow-up period [89].

Substitution analysis is an important nutrition research approach providing insights into the impacts of different foods on health outcomes. A meta-analysis by Papp et al. [2] showed a 29% decrease for CVD when substituting poultry for processed meat, and a neutral association when substituting (per 100 g/d) poultry for red meat or unprocessed red meat [2]. For CHD, substituting poultry for red meat predicted a 17% decreased risk for CHD and a neutral association when substituting poultry for processed meat or red and processed meat [2]. These observations suggest that the replacement of processed meat or red meat with poultry may reduce the risk for CVD and CHD, respectively. However, these findings should be interpreted with caution as based on the GRADE approach, the certainty of evidence was rated as low or very low. As such, more prospective cohort studies investigating associations of substituting processed or red meat with poultry are warranted.

7.2.2. Stroke

Evidence from observational studies indicates that poultry consumption has a neutral or beneficial association with stroke morbidity and mortality.

The 2021 systematic review and meta-analysis by Papp et al. [2] showed no association between the highest and lowest intakes of poultry and stroke based on nine studies. In addition, both linear and non-linear dose response meta-analysis showed no association between poultry consumption and stroke based on nine studies [2]. These findings should be interpreted with caution, due to the certainty of evidence being deemed weak for stroke using the GRADE approach. Another dose–response meta-analysis of seven prospective cohort studies assessing poultry intake and the risk of stroke showed no association for poultry intake and total stroke risk or risk of subtypes of stroke, namely, ischemic and hemorrhagic stroke [90]. In line with these observations, evidence from The JACC Study [81] and The Hiroshima/Nagasaki Life Span Study [91] showed no associations between intakes of poultry or chicken, respectively, and stroke mortality [81,91]. Evidence from both the UK Biobank study [89] and the EPIC cohort including participants from nine countries in Europe [92] found no associations between poultry intake and ischemic or hemorrhagic stroke [89,92].

Results from some prospective cohort studies indicate an inverse association between poultry consumption and stroke. A meta-analysis of prospective cohort studies showed a 13% reduction in stroke incidence when comparing the highest vs. the lowest categories of intake [93]. Analyses of women in the NHS and men from the Health Professionals Follow-up Study (HPFS) showed a dose–response association between poultry consumption and a 13% reduction in risk of stroke for men and women combined for the highest compared to the lowest quintiles of intake [94]. However, it is important to note that this decreased risk of stroke for men and women combined was largely driven by women, with a more pronounced 18% risk reduction in women alone, whereas in men alone no association was observed [94].

7.2.3. Hypertension

Evidence indicates that poultry consumption is associated with either an increase in blood pressure or neutral association with blood pressure.

Among prospective cohort studies, a meta-analysis of six studies found greater poultry consumption was associated with increased risk for hypertension: 15% greater risk for highest vs. lowest intake groups [95]. Three longitudinal cohort studies in the US—NHS I, NHS II, and HPFS—investigated the relation between long-term intake of animal meats with incident hypertension. Long term, consuming more poultry (≥1 serving/day vs. <1 serving/month of chicken and turkey, with or without skin) was associated with a 22% increased risk of hypertension [96]. The INTERnational study on MAcro/micronutrients and blood Pressure (INTERMAP), which included men and women ages 40–59 years from 17 population samples in the US, United Kingdom, China, and Japan, showed that unprocessed poultry was associated with a higher systolic blood pressure by +0.73 mmHg, but not diastolic blood pressure, in the Western population [97]. The Chicago Western

Electric Study in men, showed that the consumption of >20 servings (120 g/serving)/month compared to <4 servings/month, was associated with both higher systolic and diastolic blood pressures [98].

In contrast to these findings, both the CARDIA Study and the Tehran Lipid and Glucose Study showed no associations between poultry intake and 15-year [99] or 3-year [100] incidence of elevated blood pressure. In addition, among older women in the WHI [101] and middle-aged men in Japan [102], no associations between poultry/chicken consumption and blood pressures were observed [101,102].

8. Poultry Consumption and T2DM

Type 2 diabetes mellitus is a chronic metabolic condition affecting how the body regulates and processes glucose. Type 2 diabetes mellitus is the third leading cause of diet-related deaths worldwide and the eighth-leading cause of deaths in the US, accounting for 338,700 [70] and 102,188 [103] deaths in 2017 and 2020, respectively. The number of adults with T2DM worldwide has nearly quadrupled in the last four decades, according to the World Health Organization [104]. In the US, the number of adults diagnosed with T2DM has more than doubled in the last 20 years [103]. In the US, it is estimated that more than 32.4 million adults—approximately one in ten—have T2DM. An additional 88 million adults—greater than one in three adults—have prediabetes (when blood glucose concentrations are above the normal range but not above the threshold for a diagnosis of T2DM). Additionally, one in five people do not realize they have T2DM, while more than eight in ten do not realize they have prediabetes, negating treatment and prevention therapies [74,103].

Compared to adults without T2DM, adults with T2DM are 1.7 times more likely to die of cardiovascular-related deaths. In addition, T2DM can cause serious complications such as CVD, and T2DM is the number one cause of kidney failure, lower-limb amputations, and blindness. T2DM also comes with a significant economic burden: direct medical costs for T2DM were estimated to be $237 billion, and an additional $90 billion in indirect costs, in 2020 [103].

8.1. RCTs

Evidence from RCTs indicates that when compared to the consumption of solely a carbohydrate source, the combined ingestion of chicken or turkey with a carbohydrate source may result in beneficial effects on indices of glycemic control.

8.1.1. Acute Feeding RCTs

Two randomized cross-over controlled trials investigated the effects of lean chicken breast consumption (22–25 g of protein from chicken) on the insulinemic and glycemic responses to white rice (providing 50 g of carbohydrates) in healthy adults, with inconsistent results [105,106]. Sun et al. [105] reported that compared to white rice alone, the combination of white rice and 22.5 g of protein from chicken breast without skin lowered peak glucose and glucose incremental area under the curve (iAUC) over 120 min by 9% and 26%, respectively. The combination of rice and chicken breast also resulted in greater peak insulin and iAUC over 120 min by 22% and 30%, respectively. Quek et al. [106] reported no differences in glycemic or insulinemic responses (peak or iAUC over 120 min for both) to consuming white rice vs. white rice plus 25 g of protein from chicken breast for glycemic or insulinemic responses [106].

Similarly, another randomized cross-over trial investigated the effects of chicken breast on the glycemic and insulinemic responses to 50 g of carbohydrate from mashed potatoes [107]. Chicken breast (providing 30 g of protein) combined with potatoes, compared to potatoes alone, resulted in lower blood glucose 30 min post-ingestion by 30%, a 42% reduction in glucose iAUC, with no differences in insulinemic responses [107].

In a randomized cross-over trial involving 17 males characterized as older (mean age ± SD of 63 ± 2 years) and overweight with T2DM were assigned to consume 50 g of glucose alone or 50 g of glucose plus 25 g of protein from turkey, among other protein sources (lean beef, gelatin, egg white, cottage cheese, fish, or soy) [108]. The 5 h iAUC for glucose and insulin for the co-ingestion of glucose plus a protein source (except for egg white) were lower and higher, respectively, compared to glucose alone [108]. The findings suggest that the co-ingestion of a protein source, inclusive of turkey, with glucose can decrease the glycemic response and increase the insulinemic response in older males classified as overweight and with T2DM.

Taken together, evidence from acute feeding RCTs indicate that the co-ingestion of lean chicken breast or turkey with a carbohydrate source can improve the glycemic response and either increase or have no effect on the insulinemic response in healthy adults or older males classified as overweight and with T2DM.

8.1.2. Chronic Feeding RCTs

Diabetes can lead to reduced kidney function. While higher protein intake does not apparently impair kidney function in heathy adults [109], reduced protein intake is recommended to help manage neuropathy, also referred to as diabetic kidney disease [110–112]. In those with T2DM, the inclusion of chicken-based diets is apparently beneficial for renal function [113–115]. A randomized, cross-over, controlled trial involving 28 adults with T2DM assessed the effect of replacing red meat with chicken in participants' usual diets or a low-protein diet on cardiometabolic disease-related outcomes. The outcomes included glomerular filtration rate (GFR), urinary albumin excretion rate (UAER), blood lipids and lipoproteins, blood pressures, and blood glucose [113]. The participants were assigned to consume a low-protein diet (0.5–0.8 g/kg/d), their usual diet including red meat, or a chicken-based diet (skinless leg quarter) for periods of four weeks each, with a four-week washout between each intervention diet. Total energy intake was not different between the chicken and red meat diets, but there was a 10% lower total energy intake in the low-protein diet compared to chicken and red meat diets. Protein intake was higher in the chicken diet (1.35 g/kg/d) and usual diet with red meat (1.43 g/kg/d), compared to the low-protein diet (0.66 g/kg/d). For the analyses, participants who were normo-albuminuric (24 h UAER < 20 μg/min) and micro-albuminuric (24 h UAER 20–200 μg/min) were analyzed separately [113].

In participants classified as normo-albuminuric, GFR following the chicken and low-protein diets were 11% and 17% lower, respectively, vs. usual diet with red meat. There were no differences in GFR between the low-protein and chicken diets. Consuming the varied diets did not differentially affect UAER, measures of glycemic control, blood lipids and lipoproteins, or blood pressure among diets in normo-albuminuric participants. [113]. In participants classified as micro-albuminuric, GFR was lower by 9% and 13%, respectively, with the low-protein diet compared to the usual diet with red meat and chicken diet. UAER was lower for the chicken diet compared to the low-protein diet or usual diet with red meat by 34% and 46%. Total cholesterol and apolipoprotein B were lower for the chicken diet by 12% and 15%, respectively, and low-protein diet by 13% and 23%, respectively, compared to the usual diet with red meat. No differences in other blood lipids and lipoproteins, measures of glycemic control, or blood pressure were reported in micro-albuminuric participants [113]. These findings may suggest that incorporating lean chicken in place of red meat in a diet may represent an alternative strategy to a low protein diet for adults with T2DM to manage their renal function.

Consistent with these findings, a randomized, cross-over, controlled trial including 17 older adults (mean age ± SD of 59 ± 11 years) with T2DM and macro-albuminuria (24 h UAER ≥ 200 μg/min), found that UAER and non-HDL cholesterol were lower after the chicken diet by 14% and 7%, respectively, and low-protein diet by 27% and 7%, respectively, vs. the red meat diet. [114]. While both short-term studies [113,114] provide evidence that chicken consumption, in place of red meat, may be beneficial for renal function and some blood lipid and lipoprotein measures in individuals with T2DM, there is still the question of longer-term effects.

To address this question, Mello et al. [115] conducted a randomized, open-label, controlled clinical trial with a follow-up period of one year. They assessed the effects of consuming a chicken-based diet plus placebo compared to the angiotensin-converting enzyme inhibitor enalapril (10 mg/d) on renal function and lipid profile in 28 older aged (mean age ± SD of 54.1 ± 10.9 years) participants with T2DM and microalbuminuria. Energy and macronutrient intakes were not different between groups, with total protein intake 1.2–1.3 g/kg/d. Following one year, both diets reduced UAER and mean blood pressure, while the chicken diet reduced total and LDL cholesterol. Participants in the enalapril group had reduced GFR, with a trend for reduced GFR in the chicken group ($p = 0.069$) [115].

Taken together, evidence from these chronic feeding RCTs suggests adults with T2DM who consume chicken as the primary protein source, may experience relatively favorable changes in UAER and lipid profile, with no adverse effects on glycemic control.

8.2. Observational Studies

Observational studies on chicken/poultry consumption and diabetes risk, morbidity, and mortality provide inconsistent findings.

Two meta-analyses including 28 prospective cohort studies (accounting for duplicates) showed no associations between poultry intake and risk of T2DM [116,117]. The EPIC-InterAct Study, a case-cohort study including 340,234 adults with a 11.7-year follow-up, observed no association between poultry consumption and risk of T2DM [118]. In contrast, evidence from the UK Biobank study showed 30 g/d greater poultry consumption was associated with a 14% increased risk for diabetes over an eight-year follow-up period [89]. The Singapore Chinese Health Study, a prospective cohort study with 63,257 participants and 11-year follow-up, showed that when comparing the highest to the lowest quintiles of poultry intake, higher intakes were associated with a 15% increased risk of developing T2DM [119].

Results from several observational studies show associations between greater poultry intake and decreased risk for T2DM. The SWHS, a prospective cohort study including 74,493 middle- and older-aged women found that greater unprocessed poultry intake was associated with a decreased risk of T2DM [120]. Interestingly, the association between poultry intake and risk of developing T2DM may be modified by body weight: greater poultry intake was related to a decrease in T2DM risk for those classified as normal weight, but not for those classified with obesity [120]. Prospective evidence from the Alpha-Tocopherol, Beta-Carotene Cancer Prevention Study (ATBC) cohort also showed a reduced risk of T2DM with higher intakes of poultry [121]. Evidence from the EPIC study using a case-cohort design showed a decreased risk of T2DM mortality with higher intakes of poultry in individuals with T2DM [122].

In observational studies, there is a dearth of information assessing processed poultry intake or distinguishing between unprocessed and processed poultry. Our scoping review identified that only four of 366 (1%) observational studies assessed the influence of processed poultry on human health outcomes [4]. Steinbrecher et al. [105] using prospective data from the Hawaii population of the Multiethnic Cohort (MEC) Study, assessed associations between fresh poultry or processed poultry intake and risk of T2DM. The authors reported no association between fresh poultry consumption and T2DM risk. However, when comparing the highest vs. the lowest quintiles of processed poultry intake (≥ 1.81 vs. 0.04 g/1000 kcal/d) there was a 30% increased risk for T2DM [105]. These observations underscore the need to assess unprocessed and processed poultry separately to enhance understanding of how they influence risk for T2DM.

The substitution of poultry for red meat indicates either an inverse or neutral association with T2DM. A pooled analysis of three prospective cohort studies—the HPFS, the NHS, and the NHS II—showed that the substitution of one serving/d (4–6 oz/d) of poultry for total red meat, unprocessed red meat, or processed red meat was associated with a 15%, 15%, and 22% decreased risk for T2DM, respectively [123]. Using data from the

EPIC-InterAct case cohort, a neutral association was observed when substituting 50 g/d of poultry for red or processed meat [124]. Similarly, using data from the Danish Diet, Cancer and Health study, a neutral association was observed for substituting 150 g/week of poultry for total red meat and unprocessed red meat. A 4% decreased risk for T2DM was observed when substituting poultry for processed red meat [125].

9. Conclusions

Total chicken and poultry intakes in the US have increased over time, tripling from 1960 to 2022. The nutritional composition of chicken and other poultry products varies depending on the cut, leanness, and processing level of the meat. Chicken and other poultry products are sources of high-quality dietary protein and other essential nutrients required for human health and physiological functioning, in relatively high amounts. Chicken and other poultry products may also have other nutritive and non-nutritive components such as saturated fat, sodium, and nitrites, depending on the cut of poultry meat and/or level of processing, that should be consumed with caution. Cooking methods of chicken and other poultry products also introduce variability in the concentration of non-nutritive compounds. High-heat cooking methods can result in the formation of compounds such as advanced glycation end-products, heterocyclic aromatic amines, and polycyclic aromatic hydrocarbons that are associated with negative cardiometabolic health-related outcomes. Therefore, the nutritive and non-nutritive components of chicken and other poultry products can contribute to human health in positive and negative ways.

An important consideration regarding experimental and observational studies is that inconsistencies in the findings may, in part, be explained by discrepant definitions of poultry, a lack of distinction and specific categorizations of chicken/poultry products (e.g., unprocessed vs. processed), amounts and types consumed, and cooking methods, which influence the energy and nutrient profiles and health-related outcomes. It is also important to emphasize that the conclusions provided below apply to the specific types of poultry products included in the articles synthesized in this review and that other dietary and lifestyle factors also influence health outcomes.

Limited evidence from RCTs suggest consuming lean unprocessed animal-based protein-rich foods, inclusive of chicken, as the primary source of dietary protein favorably affects body weight or body composition concurrent with purposeful weight loss, but not weight maintenance. Observational studies provide inconsistent findings that greater chicken/poultry consumption is either unrelated or positively related to higher BMI.

Pertaining to CVD, the consumption of varying lean meats (poultry, red meat, fish) as a primary protein food source does not influence the health-promoting effects of consuming a healthy dietary pattern on multiple CVD risk factors. These findings are supported by a meta-analysis of RCTs showing no differential effects between red meat and poultry consumption on CVD risk factors [126]. In "generally healthy" adults, when the primary sources of protein foods consumed as part of a typical American diet are nonmeat, reductions in blood lipids and lipoproteins can occur compared to lean poultry or red meat. This should be interpreted with caution, due to the limited number of RCTs specifically pertaining to chicken/poultry consumption and CVD risk factors.

Evidence from observational studies indicates greater poultry consumption has either neutral or beneficial associations with CVD, CHD, ischemic heart disease, and stroke, but neutral or adverse associations with blood pressure and hypertension.

Pertaining to T2DM, results from RCTs and observational studies assessing the effects of or associations between chicken/poultry intake and T2DM seem inconsistent. Evidence from RCTs indicate the consumption of lean chicken/poultry is either beneficial or has neutral effects on T2DM risk factors in healthy individuals, those at an increased risk for T2DM, and those with T2DM. In acute feeding trials, co-ingestion of chicken/poultry with a carbohydrate source favorably affects glycemic responses, with favorable or neutral effects on insulinemic responses. Regarding renal function, lower protein diets are being used to help manage diabetic kidney disease. Limited provocative evidence suggests higher-protein intakes achieved with lean chicken as the primary dietary protein source, may have relatively beneficial or neutral effects on renal function in those with T2DM. Healthy adults may consume higher protein diets without detrimental effects on renal function. Inconsistent evidence from observational studies may be used to support beneficial, neutral, or detrimental associations between chicken/poultry consumption and T2DM-related outcomes.

Future Research Recommendations

Based on evidence identified from our comprehensive systematically searched scoping review [4] and synthesized in this narrative review on poultry consumption and body weight and body composition, CVD, or T2DM health-related outcomes, the following suggestions may be considered for future research:

(1) There is a need for future experimental and observational research to include definitions and detailed descriptions of the different types and amounts of poultry products consumed.
Rationale: The research that currently exists on poultry is complicated by the lack of a clear definition of poultry and limited descriptions of the types and forms of poultry used among studies. Importantly, "muscle food categories and descriptions are substantively different within and between experimental and observational studies and do not match regulatory definitions" [20]. New research with greater consideration and more detailed descriptions of multiple factors, including the amounts, types, and forms of chicken/poultry consumed; the health, medical, and dietary characteristics of the research cohorts; and other confounding factors will help improve our understanding of the influence of chicken/poultry on body weight and body composition, CVD, and T2DM.

(2) Chronic feeding RCTs are warranted assessing the effects of consuming unprocessed and processed poultry products in the context of healthy and unhealthy dietary patterns on body weight and body composition, CVD, and T2DM health-related outcomes.
Rationale: Of 59 RCTs identified in our scoping review [4], only seven included assessments of body weight and body composition, 17 included CVD risk factors, and 11 included T2DM risk factors. Accounting for overlap among studies, there were 26 unique RCTs. Zero RCTs specifically assessed processed chicken/poultry, 23 RCTs assessed unprocessed chicken/poultry, and 3 RCTs were indeterminate. Most chronic feeding RCTs did not document (e.g., using the Healthy Eating Index) the healthfulness of the dietary pattern.

(3) Observational studies are warranted examining associations between processed poultry consumption or poultry cooking methods and body weight and body composition, CVD, or T2DM health-related outcomes in humans across the life course.
Rationale: Our scoping review identified only four of 366 (1%) observational studies assessed the influence of processed poultry on human health outcomes [4]. Of these four observational studies identified and included in this review, three were on body weight or BMI and one was on T2DM risk. Zero observational studies were identified that included investigating associations between processed poultry consumption and CVD. In addition, only 14% of 366 observational studies reported the cooking method used [4].

Author Contributions: Conceptualization, G.C. and W.W.C.; methodology, G.C. and W.W.C.; writing—original draft preparation, G.C.; writing—review and editing, G.C. and W.W.C.; supervision, W.W.C.; funding acquisition, W.W.C. All authors have read and agreed to the published version of the manuscript.

Funding: This research was funded by the National Chicken Council. The funder had no role in the design of the research; in the collection, analyses, or interpretation of data; in the writing of the manuscript; or in the decision to publish the manuscript.

Institutional Review Board Statement: Not applicable.

Informed Consent Statement: Not applicable.

Data Availability Statement: No new data were created or analyzed in this study. Data sharing is not applicable to this article.

Conflicts of Interest: During the time this research was conducted, W.W.C. received funding for research grants, travel or honoraria for scientific presentations, or consulting services from the following organizations: National Institutes of Health, US Department of Agriculture, Beef Checkoff, Foundation for Meat and Poultry Research and Education, Pork Checkoff, North Dakota Beef Commission, Barilla Group, Mushroom Council, National Chicken Council, and the Whey Protein Research Consortium. G.C. declares no conflict of interest. The funder had no role in the design of the research; in the collection or interpretation of data; in the writing of the manuscript; or in the decision to publish the results.

References

1. National Chicken Council: Per Capita Consumption of Poultry and Livestock, 1965 to Estimated 2021, in Pounds. Available online: https://www.Nationalchickencouncil.Org/Statistic/per-Capita-Consumption-Poultry/ (accessed on 23 January 2023).
2. Papp, R.E.; Hasenegger, V.; Ekmekcioglu, C.; Schwingshackl, L. Association of Poultry Consumption with Cardiovascular Diseases and All-Cause Mortality: A Systematic Review and Dose Response Meta-Analysis of Prospective Cohort Studies. *Crit. Rev. Food Sci. Nutr.* **2023**, *63*, 2366–2387. [CrossRef] [PubMed]
3. OECD; FAO. *OECD-FAO Agricultural Outlook 2023–2032*; OECD Publishing: Paris, France, 2023. [CrossRef]
4. Connolly, G.; Clark, C.M.; Campbell, R.E.; Byers, A.W.; Reed, J.B.; Campbell, W.W. Poultry Consumption and Human Health: How Much Is Really Known? A Systematically Searched Scoping Review and Research Perspective. *Adv. Nutr.* **2022**, *13*, 2115–2124. [CrossRef] [PubMed]
5. Marangoni, F.; Corsello, G.; Cricelli, C.; Ferrara, N.; Ghiselli, A.; Lucchin, L.; Poli, A. Role of Poultry Meat in a Balanced Diet Aimed at Maintaining Health and Wellbeing: An Italian Consensus Document. *Food Nutr. Res.* **2015**, *59*, 27606. [CrossRef]
6. U.S. Department of Agriculture and U.S. Department of Health and Human Services. *Dietary Guidelines for Americans, 2020–2025*, 9th ed.; U.S. Department of Agriculture and U.S. Department of Health and Human Services: Washington, DC, USA, 2020. Available online: https://www.dietaryguidelines.gov/sites/default/files/2020-12/Dietary_Guidelines_for_Americans_2020-2025.pdf (accessed on 23 January 2023).
7. US Department of Agriculture (USDA) FoodData Central. Available online: https://fdc.nal.usda.gov/Index.Html (accessed on 25 January 2023).
8. World Cancer Research Fund/American Institute for Cancer Research. *Food, Nutrition, Physical Activity, and the Prevention of Cancer: A Global Perspective*; AICR: Washington, DC, USA, 2007.
9. Pearson, A.M.; Gillett, T.A. *Processed Meats*; Springer: New York, NY, USA, 1996. [CrossRef]
10. Pasiakos, S.M.; Agarwal, S.; Lieberman, H.R.; Fulgoni, V.L. Sources and Amounts of Animal, Dairy, and Plant Protein Intake of US Adults in 2007–2010. *Nutrients* **2015**, *7*, 7058–7069. [CrossRef] [PubMed]
11. Shan, Z.; Rehm, C.D.; Rogers, G.; Ruan, M.; Wang, D.D.; Hu, F.B.; Mozaffarian, D.; Zhang, F.F.; Bhupathiraju, S.N. Trends in Dietary Carbohydrate, Protein, and Fat Intake and Diet Quality among US Adults, 1999–2016. *JAMA* **2019**, *322*, 1178–1187. [CrossRef]
12. Hoy, K.; Clemens, J.; Moshfegh, A. Estimated Protein Intake from Animal and Plant Foods by U.S. Adults, What We Eat in America, NHANES, 2015–2016. *Curr. Dev. Nutr.* **2021**, *5*, 133. [CrossRef]
13. Phillips, S.M.; Fulgoni, V.L.; Heaney, R.P.; Nicklas, T.A.; Slavin, J.L.; Weaver, C.M. Commonly Consumed Protein Foods Contribute to Nutrient Intake, Diet Quality, and Nutrient Adequacy. *Am. J. Clin. Nutr.* **2015**, *101*, 1346S–1352S. [CrossRef]
14. Bowman, S.A.; Clemens, J.C.; Friday, J.E.; Moshfegh, A.J. *Food Patterns Equivalents Database 2017–2018: Methodology and User Guide*; Food Surveys Research Group: Beltsville, MD, USA, 2020. Available online: http://www.ars.usda.gov/nea/bhnrc/fsrg (accessed on 23 January 2023).
15. O'Connor, L.E.; Campbell, W.W. Nutritional Composition and the Value of Pig Meat. In *Achieving Sustainable Production of Pig Meat Volume 1: Safety, Quality and Sustainability*, 1st ed.; Matthew, A., Ed.; Burleigh Dodds Science Publishing: London, UK, 2017; Chapter 8; pp. 175–192. ISBN 9781351114493. [CrossRef]
16. Hébert, J.R.; Frongillo, E.A.; Adams, S.A.; Turner-McGrievy, G.M.; Hurley, T.G.; Miller, D.R.; Ockene, I.S. Perspective: Randomized Controlled Trials Are not a Panacea for Diet-Related Research. *Adv. Nutr.* **2016**, *7*, 423–432. [CrossRef]
17. Booth, C.M.; Tannock, I.F. Randomised Controlled Trials and Population-Based Observational Research: Partners in the Evolution of Medical Evidence. *Br. J. Cancer* **2014**, *110*, 551–555. [CrossRef]

18. Faraoni, D.; Schaefer, S.T. Randomized Controlled Trials vs. Observational Studies: Why Not Just Live Together? *BMC Anesthesiol.* **2016**, *16*, 102. [CrossRef]
19. Barton, S. Which Clinical Studies Provide the Best Evidence? *BMJ* **2000**, *321*, 255–256. [CrossRef]
20. O'Connor, L.E.; Gifford, C.L.; Woerner, D.R.; Sharp, J.L.; Belk, K.E.; Campbell, W.W. Dietary Meat Categories and Descriptions in Chronic Disease Research Are Substantively Different within and between Experimental and Observational Studies: A Systematic Review and Landscape Analysis. *Adv. Nutr.* **2020**, *11*, 41–51. [CrossRef] [PubMed]
21. Micha, R.; Michas, G.; Mozaffarian, D. Unprocessed Red and Processed Meats and Risk of Coronary Artery Disease and Type 2 Diabetes—An Updated Review of the Evidence. *Curr. Atheroscler. Rep.* **2012**, *14*, 515–524. [CrossRef] [PubMed]
22. Shim, J.-S.; Oh, K.; Kim, H.C. Dietary Assessment Methods in Epidemiologic Studies. *Epidemiol. Health* **2014**, *36*, e2014009. [CrossRef]
23. Gifford, C.L.; O'Connor, L.E.; Campbell, W.W.; Woerner, D.R.; Belk, K.E. Broad and Inconsistent Muscle Food Classification Is Problematic for Dietary Guidance in the U.S. *Nutrients* **2017**, *9*, 1027. [CrossRef]
24. Dalle Zotte, A. Perception of Rabbit Meat Quality and Major Factors Influencing the Rabbit Carcass and Meat Quality. *Livest. Prod. Sci.* **2002**, *75*, 11–32. [CrossRef]
25. Cavani, C.; Petracci, M.; Trocino, A.; Xiccato, G. Advances in Research on Poultry and Rabbit Meat Quality. *Ital. J. Anim. Sci.* **2009**, *8*, 741–750. [CrossRef]
26. Rimm, E.B.; Appel, L.J.; Chiuve, S.E.; Djoussé, L.; Engler, M.B.; Kris-Etherton, P.M.; Mozaffarian, D.; Siscovick, D.S.; Lichtenstein, A.H. Seafood Long-Chain n-3 Polyunsaturated Fatty Acids and Cardiovascular Disease: A Science Advisory from the American Heart Association. *Circulation* **2018**, *138*, e35–e47. [CrossRef]
27. Micha, R.; Wallace, S.K.; Mozaffarian, D. Red and Processed Meat Consumption and Risk of Incident Coronary Heart Disease, Stroke, and Diabetes Mellitus: A Systematic Review and Meta-Analysis. *Circulation* **2010**, *121*, 2271–2283. [CrossRef]
28. Förstermann, U. Oxidative Stress in Vascular Disease: Causes, Defense Mechanisms and Potential Therapies. *Nat. Clin. Pract. Cardiovasc. Med.* **2008**, *5*, 338–349. [CrossRef]
29. Kim, Y.; Keogh, J.; Clifton, P. A Review of Potential Metabolic Etiologies of the Observed Association between Red Meat Consumption and Development of Type 2 Diabetes Mellitus. *Metabolism* **2015**, *64*, 768–779. [CrossRef]
30. Abete, I.; Romaguera, D.; Vieira, A.R.; Lopez De Munain, A.; Norat, T. Association between Total, Processed, Red and White Meat Consumption and All-Cause, CVD and IHD Mortality: A Meta-Analysis of Cohort Studies. *Br. J. Nutr.* **2014**, *112*, 762–775. [CrossRef] [PubMed]
31. Ley, S.H.; Hamdy, O.; Mohan, V.; Hu, F.B. Prevention and Management of Type 2 Diabetes: Dietary Components and Nutritional Strategies. *Lancet* **2014**, *383*, 1999–2007. [CrossRef]
32. Etemadi, A.; Sinha, R.; Ward, M.H.; Graubard, B.I.; Inoue-Choi, M.; Dawsey, S.M.; Abnet, C.C. Mortality from Different Causes Associated with Meat, Heme Iron, Nitrates, and Nitrites in the NIH-AARP Diet and Health Study: Population Based Cohort Study. *BMJ* **2017**, *357*, j1957. [CrossRef] [PubMed]
33. White, D.L.; Collinson, A. Red Meat, Dietary Heme Iron, and Risk of Type 2 Diabetes: The Involvement of Advanced Lipoxidation Endproducts. *Adv. Nutr.* **2013**, *4*, 403–411. [CrossRef] [PubMed]
34. Ulrich, P.; Cerami, A. Protein Glycation, Diabetes, and Aging. *Recent. Prog. Horm. Res.* **2001**, *56*, 1–21. [CrossRef] [PubMed]
35. Liu, G.; Zong, G.; Wu, K.; Hu, Y.; Li, Y.; Willett, W.C.; Eisenberg, D.M.; Hu, F.B.; Sun, Q. Meat Cooking Methods and Risk of Type 2 Diabetes: Results from Three Prospective Cohort Studies. *Diabetes Care* **2018**, *41*, 1049–1060. [CrossRef] [PubMed]
36. Sun, Y.; Liu, B.; Snetselaar, L.G.; Robinson, J.G.; Wallace, R.B.; Peterson, L.L.; Bao, W. Association of Fried Food Consumption with All Cause, Cardiovascular, and Cancer Mortality: Prospective Cohort Study. *BMJ* **2019**, *364*, k5420. [CrossRef]
37. Krishnan, S.; Coogan, P.F.; Boggs, D.A.; Rosenberg, L.; Palmer, J.R. Consumption of Restaurant Foods and Incidence of Type 2 Diabetes in African American Women. *Am. J. Clin. Nutr.* **2010**, *91*, 465–471. [CrossRef]
38. Stierman, B.; Afful, J.; Carroll, M.D.; Chen, T.C.; Davy, O.; Fink, S.; Fryar, C.D.; Gu, Q.; Hales, C.M.; Hughes, J.P.; et al. National Health and Nutrition Examination Survey 2017–March 2020 Prepandemic Data Files-Development of Files and Prevalence Estimates for Selected Health Outcomes. *Natl. Health Stat. Rep.* **2021**, *158*, 1–21. [CrossRef]
39. Centers for Disease Control and Prevention, Childhood Obesity Facts. Available online: https://www.cdc.gov/obesity/data/childhood.html (accessed on 28 January 2023).
40. Finkelstein, E.A.; Trogdon, J.G.; Cohen, J.W.; Dietz, W. Annual Medical Spending Attributable to Obesity: Payer-and Service-Specific Estimates. *Health Aff.* **2009**, *28*, w822–w831. [CrossRef]
41. Finkelstein, E.A.; DiBonaventura, M.D.C.; Burgess, S.M.; Hale, B.C. The Costs of Obesity in the Workplace. *J. Occup. Environ. Med.* **2010**, *52*, 971–976. [CrossRef]
42. Jehan, S.; Zizi, F.; Pandi-Perumal, S.R.; McFarlane, S.I.; Jean-Louis, G.; Myers, A.K. Energy Imbalance: Obesity, Associated Comorbidities, Prevention, Management and Public Health Implications. *Adv. Obes. Weight. Manag. Control* **2020**, *10*, 141–161. [CrossRef]
43. Niemiro, G.M.; Rewane, A.; Algotar, A.M. Exercise and Fitness Effect on Obesity. In *StatPearls*; StatPearls Publishing: Treasure Island, FL, USA, 2023; Bookshelf ID: NBK539893.
44. Fock, K.M.; Khoo, J. Diet and Exercise in Management of Obesity and Overweight. *J. Gastroenterol. Hepatol.* **2013**, *28*, 59–63. [CrossRef] [PubMed]

45. Westerterp-Plantenga, M.S.; Lemmens, S.G.; Westerterp, K.R. Dietary Protein—Its Role in Satiety, Energetics, Weight Loss and Health. *Br. J. Nutr.* **2012**, *108*, S105–S112. [CrossRef] [PubMed]
46. Drummen, M.; Tischmann, L.; Gatta-Cherifi, B.; Adam, T.; Westerterp-Plantenga, M. Dietary Protein and Energy Balance in Relation to Obesity and Co-Morbidities. *Front. Endocrinol.* **2018**, *9*, 443. [CrossRef]
47. Hudson, J.L.; Wang, Y.; Bergia Iii, R.E.; Campbell, W.W. Protein Intake Greater than the RDA Differentially Influences Whole-Body Lean Mass Responses to Purposeful Catabolic and Anabolic Stressors: A Systematic Review and Meta-Analysis. *Adv. Nutr.* **2020**, *11*, 548–558. [CrossRef]
48. Kim, J.E.; O'Connor, L.E.; Sands, L.P.; Slebodnik, M.B.; Campbell, W.W. Effects of Dietary Protein Intake on Body Composition Changes after Weight Loss in Older Adults: A Systematic Review and Meta-Analysis. *Nutr. Rev.* **2016**, *74*, 210–224. [CrossRef]
49. Paddon-Jones, D.; Westman, E.; Mattes, R.D.; Wolfe, R.R.; Astrup, A.; Westerterp-Plantenga, M. Protein, Weight Management, and Satiety. *Am. J. Clin. Nutr.* **2008**, *87*, 1558S–1561S. [CrossRef]
50. Magkos, F. The Role of Dietary Protein in Obesity. *Rev. Endocr. Metab. Disord.* **2020**, *21*, 329–340. [CrossRef]
51. Murphy, K.J.; Parker, B.; Dyer, K.A.; Davis, C.R.; Coates, A.M.; Buckley, J.D.; Howe, P.R.C. A Comparison of Regular Consumption of Fresh Lean Pork, Beef and Chicken on Body Composition: A Randomized Cross-over Trial. *Nutrients* **2014**, *6*, 682–696. [CrossRef] [PubMed]
52. Mahon, A.K.; Flynn, M.G.; Stewart, L.K.; McFarlin, B.K.; Iglay, H.B.; Mattes, R.D.; Lyle, R.M.; Considine, R.V.; Campbell, W.W. Protein Intake during Energy Restriction: Effects on Body Composition and Markers of Metabolic and Cardiovascular Health in Postmenopausal Women. *J. Am. Coll. Nutr.* **2007**, *26*, 182–189. [CrossRef] [PubMed]
53. Melanson, K.; Gootman, J.; Myrdal, A.; Kline, G.; Rippe, J.M. Weight Loss and Total Lipid Profile Changes in Overweight Women Consuming Beef or Chicken as the Primary Protein Source. *Nutrition* **2003**, *19*, 409–414. [CrossRef] [PubMed]
54. Sharp, M.H.; Lowery, R.P.; Shields, K.A.; Lane, J.R.; Gray, J.L.; Partl, J.M.; Hayes, D.W.; Wilson, G.J.; Hollmer, C.A.; Minivich, J.R.; et al. The Effects of Beef, Chicken, or Whey Protein After Workout on Body Composition and Muscle Performance. *J. Strength. Cond. Res.* **2018**, *32*, 2233–2242. [CrossRef] [PubMed]
55. Keogh, C.; Li, C.; Gao, Z. Evolving Consumer Trends for Whey Protein Sports Supplements: The Heckman Ordered Probit Estimation. *Agric. Food. Econ.* **2019**, *7*, 6. [CrossRef]
56. Gilsing, A.M.J.; Weijenberg, M.P.; Hughes, L.A.E.; Ambergen, T.; Dagnelie, P.C.; Goldbohm, R.A.; van den Brandt, P.A.; Schouten, L.J. Longitudinal Changes in BMI in Older Adults Are Associated with Meat Consumption Differentially, by Type of Meat Consumed. *J. Nutr.* **2012**, *142*, 340–349. [CrossRef]
57. Linde, J.A.; Utter, J.; Jeffery, R.W.; Sherwood, N.E.; Pronk, N.P.; Boyle, R.G. Specific Food Intake, Fat and Fiber Intake, and Behavioral Correlates of BMI among Overweight and Obese Members of a Managed Care Organization. *Int. J. Behav. Nutr.Phys. Act.* **2006**, *3*, 42. [CrossRef]
58. Weinrich, S.P.; Priest, J.; Reynolds, W.; Godley, P.A.; Tuckson, W.; Weinrich, M. Body Mass Index and Intake of Selected Foods in African American Men. *Public Health Nurs.* **2007**, *24*, 217–229. [CrossRef]
59. Satija, A.; Taylor, F.C.; Khurana, S.; Tripathy, V.; Khandpur, N.; Bowen, L.; Prabhakaran, D.; Kinra, S.; Reddy, S.; Ebrahim, S. Differences in Consumption of Food Items between Obese and Normal-Weight People in India. *Natl. Med. J. India* **2012**, *25*, 10–13.
60. León-Muñoz, L.M.; García-Esquinas, E.; Soler-Vila, H.; Guallar-Castillón, P.; Banegas, J.R.; Rodríguez-Artalejo, F. Unhealthy Eating Behaviors and Weight Gain: A Prospective Study in Young and Middle-Age Adults. *Obesity* **2016**, *24*, 1178–1184. [CrossRef]
61. Giglio, B.M.; Duarte, V.I.R.; Galvão, A.F.; Marini, A.C.B.; Schincaglia, R.M.; Mota, J.F.; Souza, L.B.; Pimentel, G.D. High-Protein Diet Containing Dairy Products Is Associated with Low Body Mass Index and Glucose Concentrations: A Cross-Sectional Study. *Nutrients* **2019**, *11*, 1384. [CrossRef] [PubMed]
62. Nicklas, T.A.; Yang, S.-J.; Baranowski, T.; Zakeri, I.; Berenson, G. Eating Patterns and Obesity in Children. The Bogalusa Heart Study. *Am. J. Prev. Med.* **2003**, *25*, 9–16. [CrossRef] [PubMed]
63. Harris, C.; Buyken, A.; von Berg, A.; Berdel, D.; Lehmann, I.; Hoffmann, B.; Koletzko, S.; Koletzko, B.; Heinrich, J.; Standl, M. Prospective Associations of Meat Consumption during Childhood with Measures of Body Composition during Adolescence: Results from the GINIplus and LISAplus Birth Cohorts. *Nutr. J.* **2016**, *15*, 101. [CrossRef] [PubMed]
64. Dong, D.; Bilger, M.; van Dam, R.M.; Finkelstein, E.A. Consumption of Specific Foods and Beverages and Excess Weight Gain among Children and Adolescents. *Health Aff.* **2015**, *34*, 1940–1948. [CrossRef]
65. Gunes, F.E.; Bekiroglu, N.; Imeryuz, N.; Agirbasli, M. Relation between Eating Habits and a High Body Mass Index among Freshman Students: A Cross-Sectional Study. *J. Am. Coll. Nutr.* **2012**, *31*, 167–174. [CrossRef] [PubMed]
66. Musaiger, A.O.; Hammad, S.S.; Tayyem, R.F.; Qatatsheh, A.A. Socio-Demographic and Dietary Factors Associated with Obesity among Female University Students in Jordan. *Int. J. Adolesc. Med. Health* **2015**, *27*, 299–305. [CrossRef]
67. Mohammadbeigi, A.; Asgarian, A.; Moshir, E.; Heidari, H.; Afrashteh, S.; Khazaei, S.; Ansari, H. Fast Food Consumption and Overweight/Obesity Prevalence in Students and Its Association with General and Abdominal Obesity. *J. Prev. Med. Hyg.* **2018**, *59*, E236–E240. [CrossRef]
68. Tsao, C.W.; Aday, A.W.; Almarzooq, Z.I.; Alonso, A.; Beaton, A.Z.; Bittencourt, M.S.; Boehme, A.K.; Buxton, A.E.; Carson, A.P.; Commodore-Mensah, Y.; et al. Heart Disease and Stroke Statistics-2022 Update: A Report from the American Heart Association. *Circulation* **2022**, *145*, e153–e639. [CrossRef]

69. Joseph, J.J.; Deedwania, P.; Acharya, T.; Aguilar, D.; Bhatt, D.L.; Chyun, D.A.; Di Palo, K.E.; Golden, S.H.; Sperling, L.S. Comprehensive Management of Cardiovascular Risk Factors for Adults with Type 2 Diabetes: A Scientific Statement from the American Heart Association. *Circulation* 2022, *145*, e722–e759. [CrossRef]
70. Afshin, A.; Sur, P.J.; Fay, K.A.; Cornaby, L.; Ferrara, G.; Salama, J.S.; Mullany, E.C.; Abate, K.H.; Abbafati, C.; Abebe, Z.; et al. Health Effects of Dietary Risks in 195 Countries, 1990–2017: A Systematic Analysis for the Global Burden of Disease Study 2017. *Lancet* 2019, *393*, 1958–1972. [CrossRef]
71. Centers for Disease Control and Prevention, National Center for Health Statistics. About Multiple Cause of Death, 1999–2020. CDC WONDER Online Database Website. Centers for Disease Control and Prevention: Atlanta, GA, USA. 2022. Available online: https://wonder.cdc.gov/wonder/help/mcd.html (accessed on 28 February 2023).
72. Ahmad, F.B.; Anderson, R.N. The Leading Causes of Death in the US for 2020. *JAMA* 2021, *325*, 1829–1830. [CrossRef]
73. Virani, S.S.; Alonso, A.; Benjamin, E.J.; Bittencourt, M.S.; Callaway, C.W.; Carson, A.P.; Chamberlain, A.M.; Chang, A.R.; Cheng, S.; Delling, F.N.; et al. Heart Disease and Stroke Statistics—2020 Update a Report from the American Heart Association. *Circulation* 2020, *141*, e139–e596. [CrossRef] [PubMed]
74. Centers for Disease Control and Prevention; National Center for Health Statistics. About Underlying Cause of Death 1999–2019. CDC WONDER Online Database. Available online: https://wonder.cdc.gov/ucd-icd10.html (accessed on 28 February 2023).
75. Bergeron, N.; Chiu, S.; Williams, P.T.; M King, S.; Krauss, R.M. Effects of Red Meat, White Meat, and Nonmeat Protein Sources on Atherogenic Lipoprotein Measures in the Context of Low Compared with High Saturated Fat Intake: A Randomized Controlled Trial. *Am. J. Clin. Nutr.* 2019, *110*, 24–33. [CrossRef]
76. Beauchesne-Rondeau, É.; Gascon, A.; Bergeron, J.; Jacques, H. Plasma Lipids and Lipoproteins in Hypercholesterolemic Men Fed a Lipid-Lowering Diet Containing Lean Beef, Lean Fish, or Poultry. *Am. J. Clin. Nutr.* 2003, *77*, 587–593. [CrossRef] [PubMed]
77. Scott, L.W.; Dunn, J.K.; Pownall, H.J.; Braucht, D.J.; McMann, M.C.; Herd, J.A.; Harris, K.B.; Savell, J.W.; Cross, H.R.; Gotto, A.M. Effects of Beef and Chicken Consumption on Plasma Lipid Levels in Hypercholesterolemic Men. *Arch. Intern. Med.* 1994, *154*, 1261–1267. [CrossRef] [PubMed]
78. Mateo-Gallego, R.; Perez-Calahorra, S.; Cenarro, A.; Bea, A.M.; Andres, E.; Horno, J.; Ros, E.; Civeira, F. Effect of Lean Red Meat from Lamb v. Lean White Meat from Chicken on the Serum Lipid Profile: A Randomised, Cross-over Study in Women. *Br. J. Nutr.* 2012, *107*, 1403–1407. [CrossRef]
79. Lee, J.E.; McLerran, D.F.; Rolland, B.; Chen, Y.; Grant, E.J.; Vedanthan, R.; Inoue, M.; Tsugane, S.; Gao, Y.T.; Tsuji, I.; et al. Meat Intake and Cause-Specific Mortality: A Pooled Analysis of Asian Prospective Cohort Studies. *Am. J. Clin. Nutr.* 2013, *98*, 1032–1041. [CrossRef]
80. Takata, Y.; Shu, X.O.; Gao, Y.T.; Li, H.; Zhang, X.; Gao, J.; Cai, H.; Yang, G.; Xiang, Y.B.; Zheng, W. Red Meat and Poultry Intakes and Risk of Total and Cause-Specific Mortality: Results from Cohort Studies of Chinese Adults in Shanghai. *PLoS ONE* 2013, *8*, e56963. [CrossRef]
81. Nagao, M.; Iso, H.; Yamagishi, K.; Date, C.; Tamakoshi, A. Meat Consumption in Relation to Mortality from Cardiovascular Disease among Japanese Men and Women. *Eur. J. Clin. Nutr.* 2012, *66*, 687–693. [CrossRef]
82. Key, T.J.; Appleby, P.N.; Bradbury, K.E.; Sweeting, M.; Wood, A.; Johansson, I.; Kühn, T.; Steur, M.; Weiderpass, E.; Wennberg, M.; et al. Consumption of Meat, Fish, Dairy Products, and Eggs and Risk of Ischemic Heart Disease. *Circulation* 2019, *139*, 2835–2845. [CrossRef]
83. Haring, B.; Gronroos, N.; Nettleton, J.A.; Wyler Von Ballmoos, M.C.; Selvin, E.; Alonso, A. Dietary Protein Intake and Coronary Heart Disease in a Large Community Based Cohort: Results from the Atherosclerosis Risk in Communities (ARIC) Study. *PLoS ONE* 2014, *9*, e109552. [CrossRef]
84. Ogilvie, R.P.; Lutsey, P.L.; Heiss, G.; Folsom, A.R.; Steffen, L.M. Dietary Intake and Peripheral Arterial Disease Incidence in Middle-Aged Adults: The Atherosclerosis Risk in Communities (ARIC) Study. *Am. J. Clin. Nutr.* 2017, *105*, 651–659. [CrossRef] [PubMed]
85. Park, K.; Son, J.; Jang, J.; Kang, R.; Chung, H.K.; Lee, K.W.; Lee, S.M.; Lim, H.; Shin, M.J. Unprocessed Meat Consumption and Incident Cardiovascular Diseases in Korean Adults: The Korean Genome and Epidemiology Study (KoGES). *Nutrients* 2017, *9*, 498. [CrossRef] [PubMed]
86. Bernstein, A.M.; Sun, Q.; Hu, F.B.; Stampfer, M.J.; Manson, J.E.; Willett, W.C. Major Dietary Protein Sources and Risk of Coronary Heart Disease in Women. *Circulation* 2010, *122*, 876–883. [CrossRef] [PubMed]
87. Wang, D.; Campos, H.; Baylin, A. Red Meat Intake Is Positively Associated with Non-Fatal Acute Myocardial Infarction in the Costa Rica Heart Study. *Br. J. Nutr.* 2017, *118*, 303–311. [CrossRef]
88. Zhong, V.W.; Van Horn, L.; Greenland, P.; Carnethon, M.R.; Ning, H.; Wilkins, J.T.; Lloyd-Jones, D.M.; Allen, N.B. Associations of Processed Meat, Unprocessed Red Meat, Poultry, or Fish Intake With Incident Cardiovascular Disease and All-Cause Mortality. *JAMA. Intern. Med.* 2020, *180*, 503. [CrossRef]
89. Papier, K.; Fensom, G.K.; Knuppel, A.; Appleby, P.N.; Tong, T.Y.N.; Schmidt, J.A.; Travis, R.C.; Key, T.J.; Perez-Cornago, A. Meat Consumption and Risk of 25 Common Conditions: Outcome-Wide Analyses in 475,000 Men and Women in the UK Biobank Study. *BMC Med.* 2021, *19*, 53. [CrossRef]
90. Mohammadi, H.; Jayedi, A.; Ghaedi, E.; Golbidi, D.; Shab-bidar, S. Dietary Poultry Intake and the Risk of Stroke: A Dose–Response Meta-Analysis of Prospective Cohort Studies. *Clin. Nutr. ESPEN* 2018, *23*, 25–33. [CrossRef]

1. Sauvaget, C.; Nagano, J.; Allen, N.; Grant, E.J.; Beral, V. Intake of Animal Products and Stroke Mortality in the Hiroshima/Nagasaki Life Span Study. *Int. J. Epidemiol.* **2003**, *32*, 536–543. [CrossRef]
2. Tong, T.Y.N.; Appleby, P.N.; Key, T.J.; Dahm, C.C.; Overvad, K.; Olsen, A.; Tjønneland, A.; Katzke, V.; Kühn, T.; Boeing, H.; et al. The Associations of Major Foods and Fibre with Risks of Ischaemic and Haemorrhagic Stroke: A Prospective Study of 418 329 Participants in the EPIC Cohort across Nine European Countries. *Eur. Heart J.* **2020**, *41*, 2632–2640. [CrossRef]
93. Kim, Y.; Je, Y. Meat Consumption and Risk of Metabolic Syndrome: Results from the Korean Population and a Meta-Analysis of Observational Studies. *Nutrients* **2018**, *10*, 390. [CrossRef] [PubMed]
94. Bernstein, A.M.; Pan, A.; Rexrode, K.M.; Stampfer, M.; Hu, F.B.; Mozaffarian, D.; Willett, W.C. Dietary Protein Sources and the Risk of Stroke in Men and Women. *Stroke* **2012**, *43*, 637–664. [CrossRef] [PubMed]
95. Zhang, Y.; Zhang, D. Red Meat, Poultry, and Egg Consumption with the Risk of Hypertension: A Meta-Analysis of Prospective Cohort Studies. *J. Hum. Hypertens.* **2018**, *32*, 507–517. [CrossRef] [PubMed]
96. Borgia, L.; Curhan, G.C.; Willett, W.C.; Hu, F.B.; Satijad, A.; Forman, J.P. Long-Term Intake of Animal Flesh and Risk of Developing Hypertension in Three Prospective Cohort Studies. *J. Hypertens.* **2015**, *33*, 2231–2238. [CrossRef]
97. Griep, L.M.O.; Seferidi, P.; Stamler, J.; Van Horn, L.; Chan, Q.; Tzoulaki, I.; Steffen, L.M.; Miura, K.; Ueshima, H.; Okuda, N.; et al. Relation of Unprocessed, Processed Red Meat and Poultry Consumption to Blood Pressure in East Asian and Western Adults. *J. Hypertens.* **2016**, *34*, 1721–2729. [CrossRef]
98. Miura, K.; Greenland, P.; Stamler, J.; Liu, K.; Daviglus, M.L.; Nakagawa, H. Relation of Vegetable, Fruit, and Meat Intake to 7-Year Blood Pressure Change in Middle-Aged Men: The Chicago Western Electric Study. *Am. J. Epidemiol.* **2004**, *159*, 572–580. [CrossRef]
99. Steffen, L.M.; Kroenke, C.H.; Yu, X.; Pereira, M.A.; Slattery, M.L.; Van Horn, L.; Gross, M.D.; Jacobs, D.R. Associations of Plant Food, Dairy Product, and Meat Intakes with 15-y Incidence of Elevated Blood Pressure in Young Black and White Adults: The Coronary Artery Risk Development in Young Adults (CARDIA) Study. *Am. J. Clin. Nutr.* **2005**, *82*, 1169–1177. [CrossRef]
100. Golzarand, M.; Bahadoran, Z.; Mirmiran, P.; Azizi, F. Protein Foods Group and 3-Year Incidence of Hypertension: A Prospective Study from Tehran Lipid and Glucose Study. *J. Ren. Nutr.* **2016**, *26*, 219–225. [CrossRef]
101. Wang, L.; Manson, J.E.; Buring, J.E.; Sesso, H.D. Meat Intake and the Risk of Hypertension in Middle-Aged and Older Women. *J. Hypertens.* **2008**, *26*, 215–222. [CrossRef]
102. Takashima, Y.; Iwase, Y.; Yoshida, M.; Kokaze, A.; Takagi, Y.; Tsubono, Y.; Tsugane, S.; Takahashi, T.; Litoi, Y.; Akabane, M.; et al. Relationship of Food Intake and Dietary Patterns with Blood Pressure Levels among Middle-Aged Japanese Men. *J. Epidemiol.* **1998**, *8*, 106–115. [CrossRef]
103. Centers for Disease Control and Prevention. National Diabetes Statistics Report Website. Available online: https://www.cdc.gov/diabetes/data/statistics-report/index.html (accessed on 18 February 2023).
104. Zhou, B.; Lu, Y.; Hajifathalian, K.; Bentham, J.; Di Cesare, M.; Danaei, G.; Bixby, H.; Cowan, M.J.; Ali, M.K.; Taddei, C.; et al. Worldwide Trends in Diabetes since 1980: A Pooled Analysis of 751 Population-Based Studies with 4.4 Million Participants. *Lancet* **2016**, *387*, 1513–1530. [CrossRef]
105. Sun, L.; Ranawana, D.V.; Leow, M.K.S.; Henry, C.J. Effect of Chicken, Fat and Vegetable on Glycaemia and Insulinaemia to a White Rice-Based Meal in Healthy Adults. *Eur. J. Nutr.* **2014**, *53*, 1719–1726. [CrossRef]
106. Quek, R.; Bi, X.; Henry, C.J. Impact of Protein-Rich Meals on Glycaemic Response of Rice. *Br. J. Nutr.* **2016**, *115*, 1194–1201. [CrossRef]
107. Hätönen, K.A.; Virtamo, J.; Eriksson, J.G.; Sinkko, H.K.; Sundvall, J.E.; Valsta, L.M. Protein and Fat Modify the Glycaemic and Insulinaemic Responses to a Mashed Potato-Based Meal. *Br. J. Nutr.* **2011**, *106*, 248–253. [CrossRef] [PubMed]
108. Gannon, M.C.; Nuttall, F.Q.; Neil, B.J.; Westphal, S.A. The Insulin and Glucose Responses to Meals of Glucose plus Various Proteins in Type II Diabetic Subjects. *Metabolism* **1988**, *37*, 1081–1088. [CrossRef] [PubMed]
109. Devries, M.C.; Sithamparapillai, A.; Brimble, K.S.; Banfield, L.; Morton, R.W.; Phillips, S.M. Changes in Kidney Function Do Not Differ between Healthy Adults Consuming Higher- Compared with Lower- or Normal-Protein Diets: A Systematic Review and Meta-Analysis. *J. Nutr.* **2018**, *148*, 1760–1775. [CrossRef]
110. Walker, J.D.; Dodds, R.A.; Murrells, T.J.; Bending, J.J.; Mattock, M.B.; Keen, H.; Viberti, G.C. Restriction of Dietary Protein and Progression of Renal Failure in Diabetic Nephropathy. *Lancet* **1989**, *334*, 1411–1415. [CrossRef]
111. Hansen, H.P.; Christensen, P.K.; Tauber-Lassen, E.; Klausen, A.; Jensen, B.R.; Parving, H.H. Low-Protein Diet and Kidney Function in Insulin-Dependent Diabetic Patients with Diabetic Nephropathy. *Kidney Int.* **1999**, *55*, 621–628. [CrossRef]
112. Ko, G.J.; Rhee, C.M.; Kalantar-Zadeh, K.; Joshi, S. The Effects of High-Protein Diets on Kidney Health and Longevity. *J. Am. Soc. Nephrol.* **2020**, *31*, 1667–1679. [CrossRef]
113. Gross, J.L.; Zelmanovitz, T.; Moulin, C.C.; De Mello, V.; Perassolo, M.; Leitao, C.; Hoefel, A.; Paggi, A.; Azevedo, M.J. Effect of a Chicken-Based Diet on Renal Function and Lipid Profile in Patients with Type 2 Diabetes: A Randomized Crossover Trial. *Diabetes Care* **2002**, *25*, 645–651. [CrossRef]
114. De Mello, V.D.F.; Zelmanovitz, T.; Perassolo, M.S.; Azevedo, M.J.; Gross, J.L. Withdrawal of Red Meat from the Usual Diet Reduces Albuminuria and Improves Serum Fatty Acid Profile in Type 2 Diabetes Patients with Macroalbuminuria. *Am. J. Clin. Nutr.* **2006**, *83*, 1032–1038. [CrossRef]
115. de Mello, V.D.F.; Zelmanovitz, T.; Azevedo, M.J.; de Paula, T.P.; Gross, J.L. Long-Term Effect of a Chicken-Based Diet Versus Enalapril on Albuminuria in Type 2 Diabetic Patients with Microalbuminuria. *J. Ren. Nutr.* **2008**, *18*, 440–447. [CrossRef]

116. Fan, M.; Li, Y.; Wang, C.; Mao, Z.; Zhou, W.; Zhang, L.; Yang, X.; Cui, S.; Li, L. Dietary Protein Consumption and the Risk of Type 2 Diabetes: Adose-Response Meta-Analysis of Prospective Studies. *Nutrients* **2019**, *11*, 2783. [CrossRef] [PubMed]
117. Feskens, E.J.M.; Sluik, D.; van Woudenbergh, G.J. Meat Consumption, Diabetes, and Its Complications. *Curr. Diab. Rep.* **2013**, *13*, 298–306. [CrossRef] [PubMed]
118. The InterAct Consortium. Association between Dietary Meat Consumption and Incident Type 2 Diabetes: The EPIC-InterAct Study. *Diabetologia* **2013**, *56*, 47–59. [CrossRef] [PubMed]
119. Talaei, M.; Wang, Y.L.; Yuan, J.M.; Pan, A.; Koh, W.P. Meat, Dietary Heme Iron, and Risk of Type 2 Diabetes MellitusThe Singapore Chinese Health Study. *Am. J. Epidemiol.* **2017**, *186*, 824–833. [CrossRef]
120. Villegas, R.; Xiao, O.S.; Gao, Y.T.; Yang, G.; Cai, H.; Li, H.; Zheng, W. The Association of Meat Intake and the Risk of Type 2 Diabetes May Be Modified by Body Weight. *Int. J. Med. Sci.* **2006**, *3*, 152–159. [CrossRef]
121. Montonen, J.; Järvinen, R.; Heliövaara, M.; Reunanen, A.; Aromaa, A.; Knekt, P. Food Consumption and the Incidence of Type II Diabetes Mellitus. *Eur. J. Clin. Nutr.* **2005**, *59*, 152–159. [CrossRef]
122. Sluik, D.; Boeing, H.; Li, K.; Kaaks, R.; Johnsen, N.F.; Tjønneland, A.; Arriola, L.; Barricarte, A.; Masala, G.; Grioni, S.; et al. Lifestyle Factors and Mortality Risk in Individuals with Diabetes Mellitus: Are the Associations Different from Those in Individuals without Diabetes? *Diabetologia* **2014**, *57*, 63–72. [CrossRef]
123. Würtz, A.M.L.; Jakobsen, M.U.; Bertoia, M.L.; Hou, T.; Schmidt, E.B.; Willett, W.C.; Overvad, K.; Sun, Q.; Manson, J.A.E.; Hu, F.B.; et al. Replacing the Consumption of Red Meat with Other Major Dietary Protein Sources and Risk of Type 2 Diabetes Mellitus: A Prospective Cohort Study. *Am. J. Clin. Nutr.* **2021**, *113*, 612–621. [CrossRef]
124. Ibsen, D.B.; Steur, M.; Imamura, F.; Overvad, K.; Schulze, M.B.; Bendinelli, B.; Guevara, M.; Agudo, A.; Amiano, P.; Aune, D.; et al. Replacement of Red and Processed Meat with Other Food Sources of Protein and the Risk of Type 2 Diabetes in European Populations: The EPIC-InterAct Study. *Diabetes Care* **2020**, *43*, 2660–2667. [CrossRef] [PubMed]
125. Ibsen, D.B.; Warberg, C.K.; Würtz, A.M.L.; Overvad, K.; Dahm, C.C. Substitution of Red Meat with Poultry or Fish and Risk of Type 2 Diabetes: A Danish Cohort Study. *Eur. J. Nutr.* **2019**, *58*, 2705–2712. [CrossRef] [PubMed]
126. Guasch-Ferré, M.; Satija, A.; Blondin, S.A.; Janiszewski, M.; Emlen, E.; O'Connor, L.E.; Campbell, W.W.; Hu, F.B.; Willett, W.C.; Stampfer, M.J. Meta-Analysis of Randomized Controlled Trials of Red Meat Consumption in Comparison with Various Comparison Diets on Cardiovascular Risk Factors. *Circulation* **2019**, *139*, 1828–1845. [CrossRef] [PubMed]

Disclaimer/Publisher's Note: The statements, opinions and data contained in all publications are solely those of the individual author(s) and contributor(s) and not of MDPI and/or the editor(s). MDPI and/or the editor(s) disclaim responsibility for any injury to people or property resulting from any ideas, methods, instructions or products referred to in the content.

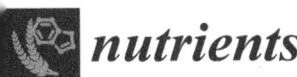

Article

Novel α-Glucosidase Inhibitory Peptides Identified In Silico from Dry-Cured Pork Loins with Probiotics through Peptidomic and Molecular Docking Analysis

Paulina Kęska, Joanna Stadnik *, Aleksandra Łupawka and Agata Michalska

Department of Animal Food Technology, Faculty of Food Science and Biotechnology, University of Life Sciences in Lublin, Skromna 8, 20-704 Lublin, Poland
* Correspondence: joanna.stadnik@up.lublin.pl

Abstract: Diabetes mellitus is a serious metabolic disorder characterized by abnormal blood glucose levels in the body. The development of therapeutic strategies for restoring and maintaining blood glucose homeostasis is still in progress. Synthetic alpha-amylase and alpha-glucosidase inhibitors can improve blood glucose control in diabetic patients by effectively reducing the risk of postprandial hyperglycemia. Peptides of natural origin are promising compounds that can serve as alpha-glucosidase inhibitors in the treatment of type 2 diabetes. Potential alpha-glucosidase-inhibiting peptides obtained from aqueous and saline extracts from dry-cured pork loins inoculated with probiotic LAB were evaluated using in vitro and in silico methods. To identify the peptide sequences, liquid chromatography-mass spectrometry was used. For this purpose, in silico calculation methods were used, and the occurrence of bioactive fragments in the protein followed the ADMET approach. The most promising sequences were molecularly docked to test their interaction with the human alpha-glycosidase molecule (PDB ID: 5NN8). The docking studies proved that oligopeptides VATPPPPPPK, DIPPPPM, TPPPPPPG, and TPPPPPPK obtained by hydrolysis of proteins from ripening dry-cured pork loins showed the potential to bind to the human alpha-glucosidase molecule and may act effectively as a potential antidiabetic agent.

Keywords: probiotics; bioactive peptides; dry-cured meat; fermentation

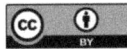

1. Introduction

Diabetes mellitus is a metabolic disorder characterized by impaired insulin secretion and/or action leading to chronic hyperglycemia, as well as alterations in carbohydrate, lipid, and protein metabolism. Diabetes, both type 1 (T1D) and type 2 (T2D), are an important problem, but are also a priority for public health agencies, the pharmaceutical and food industry, and scientists to solve, as the number of diseases and the percentage of deaths caused by diabetes increases every year. In particular, T2D accounts for more than 90% of all diabetes cases worldwide. Currently, different classes of hypoglycemic drugs are used in the treatment of type 2 diabetes, including dipeptidyl peptidase inhibitors. They act by prolonging the action of human incretin glucagon-like peptide 1 (GLP-1) and gastric inhibitory polypeptide (GIP), thereby increasing postprandial insulin secretion from pancreatic beta cells. Incretins additionally inhibit the secretion of glucagon, a hormone that increases the concentration of glucose in the blood, and inhibit the motility of the gastrointestinal tract, delaying gastric emptying. Other drugs used in pharmacology against the effects of diabetes are alpha-amylase and alpha-glucosidase inhibitors [1,2]. This class of drugs inhibits the digestion of carbohydrates by targeting these enzymes, thereby reducing postprandial hyperglycemia by delaying the hydrolysis of complex carbohydrates. The first, α-Amylase, catalyzes the initial stage of hydrolysis of polysaccharides, mainly starch, to maltose, while α-glucosidase, an enzyme associated with the small intestinal epithelium, catalyzes the hydrolysis of maltose and other disaccharides to release free glucose molecules.

Thus, the strategy in which inhibitors act for these enzymes prevents glucose from being derived from complex dietary carbohydrates and released into the bloodstream [1,2]. In this way, the risk of postprandial hyperglycemia is effectively reduced.

In response to the needs of patients reporting additional, negative effects of the use of synthetic drugs, such as nausea, vomiting, or diarrhea, a new direction of research has become the search for alternatives among natural compounds that would equally effectively inhibit the action of human enzymes. A promising class of drugs that can serve as α-glucosidase inhibitors in the treatment of type 2 diabetes are bioactive compounds, such as peptides of natural origin. According to Ibrahim et al. [2], a total of 43 fully sequenced α-glucosidase inhibitory peptides have been described so far, and 13 of them had IC_{50} values several times lower than acarbose—a popular, synthetic antidiabetic drug that is an α-glucosidase inhibitor. Little is known about the bioactive compounds in food that act as a preventative or supportive factor in the treatment of diabetes when consumed in the daily diet. Although there are reports of alpha-glucosidase inhibitors in foods of plant origin, such as wheat bran and germ [3], grape pomace [4], and other plants containing bioactive ingredients, i.e., flavonoids, phenolic acids, tannins, and anthocyanins [5,6], there are only a few reports on meat as an example of food of animal origin as a source of antidiabetic ingredients. Recently, studies by Martínez-Sánchez et al. [7] assessed the cause-and-effect relationship between the consumption of dry-cured ham and cardiovascular effects, showing that consumption of dry-cured ham improves inflammatory responses and regulates thrombotic status in human clinical trials. In turn, Montoro-García et al. [8], in a similar study, showed no negative impact on the blood pressure of patients who consumed 80 g of dried ham daily. Additionally, the authors observed that total cholesterol, LDL, and basal glucose levels decreased [8], suggesting the potential of ripening meat products as a source of natural antidiabetic peptides. Previous studies have shown that raw ripened meat products are carriers of bioactive peptides with DPP-IV inhibitory activity, which may act as a strategy against type 2 diabetes mellitus [9–12]. In turn, in the study by Mora et al. [13], the α-glucosidase inhibitory potential of the peptides obtained in the water fraction of proteins extracted from traditional Spanish dry-cured ham was described for the first time. This study identified two new and active α-glucosidase inhibiting peptides that can resist digestion in the human digestive system and therefore can delay postprandial hyperglycemia in diabetic patients.

In this study, α-glucosidase-inhibiting peptides obtained from extracts (aqueous and saline) of dry-cured pork loin inoculated with LAB strains after 6 months of aging were evaluated using in vitro and in silico methods. The extracts were subjected to pepsin and pancreatin hydrolysis to obtain fragments of peptides that were potentially resistant to gastrointestinal digestion. Liquid chromatography-mass spectrometry was then used to identify the peptide sequences. Their potential for α-glucosidase inhibition was also tested in an in silico study, and pharmacokinetic properties were assessed using the ADMET approach. The most promising sequences were molecularly docked to test their interaction with the human α-glycosidase molecule (PDB ID: 5NN8).

2. Materials and Methods

2.1. Preparation of Dry-Cured Meat Products

The meat (*m. longissimus thoracis*) was cut 24 h after slaughter in a local slaughterhouse from half-carcasses of Polish large white pigs chilled to 4 °C. The next day, all loins (12) were cured with a curing mixture (20 g NaCl, 9.7 g cured salt, and 0.3 g $NaNO_3$/kg loin) by surface massage. All cured batches were kept at 4 °C for 24 h to allow the curing salt to diffuse. After curing, the loin was portioned into pieces weighing about 1 kg, which were randomly divided into four experimental groups: control variant (C—not inoculated with LAB strain), LOCK (probiotic strain *Lacticaseibacillus rhamnosus* LOCK900 was used, strain deposit number: CP00548), BB12 (probiotic strain *Bifidobacterium animalis* ssp. *lactis* BB-12, strain deposit number: DSM15954), and BAUER (potentially probiotic strain *L. acidophilus* Bauer Ł0938 was used). The inoculum was applied on the surface in the amount of 0.2%

(v/w) to obtain 10^6–10^7 CFU/g of meat, then the meat portions were suspended in a laboratory maturing chamber at a temperature of 16 ± 1 °C and relative air humidity of $75 \pm 5\%$ for 21 days, then whole loins were vacuum packed and matured at 4 ± 1 °C for 6 months (180 days).

2.2. Meat Protein Extraction and Hydrolysis

The water-soluble fraction (S) of meat proteins was extracted by homogenizing 10 g of meat for 5 min (T25 Basic ULTRA-TURRAX; IKA, Staufen, Germany) and distilled water (1:10 w/v) on ice and subjecting the resulting homogenate to centrifugation (10,000× g, 4 °C for 10 min) [14]. To prepare the salt soluble fraction (M), the precipitate resulting from the S extraction was resuspended in 0.6 M NaCl in 0.1 M phosphate buffer (pH 6.2) at a ratio of 1:6 and homogenized for 1 min on ice [15]. The resulting homogenate was kept for 18 h at 4 °C for degassing. After this time, the homogenate was subjected to centrifugation (10,000× g, 4 °C for 10 min), and the supernatant was filtered through Whatman No. 1 filter paper. The protein fractions obtained in this way were subjected to in vitro hydrolysis using pepsin and pancreatin [16]. In the first step, the protein extracts were adjusted to pH 2.0 with 1 M HCl and a solution of pepsin HCl (pH 2.0; 6 M) was added in an enzyme to substrate ratio of 1:100. The hydrolysis process was carried out for 120 min under the following conditions: temperature 37 °C in the dark and with continuous stirring. After the pepsin digestion step, its effect was inhibited by neutralizing the solution to pH 7.0 with 1 M NaOH. Pancreatin was then added in an enzyme to substrate ratio of 1:50 for 180 min with the conditions as before. The process of enzymatic hydrolysis was stopped by heating at 95 °C for 10 min. The hydrolysates were then dialyzed using membrane tubes (7 kDa molecular weight cutoff, Spectra/Por®) (Repligen Europe B.V.; Breda, The Netherlands) against phosphate-buffered saline (PBS; pH 7.4; 1:4, v/v) for 1 h at 37 °C. Obtained hydrolysates were concentrated in the evaporator and dissolved in 2 mL of 0.01 M HCl prior to chromatographic analysis.

2.3. Peptidomic Characteristic

2.3.1. Peptide Identification by LC-MS/MS

Before the analysis, the samples were concentrated and desalted on an RP-C18 pre-column (Waters Corp., Milford, MA, USA). Separation was performed on an RP-C18 nano-Ultra Performance column (Waters, BEH130 C18 column, 75 µm i.d., 250 mm long) of a nanoACQUITY UPLC system (Warsaw, Poland) using a 180 min linear acetonitrile gradient (0–35%) at a flow rate of 250 nL/min. The column outlet was directly connected to a mass spectrometer (Orbitrap Velos, Thermo Fisher Scientific Inc., Waltham, MA, USA) for the analysis. The raw data files were preprocessed using Mascot Distiller software (version 2.4.2.0, Matrix Science Inc., Boston, MA, USA). The obtained peptide masses and their identified fragmentation pattern were compared with the protein sequence database (UniProt KB) [17] using the Mascot search engine (Mascot Daemon v. 2.4.0, Mascot Server v.2.4.1, Matrix Science, London, UK). The "mammals" option was chosen as the taxonomy constraint parameter. The search parameters applied were as follows: enzyme specificity, none; peptide mass tolerance, 5×10^{-6}; fragment mass tolerance, 0.01 Da. The protein mass was left unrestricted, and the mass values were assumed as monoisotopic with a maximum of two missed cleavages allowed. Methylthiolation, oxidation, and carbamidomethylation were set as fixed and variable modifications. The peptide sequences from unknown original proteins were excluded. Peptide identification was performed using the Mascot search engine (Matrix Science), with a probability-based algorithm. The expected value threshold was set at 0.05 for the analysis (all peptide identification had <0.05% chance of being a random match).

2.3.2. α-Glucosidase Inhibitory Activity Peptides Search

Spectrometric analysis resulted in a list of peptide sequences (a total of 8 searches: 4 for the water-soluble fraction and 4 for the salt-soluble fraction). All were tested for the presence of sequences that are potential α-glucosidase inhibitors. The search was carried out using the BIOPEP-UWM database [18]. For this purpose, in the "Calculations" tab, the frequency of occurrence of bioactive fragments in the protein sequence (parameter A) was used, which is described by the formula:

$$A = a/N$$

where: a—the number of fragments with a given activity in the protein sequence and N—the number of protein amino acid residues.

2.3.3. Allergenic and ADMET Prediction

The potential effectiveness of selected peptide sequences from dry-cured pork loins was estimated by ADMET (absorption, distribution, metabolism, excretion, and toxicity) analysis. The analysis was performed using an internet platform called ADMETlab [19]. ADMET analysis included Caco-2 permeability log and human intestinal absorption (HIA) as adsorption steps, plasma protein binding (PPB), and blood–brain barrier (BBB) penetration as distribution steps, the prediction of cytochrome P450 (CYP450) 2D6 inhibition as a metabolic step, the determination of the half-life ($T_{1/2}$) as the step of excretion, and finally the acute toxicity (LD_{50}), human hepatotoxicity (H-HP), and maximum recommended daily dose (FDAMDD) was determined as the stage of toxicity. Their potential allergenicity was also tested using the AllerTOP v. 2.0 tool [20].

2.4. Molecular Docking

2.4.1. Receptor Structure and Preparation

The receptor utilized in the molecular docking method was chain A of the crystal structure of human lysosomal acid α-glucosidase, GAA (PDB ID: 5NN8) [21–23]. This enzyme is essential for the degradation of glycogen within lysosomes. It exhibits the highest activity on α-1,4-glycosidic bonds, but is also capable of hydrolyzing glucans linked by α-1,6 bonds. This transmembrane protein, which is composed of 872 amino acid residues, was obtained via X-ray diffraction. The first step was to remove from the structure all entities that were not a protein receptor, and which could interfere with the course of molecular docking, including water molecules, S-hydroxycysteine, α-L-fucopyranose, 2-acetamido-2-deoxy-β-D-gluxopyranose, β-D-mannopyranose, α-D-glucopyranose, 4,6-dideoxy-4-{[{1S, 4R, 5S, 6S)-4,5,6-trihydroxy-3-(hydroxymethyl) cyclohex-2-en-1-yl]amino}-α-D-gluxopyranose, sulfate ions, chloride ions, glycerol, 1,2-ethanediol, triethylene glycol, ethylene glyxol, N-[4-hydroxymethyl-cyclohexan-6-yl-1,2,3-triol]-4,6-dideoxy-4-aminoglucopyranoside, and glycerin. The subsequent step involved preparing the receptor for molecular docking. This entailed adding hydrogen atoms and partial charges to the receptor's structure, as well as optimizing it. To accomplish this, the AutoDockTools package, which is part of the MGLTools software (version 1.5.7) suite, was utilized [24,25]. Hydrogen atoms and partial charges (Gasteiger) were added using this package. Additionally, energy minimization was performed using General Amber Force Field (GAFF) in the Open Babel software (version 3.0.0) [26]. The file format was also appropriately converted to the one required by the QuickVina-W docking engine [27]. The prepared structure used for the study is presented in Figure 1.

2.4.2. Ligand Structures and Preparation

The three-dimensional structures of the peptides were predicted based on their amino acid sequences using the ECEPP software (ECEPP-05 version) [28], using an Electrostatically Driven Monte Carlo (EDMC) method for peptide structure determination. The simulation proceeds through a series of Monte Carlo steps, driven by the electrostatic interaction energy between the charged residues, to pick up different variants of the peptide conformation. Finally, the resulting conformations were ranked based on their energies, and the lowest energy conformations were selected as potential 3D structures for peptide. The generated structures of each peptide were subjected to a short optimization process using GAFF force field [26]. The subsequent step involved adding partial charges to the ligand structures. Similar to the receptor, the AutoDockTools package was employed for this task. The file format was also converted to the format required by the QuickVina-W docking engine (see Figure 2).

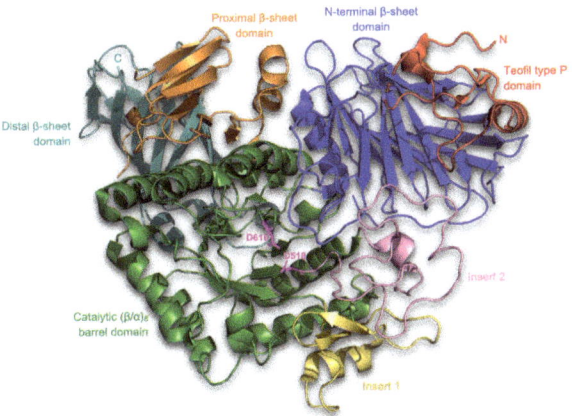

Figure 1. Cartoon representation of the three-dimensional structure of human lysosomal acid α-glucosidase (PDB ID: 5NN8), consisting of the N-terminal β-sheet domain (blue), trefoil type P domain (red), the proximal (orange) and distal (teal) β-sheet domains, and the catalytic (β/α)$_8$ barrel domain (green) with insert I (yellow) and insert II (pink). Catalytic amino acid residues such as D616 and D518 are marked in magenta.

2.4.3. Molecular Docking Analysis

To determine the binding affinity of the defined peptides to protein 5NN8 in its selected 10 binding pockets, we utilized molecular docking. We used three different types of computational software to predict the potential binding poses on the surface of the studied peptide: fpocket [29], CAVITY [30], and open-source GHECOM software (version 1.0) [31]. Peptide docking was carried out using QuickVina-W. Docking analyses were performed for the 10 selected cavities. For each cavity, the search space was set to include all atoms belonging to the cavity with some extra margin. Each of the four considered ligands were docked separately into each cavity. All analyses were performed with the exhaustiveness parameter set to 100, while all other settings were kept at their default values.

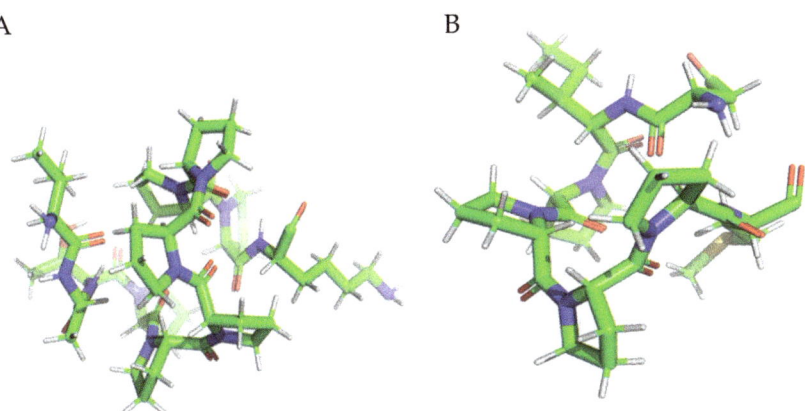

Figure 2. *Cont.*

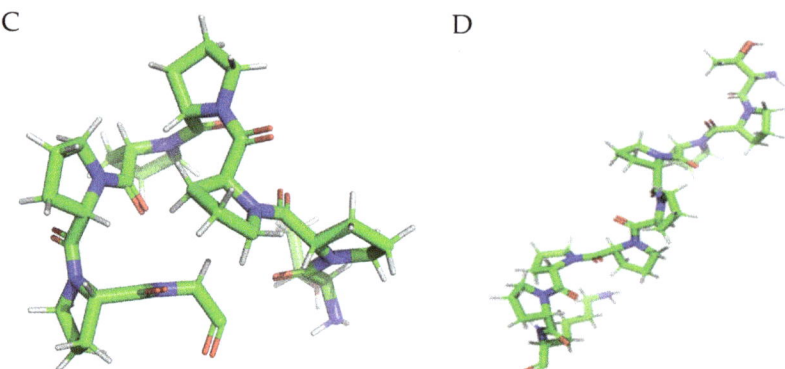

Figure 2. Minimized 3D structure of a peptide with the sequence VATPPPPPPPK (**A**), DIPPPPM (**B**), TPPPPPPG (**C**), and TPPPPPPPK (**D**). The color green represents C atoms, blue represents N atoms, white represents H atoms, and red represents O atoms.

3. Results and Discussion
3.1. Peptide Characteristics

In accordance with the peptidomic approach, peptides derived from variant assays (C, LOCK, BB12, BAUER, both from the S and M fraction) were analyzed by mass spectrometry, measuring their amino acid composition, molecular mass, and the type of protein from which bioinforma that are potential α-glucoside inhibitors, along with their place of occurrence, are presented in Supplement Materials (Table S1). As shown in Figure 3, both within the S fraction (extracted from the meat product with a water solvent) and the M fraction (extraction of proteins with a saline solution), a relatively equal number of sequences potentially inhibiting the activity of α-glucosidase were identified.

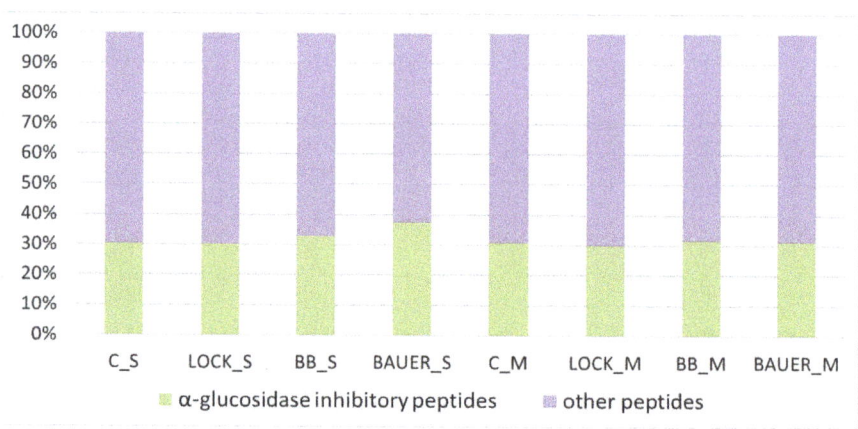

Figure 3. Cumulative distribution of peptides identified in test variants, including sequences potentially inhibiting α-glucosidase activity. S—peptides obtained from water-soluble fraction; M—peptides obtained from salt-soluble fraction; C, control sample; LOCK, sample inoculated with *Lacticaseibacillus rhamnosus* LOCK900; BB12, sample inoculated with *Bifidobacterium animalis* ssp. *lactis* BB-12; BAUER, sample inoculated with *Lactobacillus acidophilus* Bauer Ł0938.

Taking into account the influence of the LAB strain used, an increased number of peptide sequences with the discussed bioactivity was observed in the sample inoculated with the potentially probiotic strain *L. acidophilus* Bauer Ł0938, when the extraction of proteins from the product after 6 months of maturation was carried out with water (S).

The obtained sequences of peptides that are potential α-glucosidase inhibitors were characterized by a different value of parameter A [32]. The higher the value of parameter A, the greater part of the peptide sequence has a chance to act by interacting with the receptor present on the α-glucosidase molecule, limiting the range of its action and inhibiting the breakdown of α bonds of carbohydrates, reducing the absorption of glucose into the blood from the digestive tract, which in turn reduces glycemia after meals. Of all the sequences obtained in this analysis, only those with an A value of <0.400 were selected for further testing. Their list is presented in Table 1. The best source turned out to be the protein Phosphoglycerate mutase (B5KJG2) It is an enzyme involved in glycolysis, and its shorter fragments (peptides) can be found in the meat matrix [33]. Taking into account the method of obtaining the protein fraction, a greater number of peptide sequences with parameter A > 0.400 were associated with S than with M. Moreover, within the S fraction, the research variant subjected to spontaneous fermentation (C) was characterized by a lower number of peptides acting as potential α-glucosidase inhibitors than the variants vaccinated with the LAB starter culture. In particular, the sample inoculated with the strain *L. acidophilus* Bauer Ł0938 (BAUER_S) was characterized by almost 70% share of peptide sequences selected for further analysis.

Table 1. List of peptide sequences (*A* parameter > 0.400) from dry-cured pork loins after hydrolysis.

No.	Peptides	A Parameter	MW [Da]	Protein ID	C_S	LOCK_S	BB_S	BAUER_S	C_M	LOCK_M	BB_M	BAUER_M
1	DIPPPPMDEK	0.400	1137.54	B5KJG2	+	+	+	+	−	−	+	−
2	EAPPPPAEVH	0.400	1042.51	Q75NG9	−	−	−	−	−	+	+	+
3	FDIPPPPMDE	0.400	1156.51	B5KJG2	−	−	−	+	−	−	−	−
4	SFDIPPPPMD	0.400	1114.50	B5KJG2	−	+	+	+	−	−	+	−
5	DLFPPPP	0.429	781.40	F1RYS7	−	−	−	+	−	−	−	−
6	IIAPPER	0.429	794.46	B6VNT8; C7AI81; F1SLG5; I3LVD5; P68137; Q6QAQ1	−	+	+	+	+	+	+	+
7	PPLIPPK	0.429	760.48	Q75ZZ6	−	−	−	−	+	−	−	−
8	FDIPPPPMD	0.444	1027.47	B5KJG2	−	−	−	+	−	−	−	−
9	IPPPPMDEK	0.444	1022.51	B5KJG2	−	−	−	+	−	−	−	−
10	RPPPISPPP	0.444	956.54	F1RNQ0; I3LH78; I3LL74	−	−	−	+	−	−	−	−
11	SFDIPPPPM	0.444	999.47	B5KJG2	−	+	−	−	−	−	−	−
12	KSLRSGLL GDTLTEGGLS QLGRALREL	0.476	2839.59	F1RGE5	+	−	−	−	−	−	−	−
13	VATPPPPPPK	0.546	1096.63	I3LNG8	−	−	+	−	−	−	−	−
14	DIPPPPM	0.571	765.373	B5KJG2	−	−	−	+	−	−	−	−
15	TPPPPPPG	0.625	758.40	F1STN6	−	−	−	+	−	−	−	−
16	TPPPPPPPK	0.667	926.52	I3LNG8	−	−	−	+	−	−	−	−
				Total number	2	4	4	11	2	2	4	2

The ADMET profile is a useful tool for predicting the pharmacological and toxicological properties of drug candidates, especially at preclinical stages, but it has also been increasingly used for bioactive food ingredients to confirm their functional action and the role of nutrition in preventing incidence of non-communicable diseases [9,34–36]. Table 2 shows the pharmacokinetic properties of selected peptide sequences potentially inhibiting α-glucosidase activity by the ADMET approach.

Table 2. Allergenicity and ADMET characteristics of selected peptide sequences with α-glucosidase inhibitor activity.

No.	Peptides	Allergencity [1]	A Caco-2 Permeability [2]	HIA [3]	PPB [4]	D BBB [5]	VD [6]	M Cyp450 2D6 [7] [I/S]	E $T_{1/2}$ [8]	LD_{50} [9]	T H-HT [10]	FDA [11]
1	DIPPPPMDEK	Probable Non-Allergen	−6.522	0.270	52.70	0.076	−0.78	0.336/0.521	1.99	3.125	0.0	0.478
2	EAPPPPAEVH	Probable Allergen	−6.576	0.220	51.77	0.178	−0.74	0.376/0.473	1.92	3.226	0.0	0.31
3	FDIPPPPMDE	Probable Non-Allergen	−6.526	0.284	61.95	0.119	−0.87	0.407/0.488	1.95	3.157	0.0	0.346
4	SFDIPPPPMD	Probable Non-Allergen	−3.223	0.262	60.42	0.052	−0.85	0.375/0.479	1.93	3.178	0.0	0.308
5	DLFPPPP	Probable Non-Allergen	−3.185	0.208	62.08	0.256	−0.43	0.344/0.494	1.83	2.821	0.176	0.284
6	IIAPPER	Probable Allergen	−6.383	0.288	49.89	0.105	−0.52	0.359/0.526	1.68	2.838	0.056	0.418
7	PPLIPPK	Probable Non-Allergen	−5.963	0.312	56.01	0.079	−0.14	0.382/0.481	1.76	2.772	0.104	0.388
8	FDIPPPPMD	Probable Non-Allergen	−6.511	0.284	58.38	0.110	−0.80	0.384/0.499	1.88	3.143	0.0	0.324
9	IPPPPMDEK	Probable Non-Allergen	−3.292	0.270	50.21	0.094	−0.71	0.315/0.512	1.92	3.08	0.002	0.484
10	RPPPISPPP	Probable Non-Allergen	−6.631	0.280	51.28	0.024	−0.56	0.327/0.475	1.94	3.179	0.01	0.448
11	SFDIPPPPM	Probable Non-Allergen	−6.483	0.262	58.47	0.052	−0.76	0.387/0.478	1.90	3.102	0.0	0.306
12	KSLRSGLLGDTLTEGGLSQLGRALREL	Probable Allergen	−6.221	0.161	59.80	0.041	−0.25	0.445/0.437	2.15	3.239	0.0	0.44
13	VATPPPPPPPK	Probable Non-Allergen	−6.352	0.197	50.76	0.084	−0.30	0.343/0.518	2.08	3.314	0.0	0.428
14	DIPPPPM	Probable Non-Allergen	−6.122	0.278	47.39	0.175	−0.74	0.303/0.488	1.70	2.685	0.128	0.43
15	TPPPPPPG	Probable Non-Allergen	−6.132	0.165	43.80	0.548	−0.48	0.252/0.501	1.83	2.892	0.100	0.492
16	TPPPPPPPK	Probable Non-Allergen	−6.246	0.173	46.57	0.137	−0.34	0.270/0.548	1.99	3.218	0.024	0.472

[1]—allergenicity based on AllerTop 2.0; [2]—Caco-2 Permeability [Expressed in cm × s^{-1}], optimal: higher than −5.15 Log unit; [3]—Human Intestinal Absorption, criteria: 0: HIA−(HIA < 30%), 1: HIA+ (HIA > 30%); [4]—Plasma Protein Binding [%], optimal: <90%, significant with drugs that are highly protein-bound and have a low therapeutic index; [5]—Blood–Brain Barrier (BBB), range: BB ratio ≥ 0.1: BBB+, BB ratio < 0.1: BBB−; [6]—Value Distribution [L × kg^{-1}], optimal: 0.04–20; [7]—Cyp 450 inhibitor or substrate, criteria: 0: non-inhibitor/substrate, category 1: inhibitor/substrate; [8]—Half Life, criteria: >8 h: high, from 3 h to 8 h: moderate, <3 h: low; [9]—LD50 of acute toxicity [−log mol kg^{-1}]; [10]—Human Hepatotoxicity (H-HP), category 0: H-HT negative (−); Category 1: H-HT positive (+); [11]—Maximum Recommended Daily Dose (FDAMDD), Category 0: FDAMDD negative (−); Category 1: FDAMDD positive (+).

For bioactive peptides, as well as drugs, to be effective in action they should be characterized by several features after consumption, i.e., be resistant to the action of digestive enzymes without losing biological activity, quickly and effectively absorbed (A) and distributed (D), and minimally degraded metabolically (M). There is a high probability that it will quickly reach peak blood concentration and maintain the desired level for a longer period of time before being excreted (E) [37]. Through this approach, it is possible to analyze the additional processes that peptides from food may undergo after passing through the intestinal walls into the bloodstream. Such an approach is relatively difficult to perform on humans or animals, therefore it can be performed using methods offered by in silico analysis, e.g., by using bioinformatics tools available on the ADMETlab internet platform [19].

The results of the allergenicity assessment (based on AllerTop v. 2.0) of these peptides were also presented, which showed a probable lack of allergenicity, with the exception of three sequences, i.e., EAPPPPAEVH, IIAPPER, and KSLRSGLLGDTLTEGGLSQLGRAL-

REL, for which the "probable allergen" status was determined (Table 2). It should be clarified that this result does not determine their potential allergenicity (this result was not confirmed by an additional analysis carried out in the BIOPEP-UWM database), but additional analyses in this direction should be performed. In the ADMET approach the Caco-2 permeability analysis and human intestinal absorption (HIA) of peptides obtained by hydrolyzing protein extracts from dry-curing pork loin after 6 months of aging were considered as adsorption (A) steps. In this study predicted Caco-2 permeability of isolated peptides averaged -6.356, and this is lower than the optimal value according to the program criteria, i.e., the optimal logarithm of permeability should exceed -5.15, which proves the average permeability of this peptides. The exception was three peptides, i.e., SFDIPPPPMD, DLFPPPP, and IPPPPMDEK, for which the value of Caco-2 permeability was -3.223, -3.185, and -3.292, respectively. Other parameters such as human intestinal adsorption (HIA) have been used to describe parameters of feasibility of intestinal absorption, where a higher HIA means that the compound may be more efficiently absorbed by the intestine after oral administration. All analyzed sequences have a positive HIA value, on average 0.245 (Table 2). This result is lower than that reported by other food peptide researchers. As an example, 17 of the 20 analyzed sequences obtained by in silico hydrolysis of proteins from Chickpea had an HIA value > 0.3 [34]. Also, Borawska-Dziadkiewicz et al. [36] pointed out that 25 out of the 30 peptide sequences from salmon and carp revealed high predicted intestinal absorption probability with HIA > 0.3. Comparing these data, the intestinal absorption capacity of these peptides is average, and it may be a problem when we want to deliver them by food. The probable cause may be the size of the analyzed sequences. However, it should be noted that in the analysis conditions used (hydrolysis with pepsin and pancreatin) the hydrolysis of the brush border enzymes in vitro was not included, which could have affected the presented results. In addition, the examples cited were based on the in silico analysis of peptides obtained by simulating the hydrolysis of selected sequences, resulting mainly in tri-peptides and dipeptides. This approach, however, is not fully replicable in the in vitro conditions used in this study, where additional factors (e.g., intermolecular interactions in hydrolysates) may interfere with ideal hydrolysis conditions. In terms of the distribution (D) of peptides in the living organism, plasma protein binding (PPB) was also analyzed. Binding to plasma proteins may increase or decrease the bioactive effect of the drug (peptide). Therefore, the free drug concentration is a critical factor in evaluating pharmaceutical activity; the likely binding of the compounds to plasma proteins should be determined. All biopeptides are expected to be less than 90% PPB. As can be seen from the data presented in Table 2, the PPB value in this study ranged from 43.80 to 62.08%. Low molecular weight peptides can penetrate the blood–brain barrier (BBB) by slow diffusion through lipids, causing a variety of effects, including, for example, opioid side effects. The acceptable range of BBB for health promotion of candidate compounds (including drugs) is from -3.0 to 1.2 [38], which was met by all analyzed peptide fragments. The BBB coefficient value obtained in this study ranged from 0.024 (for RPPPISPPP) to 0.548 (for TPPPPPPG), which gives good safety properties of these peptides in terms of BBB penetration. The low permeability of the BBB reduces the likelihood of undesirable side effects related to the central nervous system.

In addition, all peptides were predicted to be restricted to blood (VD assumed "minus" values), which, however, does not fall within the optimal range for this parameter (i.e., 0.04–20). On the other hand, the results reported in [39] showed that acarbose, which is used as a commercial α-amylase inhibitor (same as α-glucosidase inhibitors) in the treatment of diabetes, is VD-negative. This means that the compound has some problems with intestinal absorption, however, it is effective and commercially used as a pharmacological agent. Also, peptide dipeptidyl peptidase IV inhibitors helpful in preventing the onset of diabetes derived from meat products had a negative VD determined in silico [9]. Thus, a negative VD value cannot be considered a factor that disqualifies peptides as potential antidiabetic drugs.

CYP enzymes are the main and most studied enzymes involved in various physiological and pathophysiological processes, including detoxification of xenobiotic compounds. It is estimated that only every fourth drug available on the market is not metabolized by CYP. The remaining percentage is metabolized by five major CYP isoforms, of which CYP4502D6 is involved in the metabolism of up to 75–90% of drugs [40]. In this study, metabolization (M) was assessed through potential interactions between the analyzed peptides and CYP4502D6. Cytochrome CYP24502D6 is an important enzyme in the metabolism of many xenobiotics, and therefore its inhibition may result in uncontrolled drug–drug interactions or drug lifespan. Therefore, the assessment of CYP2D6 inhibition is a key part of the discovery and development of compounds such as drugs [41]. As presented in Table 2, the analyzed peptides had both substrate and inhibitor status in relation to the CYP4502D6 enzyme. Consistent with this observation, peptide molecules have the potential to be metabolized by CYP450 enzymes. In turn, the CYP450 inhibitor status means that the molecule may hinder the biotransformation of drugs metabolized by the CYP450 enzyme. It is important that for, all analyzed peptide sequences, a stronger role as an inhibitor than a substrate was observed.

The excretion (E) capacity of the peptides was determined by determining their theoretical half-life ($T_{1/2}$). The calculated half-life of less than 2 h was observed, which, according to the adopted criterion (>3 h), proves their low stability in the environment of the human body and high susceptibility of the peptides to degradation. However, as noted by Arámburo-Gálvez et al. [34] on the example of ACE-I inhibitors, drugs with a short serum half-life are not uncommon, although their effect can persist for hours after their consumption. The author explains that the capacity of ACE-I inhibitors to form reversible complexes with plasma proteins can serve as drug reservoirs [34,42]. It is suspected that this mechanism may also apply to other proteins acting as enzyme inhibitors, such as α-glucosidase.

The toxicity of peptides acting as potential α-glucosidase inhibitors was assessed on the basis of three independent parameters, i.e., median lethal dose (LD50), human hepatotoxicity (H-HP), and maximum recommended daily dose (FDAMDD). LD50 usually represents the acute toxicity of chemicals. It is the dose amount of a tested molecule to kill 50% of the treated animals within a given period. When comparing LD50 doses, the compound at the lower dose is more lethal than the compound at the higher LD50 dose [43]. Based on the obtained results (Table 2), the mean LD50 level was 3.060 [$-\log$ mol kg^{-1}]. Taking into account the hepatotoxicity index, half of the analyzed sequences had a non-hepatotoxic status, while the other half showed a relatively low value of this index, with the highest value of 0.128 for the DIPPPPM peptide. The maximum recommended daily dose of a peptide (drug) molecule averaged 0.379 for the sequences analyzed in this study (Table 2).

3.2. Molecular Docking

Molecular docking is a very important approach used to better understand the binding mode between a ligand and a protein, thus determining the molecule that has the best interactions with the receptor. According to literature data, the binding pose for the 5NN8 receptor is situated in the following regions: Trp376, Tyr378, Leu405, Trp481, Asp518, Met519, Phe525, Asp616, Trp618, Phe649, Leu650, His674, and Leu678 [44]. In addition, we used three different types of computational software to predict the potential binding poses on the surface of the studied protein. The first software used was fpocket, which is an open-source package for detecting pockets in proteins. It is based on Voronoi tessellation and α spheres, built on top of the publicly available Qhull package. Given the structure of a protein, it enables the identification of potential binding sites. The fpocket analysis was performed using default settings, identifying 41 potential binding sites. The second program utilized was CAVITY software (version 1.0), which is specifically designed for the detection and analysis of ligand-binding sites. CAVITY is a geometry-based method that incorporates a spherical probing of the protein surface to detect potential binding sites. The CAVITY analysis was performed using the 'whole protein detection mode' and a 'large' option of the detection mode, which is used for large and complex cavity detection. CAVITY identified 35 potential binding sites. The open-source GHECOM software (version 1.0) was also used in this study, which is designed for finding multi-scale pockets on the protein surface using mathematically derived morphology. It is based on an algorithm for the simultaneous calculation of multiscale pockets, using several different sizes of spherical probes. Based on the literature data and obtained computational results, we identified the top ten binding sites (Figure 4). The molecular surface of the receptor, to which the peptide was docked, displays the top ten binding sites. The choice of the cavity was arbitrary and was dictated by its size, shape, and the size of the peptide molecule. Target binding/catalytic residues in both ligands and receptor-active sites that dynamically interact with each other are shown in the supplement (Figure S1).

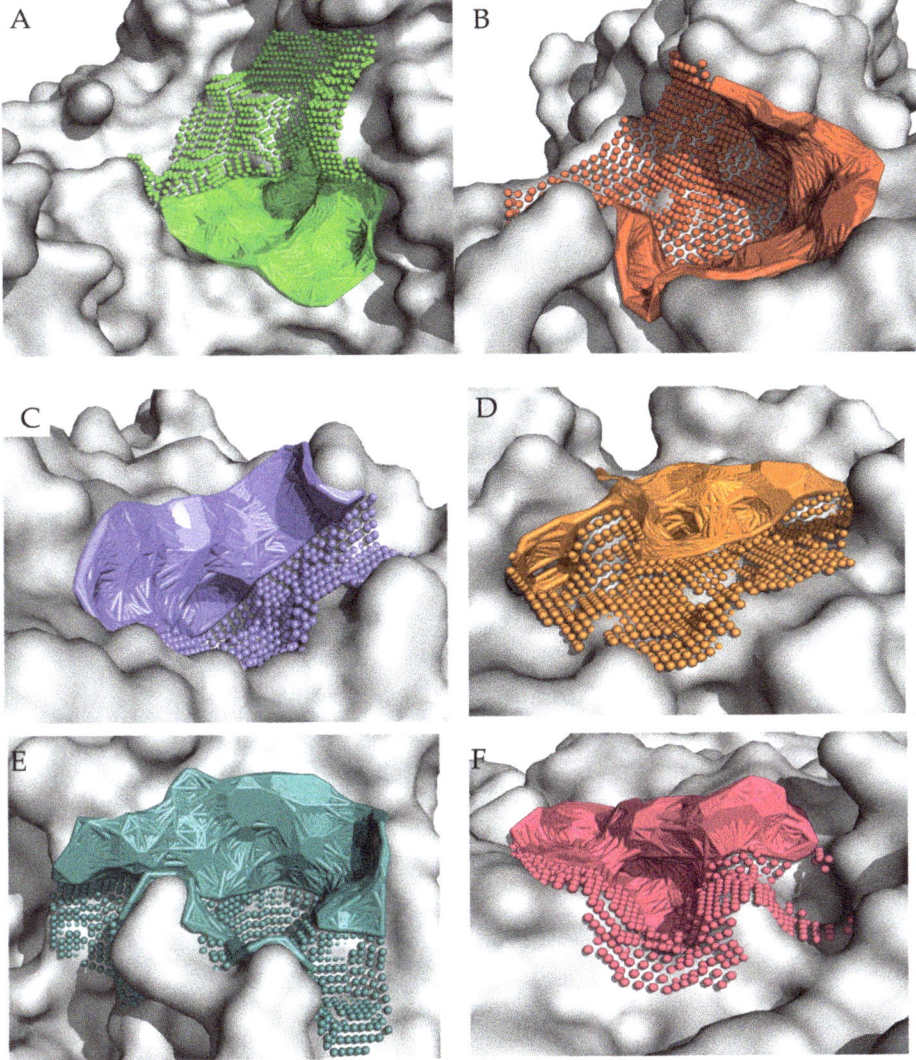

Figure 4. *Cont.*

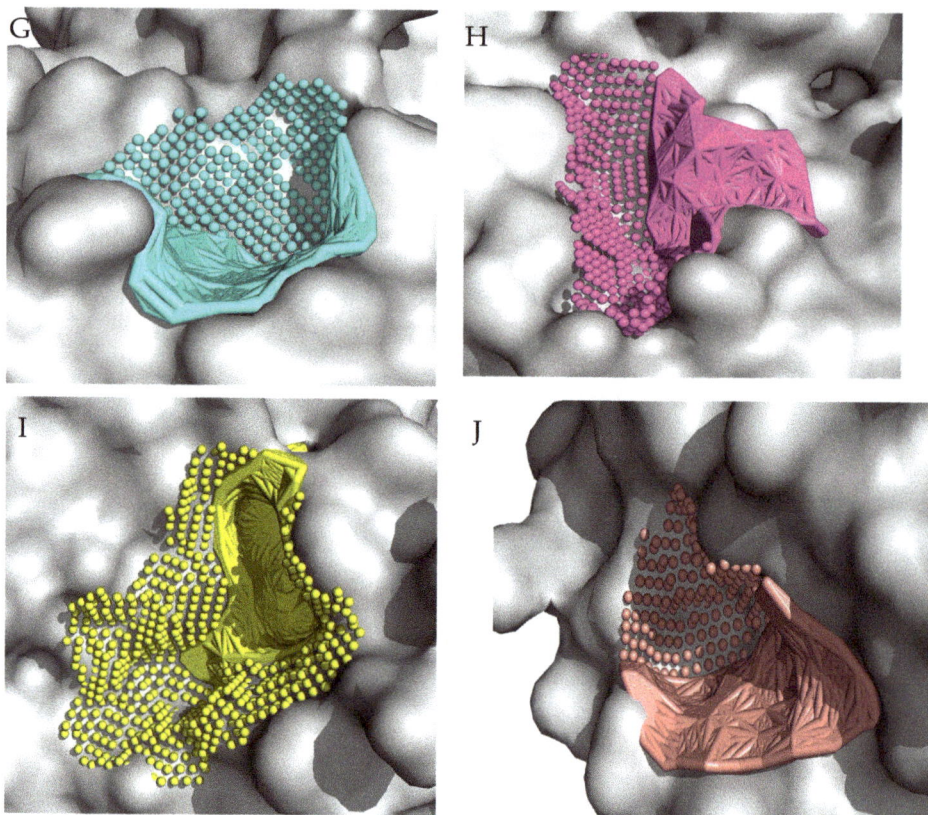

Figure 4. The best ten identified binding regions (**A**–**J**) on the molecular surface of the receptor. (**A**) The binding pocket is formed by the following amino acid residues: E346, P347, K348, S349, V350, Q352, Y360, H708, T711, L712, F713, H714, Q715, A716, V718, A719, G720, E721, T722, V723, R725, L729, E730, F731, P732, K733, W746, G747, E748, A749, L750, L769, G770, T771, L818, R819, A820, G821, Y822, I823, I824, P825, A846, L847, T848, G851, E852, A853, R854, G855, E856, L857, F858, L868, Y873, Q875, V876, I877, F878, L879, A880, Arg881, and V890; (**B**) The binding pocket is formed by the following amino acid residues: E196, Q352, Y354, L355, D356, V357, V358, G359, Y360, P361, F362, M363, P364, P365, I581, H584, R585, A586, L587, V588, K589, G592, T593, R594, P595, G607, R608, Y609, Y710, F713, H714, H717, V718, A719, G720, F858, D860, E863, S864, L865, E866, V867, L868, E869, R870, A872, and Y873; (**C**) The binding pocket is formed by the following amino acid residues: R281, D282, L283, A284, P285, Y292, W376, D404, L405, R411, I441, D443, K479, W481, W516, D518, M519, S523, N524, F525, I526, A554, A555, T556, R600, W613, G615, D616, V617, W618, D645, F649, L650, G651, N652, R672, H674, N675, S676, L677, L678, and S679; (**D**) The binding pocket is formed by the following amino acid residues: M146, Y148, R168, L169, D170, V171, M172, M173, E174, T175, R178, H180, F181, T182, I183, K184, R189, R190, Y191, E192, V193, P194, L195, E196, L246, L312, L313, N314, S315, N316, S332, G334, G335, I336, L337, D338, Y340, Q353, L355, D356, V357, V358, G359, Y360, N570, G605, R608, and Y609; (**E**) The binding pocket is formed by the following amino acid residues: P161, K162, D163, I164, L165, T166, K184, D185, A187, N188, R189, R190, Y191, E192, V193, P194, L195, F241, A242, D243, Q244, N316, T333, G334, G335, I336, T491, N536, E537, L538, E539, A559, S560, S561, H562, Q563, F564, L565, S566, T567, H568, Y569, N570, L571, and L574; (**F**) The binding pocket is formed by the following amino acid residues: G123, Q255, I257, T258, G259, L260, A261, E262, H263, L264, S265, P266, L267, M268, L269, S270, T271, S272, W273, T274, R275, I276, T277, L278, T286, P287, G288, A289, N290, L291, D319, V320, L322, P545, G546, V547, V548, E622, Q623, A625, S626, V628, P629, E630, I631, L632, Q633, F634, L637, T739, D741, and H742; (**G**) The binding pocket

is formed by the following amino acid residues: W376, G377, Y378, S379, S380, D404, L405, D406, Y407, M408, D409, S410, R411, R412, F416, N417, K418, D419, G420, F421, W481, and L677; (**H**) The binding pocket is formed by the following amino acid residues: P266, W621, E622, A625, S626, S736, T737, W738, T739, V740, D741, H742, Gln743, Ile752, T753, P754, V755, L756, Q757, A758, K760, A761, E762, V763, T764, G765, Y766, W804, T806, L807, and A809; (**I**) The binding pocket is formed by the following amino acid residues: F128, F129, P130, P131, S132, Y133, P134, S135, R154, S214, E216, P217, F218, V230, N233, T234, T235, V236, A237, P238, L239, T250, S251, L252, P53, S254, Q255, Q323, P324, S325, P326, A327, L328, Q81, C82, D83, V84, P85, N87, S88, R89, and F90; (**J**) The binding pocket is formed by the following amino acid residues: R375, W376, G377, Y378, S379, A382, I383, T384, R385, Q386, V387, V388, N390, D406, N675, S676, L677, L678, S679, L680, P681, Q682, E683, Y685, S686, and F687.

For each of the peptides, the lowest ΔG binding energy was obtained for cavity pocket no. 2 (Table 3). This suggests that in this location, the peptides are most strongly attracted to the amino acid residues of the protein binding pocket. The projection of the best binding pocket of protein PDB ID: 5NN8 with docked ligands of sequence VATPPPPPPPK (A), DIPPPPM (B), TPPPPPPG (C), and TPPPPPPPK (D) is presented in Figure 5 with ΔG binding energy −6.6 kcal/mol, −6.7 kcal/mol, −7.0 kcal/mol, and −8.0 kcal/mol, respectively.

Table 3. Free energy values for peptide binding to protein PDB ID 5NN8.

Cavity Number	$\Delta G_{binding}$ [kcal/mol]			
	VATPPPPPPPK	DIPPPPM	TPPPPPPG	TPPPPPPPK
1	−4.7	−5.7	−6.7	−6.8
2	−6.6	−6.7	−7.0	−8.0
3	−4.2	−6.6	−6.9	−6.9
4	−4.3	−4.8	−5.7	−6.3
5	−5.8	−6.2	−6.7	−6.8
6	−5.3	−5.1	−6.7	−6.1
7	−2.2	−5.4	−5.5	−5.3
8	−4.8	−5.4	−5.8	−4.9
9	5.0	−5.8	−6.1	−5.5
10	36.9	−1.9	−1.4	−1.9

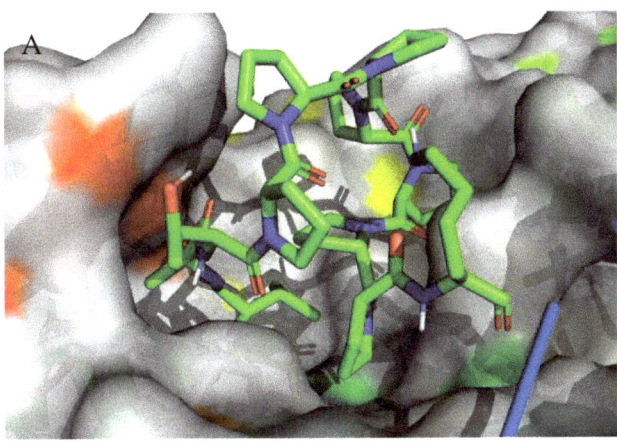

Figure 5. *Cont.*

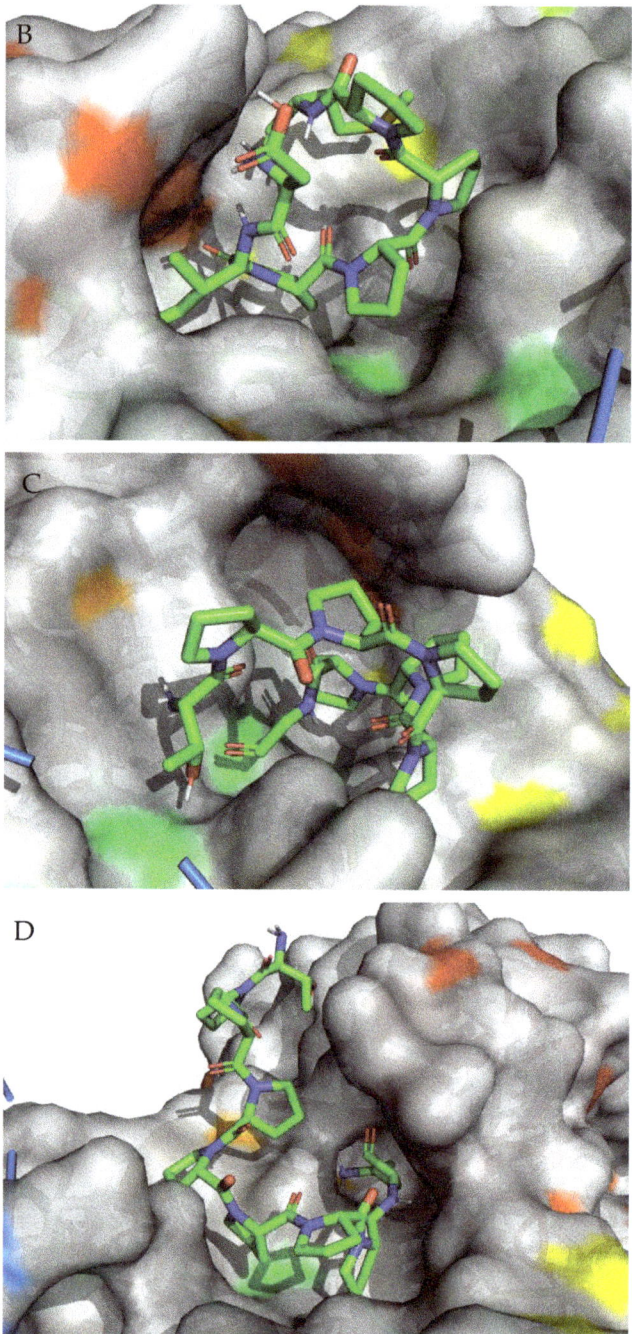

Figure 5. Projection of the best binding pocket of protein PDB ID: 5NN8 with docked ligands of sequence VATPPPPPPPK (**A**), DIPPPPM (**B**), TPPPPPPG (**C**), and TPPPPPPPK (**D**). In the peptide structure, the color green represents C atoms, blue represents N atoms, white represents H atoms, and red represents O atoms (Target binding/catalytic residues in both ligands and receptor active sites that dynamically interact with each other are shown in the supplement (Figure S2)).

These results are close to those reported by Hu et al. [21]. The authors docked a promising molecular peptide from fermented rice bran, i.e., GLLGY, on human α-glucosidase (PDB ID 5NN8), and presented a binding energy of −7.1 kcal/mol. In addition, the authors of the study proved that this oligopeptide showed the greatest inhibitory activity in vitro, further highlighting the potential of the peptides presented in this study, obtained by hydrolysis of proteins from ripening raw loin, to bind to the human α-glucosidase molecule and act effectively as a potential antidiabetic agent.

The best binding site that was identified on the protein surface, with PDB ID: 5NN8, does not fully coincide with the literature data [44]. However, in the studies described in the cited source, protein 5NN8 interacted with a completely different ligand (i.e., the iridoid, Arbortristoside-C from Nyctanthes arbor-tristis Linn., which is a potential drug candidate for diabetes targeting α-glucosidase). Depending on the type of chemical compound, different binding pockets on the protein structure may be preferred. Furthermore, it should be noted that each computational program dedicated to molecular docking is based on different mathematical algorithms and scoring functions, which may lead to certain discrepancies in the resulting data.

4. Conclusions

The results indicate that peptides obtained by the hydrolysis of proteins for dry-cured pork loins may have potential as functional food ingredients in the prevention and/or treatment of type 2 diabetes mellitus. In particular, the docking studies on human α-glucosidase revealed that VATPPPPPPPK, DIPPPPM, TPPPPPPG, and TPPPPPPPK sequences are promising anti-diabetic candidates. These in vitro findings need further in vivo investigations to determine whether α-glucosidase inhibitory peptides could be used as agents for the prevention or treatment of type 2 diabetes.

Supplementary Materials: The following supporting information can be downloaded at: https://www.mdpi.com/article/10.3390/nu15163539/s1, Table S1: List of peptides with α-glucosidase inhibiting activity from dry-cured pork loins with strain of LAB.

Author Contributions: Conceptualization, P.K. and J.S. methodology, P.K.; validation, P.K.; investigation, P.K., A.Ł. and A.M.; writing—original draft preparation, P.K.; writing—review and editing, P.K. and J.S.; visualization, P.K.; supervision, J.S. All authors have read and agreed to the published version of the manuscript.

Funding: This research received no external funding.

Institutional Review Board Statement: Not applicable.

Informed Consent Statement: Not applicable.

Data Availability Statement: All data are available in this study.

Conflicts of Interest: The authors declare no conflict of interest.

References

1. Di Stefano, E.; Oliviero, T.; Udenigwe, C.C. Functional significance and structure–activity relationship of food-derived α-glucosidase inhibitors. *Curr. Opin. Food Sci.* **2018**, *20*, 7–12. [CrossRef]
2. Ibrahim, M.A.; Bester, M.J.; Neitz, A.W.; Gaspar, A.R. Structural properties of bioactive peptides with α-glucosidase inhibitory activity. *Chem. Biol. Drug Des.* **2018**, *91*, 370–379. [CrossRef] [PubMed]
3. Liu, B.; Kongstad, K.T.; Wiese, S.; Jäger, A.K.; Staerk, D. Edible seaweed as future functional food: Identification of α-glucosidase inhibitors by combined use of high-resolution α-glucosidase inhibition profiling and HPLC–HRMS–SPE–NMR. *Food Chem.* **2016**, *203*, 16–22. [CrossRef] [PubMed]
4. Cisneros-Yupanqui, M.; Lante, A.; Mihaylova, D.; Krastanov, A.I.; Rizzi, C. The α-Amylase and α-Glucosidase Inhibition Capacity of Grape Pomace: A Review. *Food Bioproc. Tech.* **2022**, *30*, 691–703. [CrossRef] [PubMed]
5. Kumar, S.; Narwal, S.; Kumar, V.; Prakash, O. α-glucosidase inhibitors from plants: A natural approach to treat diabetes. *Pharmacogn. Rev.* **2011**, *5*, 19. [CrossRef] [PubMed]
6. Dirir, A.M.; Daou, M.; Yousef, A.F.; Yousef, L.F. A review of alpha-glucosidase inhibitors from plants as potential candidates for the treatment of type-2 diabetes. *Phytochem. Rev.* **2022**, *21*, 1049–1079. [CrossRef]

7. Martínez-Sánchez, S.M.; Minguela, A.; Prieto-Merino, D.; Zafrilla-Rentero, M.P.; Abellán-Alemán, J.; Montoro-García, S. The effect of regular intake of dry-cured ham rich in bioactive peptides on inflammation, platelet and monocyte activation markers in humans. *Nutrients* **2017**, *9*, 321. [CrossRef]
8. Montoro-García, S.; Zafrilla-Rentero, M.P.; Celdrán-de Haro, F.M.; Piñero-de Armas, J.J.; Toldrá, F.; Tejada-Portero, L.; Abellan-Aleman, J. Effects of dry-cured ham rich in bioactive peptides on cardiovascular health: A randomized controlled trial. *J. Funct. Foods* **2017**, *38*, 160–167. [CrossRef]
9. Kęska, P.; Stadnik, J. Potential DPP IV inhibitory peptides from dry-cured pork loins after hydrolysis: An in vitro and in silico study. *Curr. Issues Mol. Biol.* **2021**, *43*, 1335–1349. [CrossRef]
10. Kęska, P.; Stadnik, J. Dipeptidyl Peptidase IV Inhibitory Peptides Generated in Dry-Cured Pork Loin during Aging and Gastrointestinal Digestion. *Nutrients* **2022**, *14*, 770. [CrossRef]
11. Kęska, P.; Stadnik, J.; Bąk, O.; Borowski, P. Meat proteins as dipeptidyl peptidase iv inhibitors and glucose uptake stimulating peptides for the management of a type 2 diabetes mellitus in silico study. *Nutrients* **2019**, *11*, 2537. [CrossRef] [PubMed]
12. Kęska, P.; Stadnik, J. Structure–activity relationships study on biological activity of peptides as dipeptidyl peptidase IV inhibitors by chemometric modeling. *Chem. Biol. Drug Des.* **2020**, *95*, 291–301. [CrossRef] [PubMed]
13. Mora, L.; González-Rogel, D.; Heres, A.; Toldrá, F. Iberian dry-cured ham as a potential source of α-glucosidase-inhibitory peptides. *J. Funct. Foods* **2020**, *67*, 103840. [CrossRef]
14. Molina, I.; Toldrá, F. Detection of proteolytic activity in microorganisms isolated from dry-cured ham. *J. Food Sci.* **1992**, *57*, 1308–1310. [CrossRef]
15. Fadda, S.; Sanz, Y.; Vignolo, G.; Aristoy, M.C.; Oliver, G.; Toldrá, F. Characterization of muscle sarcoplasmic and myofibrillar protein hydrolysis caused by Lactobacillus plantarum. *Appl. Environ. Microbiol.* **1999**, *65*, 3540–3546. [CrossRef] [PubMed]
16. Escudero, E.; Mora, L.; Toldrá, F. Stability of ACE inhibitory ham peptides against heat treatment and in vitro digestion. *Food Chem.* **2014**, *161*, 305–311. [CrossRef] [PubMed]
17. UniProt KB. Available online: www.uniprot.org (accessed on 10 April 2023).
18. BIOPEP-UWM. Available online: https://biochemia.uwm.edu.pl/biopep-uwm (accessed on 10 April 2023).
19. ADMET. Available online: https://admet.scbdd.com (accessed on 10 April 2023).
20. AllerTOP. Available online: https://www.ddg-pharmfac.net/AllerTOP/ (accessed on 10 April 2023).
21. Hu, J.; Lai, X.; Wu, X.; Wang, H.; Weng, N.; Lu, J.; Lyu, M.; Wang, S. Isolation of a Novel Anti-Diabetic α-Glucosidase Oligo-Peptide Inhibitor from Fermented Rice Bran. *Foods* **2023**, *12*, 183. [CrossRef]
22. Wairata, J.; Sukandar, E.R.; Fadlan, A.; Purnomo, A.S.; Taher, M.; Ersam, T. Evaluation of the antioxidant, antidiabetic, and antiplasmodial activities of xanthones isolated from Garcinia forbesii and their in silico studies. *Biomedicines* **2021**, *9*, 1380. [CrossRef]
23. Roig-Zamboni, V.; Cobucci-Ponzano, B.; Iacono, R.; Ferrara, M.C.; Germany, S.; Bourne, Y.; Parenti, G.; Moracci, M.; Sulzenbacher, G. Structure of human lysosomal acid α-glucosidase—A guide for the treatment of Pompe disease. *Nat. Commun.* **2017**, *8*, 1111. [CrossRef]
24. Sanner, M. Python: A Programming Language for Software Integration and Development. *J. Mol. Graph. Model.* **1999**, *17*, 57.
25. Morris, G.; Huey, R.; Lindstrom, W.; Sanner, M.; Belew, R.; Goodsell, D.; Olson, A. Autodock4 and AutoDockTools4: Automated docking with selective receptor flexibility. *J. Comput. Chem.* **2009**, *30*, 2785. [CrossRef] [PubMed]
26. O'Boyle, N.M.; Banck, M.; James, C.A.; Morley, C.; Vandermeersch, T.; Hutchison, G. Open Babel: An open chemical toolbox. *J. Chem. Inform.* **2011**, *3*, 33. [CrossRef] [PubMed]
27. Hassan, N.M.; Alhossary, A.A.; Mu, Y.; Kwoh, C.-K. Protein-Ligand Blind Docking Using QuickVina-W With Inter-Process Spatio-Temporal Integration. *Sci. Rep.* **2017**, *7*, 15451. [CrossRef] [PubMed]
28. Arnautova, Y.A.; Jagielska, A.; Scheraga, H.A. A new force field (ECEPP-05) for peptides, proteins, and organic molecules. *J. Phys. Chem. B* **2006**, *110*, 5025–5044. [CrossRef]
29. Le Guilloux, V.; Schmidtke, P.; Tuffery, P. Fpocket: An open source platform for ligand pocket detection. *BMC Bioinform.* **2009**, *10*, 168. [CrossRef] [PubMed]
30. Zhang, W.; Yuan, Y.; Pei, J.; Lai, L. CAVITY: Mapping the Druggable Binding Site. In *Computer-Aided Drug Discovery. Methods in Pharmacology and Toxicology*; Zhang, W., Ed.; Humana Press: New York, NY, USA, 2015.
31. Kawabata, T. Detection of multiscale pockets on protein surfaces using mathematical morphology. *Proteins* **2010**, *78*, 1195. [CrossRef]
32. Minkiewicz, P.; Iwaniak, A.; Darewicz, M. BIOPEP-UWM database of bioactive peptides: Current opportunities. *Int. J. Mol. Sci.* **2019**, *20*, 5978. [CrossRef]
33. Kęska, P.; Stadnik, J. Peptidomic Characteristic of Peptides Generated in Dry-Cured Loins with Probiotic Strains of LAB during 360-Days Aging. *Appl. Sci.* **2022**, *12*, 6036. [CrossRef]
34. Arámburo-Gálvez, J.G.; Arvizu-Flores, A.A.; Cárdenas-Torres, F.I.; Cabrera-Chávez, F.; Ramírez-Torres, G.I.; Flores-Mendoza, L.K.; Gastelum-Acosta, P.E.; Figueroa-Salcido, O.G.; Ontiveros, N. Prediction of ACE-I inhibitory peptides derived from chickpea (*Cicer arietinum* L.): In silico assessments using simulated enzymatic hydrolysis, molecular docking and ADMET evaluation. *Foods* **2022**, *11*, 1576. [CrossRef]
35. Barrero, J.A.; Cabrera, F.; Cruz, C.M. Gliptins vs. Milk-derived Dipeptidyl-Peptidase IV Inhibiting Biopeptides: Physicochemical Characterization and Pharmacokinetic Profiling. *Vitae* **2021**, *28*, 346531. [CrossRef]

36. Borawska-Dziadkiewicz, J.; Darewicz, M.; Tarczyńska, A.S. Properties of peptides released from salmon and carp via simulated human-like gastrointestinal digestion described applying quantitative parameters. *PLoS ONE* **2021**, *16*, e0255969. [CrossRef] [PubMed]
37. Kumar, N.; Goel, N.; Yadav, T.C.; Pruthi, V. Quantum chemical, ADMET and molecular docking studies of ferulic acid amide derivatives with a novel anticancer drug target. *Med. Chem. Res.* **2017**, *26*, 1822–1834. [CrossRef]
38. Nisha, C.M.; Kumar, A.; Nair, P.; Gupta, N.; Silakari, C.; Tripathi, T.; Kumar, A. Molecular docking and in silico ADMET study reveals acylguanidine 7a as a potential inhibitor of β-secretase. *Adv. Bioinform.* **2016**, *2016*, 9258578. [CrossRef] [PubMed]
39. Altuner, E.M. In Silico Proof of the Effect of Quercetin and Umbelliferone as Alpha-Amylase Inhibitors, Which Can Be Used in the Treatment of Diabetes. *Kastamonu Univ. J. For.* **2022**, *22*, 202–216. [CrossRef]
40. Guengerich, F.P. Cytochrome p450 and chemical toxicology. *Chem. Res. Toxicol.* **2008**, *21*, 70–83. [CrossRef]
41. Mamadalieva, N.Z.; Youssef, F.S.; Hussain, H.; Zengin, G.; Mollica, A.; Al Musayeib, N.M.; Ashour, M.L.; Westermann, B.; Wessjohann, L.A. Validation of the antioxidant and enzyme inhibitory potential of selected triterpenes using in vitro and in silico studies, and the evaluation of their ADMET properties. *Molecules* **2021**, *26*, 6331. [CrossRef]
42. Duchin, K.L.; McKinstry, D.N.; Cohen, A.I.; Migdalof, B.H. Pharmacokinetics of captopril in healthy subjects and in patients with cardiovascular diseases. *Clin. Pharmacokinet.* **1988**, *14*, 241–259. [CrossRef]
43. Khaldan, A.; Bouamrane, S.; El Mchichi, R.E.M.L.; Maghat, H.; Lakhlifi, M.B.T.; Sbai, A. In search of new potent α-glucosidase inhibitors: Molecular docking and ADMET prediction. *Mor. J. Chem.* **2022**, *10*, 10–14. [CrossRef]
44. Vajravijayan, S.; Nandhagopal, N.; Anantha Krishnan, D.; Gunasekaran, K. Isolation and characterization of an iridoid, Arbortristoside-C from Nyctanthes arbor-tristis Linn., a potential drug candidate for diabetes targeting α-glucosidase. *J. Biomol. Struct. Dyn.* **2022**, *40*, 337–347. [CrossRef]

Disclaimer/Publisher's Note: The statements, opinions and data contained in all publications are solely those of the individual author(s) and contributor(s) and not of MDPI and/or the editor(s). MDPI and/or the editor(s) disclaim responsibility for any injury to people or property resulting from any ideas, methods, instructions or products referred to in the content.

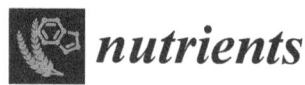 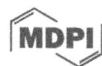

Article

Meat Consumption and Availability for Its Reduction by Health and Environmental Concerns: A Pilot Study

Andrea Turnes [1], Paula Pereira [2], Helena Cid [3] and Ana Valente [1,4,*]

[1] ATLANTIC—University Institute, 2730-036 Barcarena, Portugal
[2] Egas Moniz Interdisciplinary Research Center, Egas Moniz School of Health and Science, Quinta da Granja-Campus Universitário, 2829-511 Monte da Caparica, Portugal
[3] HeartGenetics, Genetics & Biotechnology, Av. Prof. Gama Pinto n°. 2, 1649-003 Lisbon, Portugal
[4] Ecogenetics and Human Health Research Group, Environmental Health Institute (ISAMB), Associate Laboratory TERRA, Faculty of Medicine (FMUL), University of Lisbon, 1649-028 Lisbon, Portugal
* Correspondence: ana.valente@uatlantica.pt

Abstract: (1) Background: Excessive meat consumption has raised multiple health and environmental concerns; however, there are no data on the population's willingness to reduce its intake for these reasons. The current study aims to assess the frequency of meat intake and readiness to limit consumption due to concern about the impact on health and the environment in residents of the Lisbon metropolitan region. (2) Methods: This analytical cross-sectional observational study was carried out in 197 residents in the metropolitan region of Lisbon. The participants were divided into two groups by age (GI: 20–29 years; GII: 40–64 years). Meat consumption and willingness to reduce it were assessed through a questionnaire. (3) Results: Most participants (67%) reported not having knowledge about the ecological footprint of meat. Being a less frequent meat consumer (<1 time per day) is associated with a willingness 3.6 times higher ($p < 0.001$) to reduce meat consumption due to sensitivity to the impact on health and 4.0 times higher ($p < 0.001$) due to environmental reasons. (4) Conclusions: Lower meat consumption frequency was associated with reductions in this consumption for environmental and health reasons.

Keywords: meat; consumption; health; environment; ecological footprint

Citation: Turnes, A.; Pereira, P.; Cid, H.; Valente, A. Meat Consumption and Availability for Its Reduction by Health and Environmental Concerns: A Pilot Study. *Nutrients* **2023**, *15*, 3080. https://doi.org/10.3390/nu15143080

Academic Editor: Rosa Casas

Received: 13 June 2023
Revised: 30 June 2023
Accepted: 5 July 2023
Published: 8 July 2023

Copyright: © 2023 by the authors. Licensee MDPI, Basel, Switzerland. This article is an open access article distributed under the terms and conditions of the Creative Commons Attribution (CC BY) license (https://creativecommons.org/licenses/by/4.0/).

1. Introduction

In Portugal, dietary imbalances are evident [1–3], where the consumption of meat, sugar, fat, and salt is much higher than recommended [4]. Changes in eating habits over the years have been remarkable [5]. According to recent data, just 26% of the Portuguese population adheres to the Mediterranean diet [6], indicating a noteworthy divergence from this dietary pattern known globally as a health promoter. Some studies have suggested a link between frequent and high meat consumption and noncommunicable diseases (such as cancer, diabetes, and cardiovascular disease) [7–10]. Indeed, food choices, together with other lifestyle behaviors such as smoking and lack of physical activity, have been identified as risk factors for one-third of all fatalities in Portugal [11].

More recently, environmental concerns have also been raised about excessive meat consumption [1,4,12], especially when referring to red meat, which appears to have the higher ecological footprint [13]. The emission of greenhouse gases is 57 times higher in beef when compared with tofu, while for poultry it is 4 times higher [13]. Even though there are no statistics on public knowledge of these data, this information is freely available to the public via the Our World in Statistics website. Also, the results of Sanchez-Sabaté and colleagues (2019) have shown that meat consumers are not willing to change their dietary habits for environmental reasons [12].

In Portugal, the Food Balance report published by the National Institute of Statistics for the period 2016–2020 showed an increase in meat consumption in this period, despite a decrease during the pandemic, but still 8.7% higher than the previous analysis period of 2012–2015 [1]. Currently, Portuguese society is undergoing a transformation; Europe is experiencing an energy crisis, which will certainly affect food supply, with predicted increases in meat prices and a grain shortage [14]. The pressure to modify eating habits for economic reasons is great, and this could be a chance to promote public knowledge about the need to reduce meat consumption, which has obvious health and environmental benefits. The theme of the current piece is highly timely, given the current economic downturn, social unrest, energy problem, and environmental consciousness [15]. According to current knowledge, this is the first study in Portugal that aimed to assess the frequency of meat consumption and willingness to reduce consumption due to concern about the impact on health and the environment in residents of the Lisbon metropolitan region.

2. Materials and Methods

2.1. Research Design and Sample

This cross-sectional analytical study was conducted on a sample of Lisbon metropolitan region inhabitants. From a 2,264,004 [16] population of individuals who were at least 19 years old, a minimum sample size of 97 individuals was considered with a 95% confidence level and a 10% margin of error [17]. The study was conducted from November 2022 to March 2023.

Sample Selection, Inclusion, and Exclusion Criteria

The current study used a stratified probabilistic sample with the following inclusion criteria: (1) be between the ages of 20 and 29 or 40 and 64, (2) live in the Greater Lisbon region, and (3) have an email address to obtain the self-completion questionnaire to be used in the study.

Individuals younger than 20 years old and 64 years old or older were eliminated, as were individuals who could not read or write and did not have e-mail access. Only citizens of the Lisbon metropolitan region were considered.

2.2. Variables

Several categories of variables were created:

- General and lifestyle variables: (1) age, (2) sex, (3) practice of physical exercise, (4) consumption of alcoholic beverages, (5) tobacco consumption, and (6) presence of chronic diseases.
- Socioeconomic variables: (1) place of residence, (2) household size, (3) literary qualifications, and (4) professional situation.
- Dietary variables: (1) frequency of meat consumption, (2) motivation for meat consumption, (3) willingness to change meat consumption habits due to knowledge of the associated ecological footprint, and (4) willingness to change meat consumption habits due to knowledge of the negative effects on health.

2.3. Measuring Instrument and Techniques

With the help of an online form maker [18], a questionnaire with 17 closed-ended questions was created and applied. In the beginning of the questionnaire, the project and its main goal were described. This was followed by a question in which the participant agrees to take part in the study and gives permission for the data to be used for that study. Eleven of the questions on the survey were about general information and how people live. Two questions were about how often and why people eat meat, and three questions were about why people want to change their eating habits because they know about their impact on the environment and want to improve their health. The questionnaire was sent to and shared within six companies in the Lisbon urban area that work in different fields. In these companies, data collection was performed to obtain results that were more diverse and more representative of the people who live in Lisbon.

2.4. Statistical Analysis

An operationalization table of the variables under study was constructed, in which the codification, description, valuation, and statistical categorization of the variables were carried out. The referred table was used as a tool for the construction of a database that allowed the compilation of all the results of the variables under study. The statistical analysis was performed using the statistical software for Windows, SPSS®, version 26.0 (SPSS Inc., Chicago, IL, USA). The results were expressed as a number and percentage. The frequency distribution of the qualitative variables was evaluated using the chi-square test and, in the presence of statistical significance, the Z test for proportions was applied. Contingency tables were also created, and the Mantel Haenszel test was applied to estimate associations between qualitative variables with differences in frequency distribution. For all tests, statistical significance was considered when $p < 0.05$.

3. Results

Table 1 displays the general characteristics of the sample across two distinct age groups. The sex distribution in the field of GI showed that approximately 29% of individuals identified as male, while the remaining 71% identified as female. The GII data revealed a comparatively greater proportion of female individuals within the distribution. The study did not identify any statistically significant variations between the groups with respect to the following variables: sex, household size, existence of chronic illness, existence of a chronic illness that restricts meat consumption, tobacco use, alcohol consumption, and frequency of physical activity of at least twice per week. Overall, the sample population exhibited a majority of over 50% of individuals with a household comprising three or more members. Approximately 84% of the participants reported the absence of any chronic medical conditions. With respect to smoking behaviors, a majority of 75.6% of respondents indicated that they did not engage in smoking. The data revealed that 44.2% of adults reported consuming alcohol at least once per week. Most of the participants, specifically 53.3%, reported being sedentary as they disclosed not engaging in physical exercise for a minimum of two times per week.

Table 1. Characterization of the sample by group.

Characteristics	GI (n = 94)	GII (n = 103)	Total (n = 197)	p
Sex	94 (47.7)	103 (52.3)	197 (100)	
Masculine	27 (40.9)	39 (59.1)	66 (100)	0.175
Feminine	67 (51.1)	64 (48.9)	131 (100)	
Household size	94 (47.7)	103 (52.3)	197 (100)	0.068
1 person	14 [a] (51.9)	13 [a] (48.1)	27 (13.7)	
2 persons	23 [a] (63.9)	13 [b] (36.1)	36 (18.3)	
3 persons	29 [a] (51.8)	27 [a] (48.2)	56 (28.4)	
4 persons	18 [a] (35.3)	32 [b] (64.7)	51 (25.9)	
>4 persons	10 [a] (37.0)	17 [a] (63.0)	27 (13.7)	
Literary abilities	94 (47.7)	103 (52.3)	197 (100)	<0.001 *
2nd and 3rd cycle of basic education	1 [a] (50.0)	1 [a] (50.0)	2 (1.0)	
High school	41 [a] (70.7)	17 [b] (29.3)	58 (29.4)	
University education	52 [a] (38.0)	85 [b] (62.0)	137 (69.5)	
Professional situation	94 (48.2)	101 (51.8)	195 (100)	<0.001 *
Employee	37 [a] (33.3)	74 [b] (66.7)	111 (56.9)	
Student	28 [a] (87.5)	4 [b] (12.5)	32 (16.4)	
worker—student	27 [a] (56.3)	21 [a] (43.8)	48 (24.6)	
unemployed	2 [a] (50.0)	2 [a] (50.0)	4 (2.1)	

Table 1. Cont.

Characteristics	GI (n = 94)	GII (n = 103)	Total (n = 197)	p
Presence of chronic illness	93 (47.4)	103 (52.6)	196 (100)	0.105
Yes	11 (34.4)	21 (65.6)	32 (16.3)	
No	82 (50.0)	82 (50.0)	164 (83.7)	
Presence of chronic illness that limits meat consumption	11 (34.4)	21 (65.6)	32 (100)	0.968
Yes	1 (33.3)	2 (66.7)	3 (9.4)	
No	10 (34.5)	19 (65.5)	29 (90.6)	
Smoke at least one time per week	94 (47.7)	103 (52.3)	197 (100)	0.974
Yes	23 (47.9)	25 (52.1)	48 (24.4)	
No	71 (47.7)	78 (52.3)	149 (75.6)	
Consume alcoholic beverages at least once a week	94 (47.7)	103 (52.3)	197 (100)	0.313
Yes	38 (43.7)	49 (56.3)	87 (44.2)	
No	56 (50.9)	54 (49.1)	110 (55.8)	
Exercise at least twice a week	94 (47.7)	103 (52.3)	197 (100)	0.753
Yes	45 (48.9)	47 (51.1)	92 (46.7)	
No	49 (46.7)	56 (53.3)	105 (53.3)	

The results are expressed as the number of individuals (percentage). * Statistically significant ($p < 0.05$). Frequencies in the same line marked with different letters (a,b) are statistically different according to the Z test for proportions ($p < 0.05$).

The analysis found significant differences ($p < 0.001$) in educational qualifications between the groups. A higher percentage of individuals in GII (62.0%) had higher education compared with GI (38.0%), while a higher percentage of participants in GI (70.7%) had completed secondary education compared with GII (29.3%). The statistical significance of professional status results was observed ($p < 0.001$). The distribution of employees in GI (33.3%) and GII (66.7%) and students in GI (87.5%) and GII (12.5%) showed significant differences.

The characterization of the sample by sex is shown in Table 2. Of the 66 male participants, 27 were aged between 20 and 29 (GI) years and 39 between 40 and 64 years (GII). Regarding females, 67 of the participants belonged to GI and 64 to GII. No statistically significant differences were found for the variables: household size, educational qualifications, professional situation, presence of chronic disease, presence of chronic disease that limits meat consumption, tobacco consumption, and frequency of physical exercise at least two times per week. Significant differences ($p < 0.001$) were found in relation to alcohol consumption at least once a week, and this consumption was verified in more than half of the participating males (42) and only in 45 females.

Table 2. Characterization of the sample by sex.

Characteristics	Male (n = 66)	Female (n = 131)	Total (n = 197)	p
Groups	66 (33.5)	131 (66.5)	197 (100)	0.175
GI: 20–29 (years)	27 (28.7)	67 (71.3)	94 (47.7)	
GII: 40–64 (years)	39 (37.9)	64 (62.1)	103 (52.3)	
Household size	66 (33.5)	131 (63.5)	197 (100)	0.462
1 person	13 (48.1)	14 (51.9)	27 (13.7)	
2 persons	11 (30.6)	25 (69.4)	36 (18.3)	
3 persons	16 (28.6)	40 (71.4)	56 (28.4)	
4 persons	16 (31.4)	35 (68.6)	51 (25.9)	
>4 persons	10 (37.0)	17 (63.0)	27 (13.7)	

Table 2. *Cont.*

Characteristics	Male (*n* = 66)	Female (*n* = 131)	Total (*n* = 197)	*p*
Literary abilities	66 (33.5)	131 (66.5)	197 (100)	0.759
2nd and 3rd cycle of basic education	1 (50.0)	1 (50.0)	2 (1.0)	
High school	21 (36.2)	37 (63.8)	58 (29.4)	
University education	44 (32.1)	93 (67.9)	137 (69.5)	
Professional situation	66 (33.8)	129 (66.2)	195 (100)	0.569
Employee	41 (36.9)	70 (63.1)	111 (56.9)	
Student	10 (31.3)	22 (68.8)	32 (16.4)	
Worker—student	13 (27.1)	35 (72.9)	48 (24.6)	
Unemployed	2 (50.0)	2 (50.0)	4 (2.1)	
Presence of chronic illness	66 (33.7)	130 (66.3)	196 (100)	0.617
Yes	12 (37.5)	20 (62.5)	32 (16.3)	
No	54 (32.9)	110 (67.1)	164 (83.7)	
Presence of chronic illness that limits meat consumption	12 (37.5)	20 (62.5)	32 (100)	0.273
Yes	2 (66.7)	1 (33.3)	3 (9.4)	
No	10 (34.5)	19 (65.5)	29 (90.5)	
Smoke at least one time per week	66 (33.5)	131 (66.5)	197 (100)	0.305
Yes	19 (39.6)	29 (60.4)	48 (24.4)	
No	47 (31.5)	102 (68.5)	149 (75.6)	
Consume alcoholic beverages at least once a week	66 (33.5)	131 (66.5)	197 (100)	<0.001 *
Yes	42 (48.3)	45 (51.7)	87 (44.2)	
No	24 (21.8)	86 (78.2)	110 (55.8)	
Exercise at least twice a week	66 (33.5)	131 (66.5)	197 (100)	0.957
Yes	31 (33.7)	61 (66.3)	92 (46.7)	
No	35 (33.3)	70 (66.7)	105 (53.3)	

The results are expressed as the number of individuals (percentage). * Statistically significant ($p < 0.05$).

Table 3 shows the frequency of meat intake and readiness to limit consumption by group. According to the findings, no statistically significant differences were found between the groups in terms of meat consumption frequency, reasons for never consuming meat, or willingness to reduce consumption due to health and environmental concerns. Knowledge of the ecological footprint was similarly comparable across groups. The frequency of meat consumption four to six times per week was most frequently stated by individuals (86), with 38 in GI and 48 in GII. The option of consuming more than six times per week was the second most popular, with 53 people indicating this frequency of intake, 31 in GI and 22 in GII. Only 15 people said they would never eat meat again, and the most common explanation was that they were devout vegetarians. In terms of willingness to minimize meat eating, 139 people said they were willing to do so because they were concerned about the influence on their health. This option was chosen by 66 people in GI and 73 people in GII. A large proportion of participants (67%) stated that they were unaware of the ecological footprint of meat. However, 125 (GI: 57 vs. GII: 68) reported being able to minimize their consumption due to environmental concerns.

Table 3. Assessment of meat consumption frequency and willingness to reduce this consumption by group.

Characteristics	GI (n = 94)	GII (n = 103)	Total (n = 197)	p
Frequency of meat consumption	94 (47.7)	103 (52.3)	197 (100)	0.237
Never	8 (53.3)	7 (46.7)	15 (7.6)	
One to three times per week	17 (39.5)	26 (60.5)	43 (21.8)	
Four to six times per week	38 (44.2)	48 (55.8)	86 (43.7)	
More than six times per week	31 (58.5)	22 (41.5)	53 (26.9)	
Reason to never eat meat	8 (53.3)	7 (46.7)	15 (100)	0.689
Environmental impact	4 (66.7)	2 (33.3)	6 (40.0)	
Being a strict vegetarian	3 (42.9)	4 (57.1)	7 (46.7)	
Other	1 (50.0)	1 (50.0)	2 (13.3)	
Willingness to reduce meat consumption due to health impact	85 (47.2)	95 (52.8)	180 (100)	0.898
Yes	66 (47.5)	73 (52.5)	139 (77.2)	
No	19 (46.3)	22 (53.7)	41 (22.8)	
Knowledge of the ecological footprint of meat	92 (48.2)	99 (51.8)	191 (100)	0.303
Yes	27 (42.9)	36 (57.1)	63 (33.0)	
No	65 (50.8)	63 (49.2)	128 (67.0)	
Willingness to reduce meat consumption due to environmental impact	88 (47.8)	96 (52.2)	184 (100)	0.379
Yes	57 (45.6)	68 (54.4)	125 (67.9)	
No	31 (52.5)	28 (47.5)	59 (32.1)	

The results are expressed as the number of individuals (%). Statistically significant ($p < 0.05$).

The frequency of meat consumption and willingness to reduce this consumption by sex are presented in Table 4. No significant differences were observed between males and females regarding the frequency of meat consumption, reasons for never consuming meat, and knowledge about the ecological footprint. The frequency of meat consumption four to six times per week was again the most described by both sexes, with 34 of the 66 males evaluated consuming meat four to six times per week. Only one male indicated never eating meat, while 14 females chose this frequency. In addition, 57.8% of females indicated that they were unaware of the ecological footprint of meat, and 42.2% of the males indicated the same. Statistically significant differences were observed in terms of willingness to reduce meat consumption due to its impact on health, with females be more willing (73.9%) to make this reduction than males (26.6%). The same was verified in relation to the willingness to reduce meat consumption based on knowledge of the environmental impact ($p < 0.001$), in which 74.4% of females responded that they were available to reduce meat consumption against 25.6% of males.

Table 4. Characterization of meat consumption and willingness to reduce its consumption by sex.

Characteristics	Male (n = 66)	Female (n = 131)	Total (n = 197)	p
Frequency of meat consumption	66 (35.5)	131 (66.5)	197 (100)	0.072
Never	1 (6.7)	14 (93.3)	15 (7.6)	
One to three times per week	12 (27.9)	31 (72.1)	43 (21.8)	
Four to six times per week	34 (39.5)	52 (60.5)	86 (43.7)	
More than six times per week	19 (35.8)	34 (64.2)	53 (26.9)	

Table 4. Cont.

Characteristics	Male (n = 66)	Female (n = 131)	Total (n = 197)	p
Reason to never eat meat	1 (6.7)	14 (93.3)	15 (100)	0.448
Environmental impact	1 (16.7)	5 (83.3)	6 (40.0)	
Being a strict vegetarian	0 (0.0)	7 (100)	7 (46.7)	
Other	0 (0.0)	2 (100)	2 (13.3)	
Willingness to reduce meat consumption due to health impact	61 (33.9)	119 (66.1)	180 (100)	<0.001 *
Yes	37 [a] (26.6)	102 [b] (73.9)	139 (77.2)	
No	24 [a] (39.3)	17 [b] (14.3)	41 (22.8)	
Knowledge of the ecological footprint of meat	65 (34.0)	126 (66.0)	191 (100)	0.428
Yes	19 (30.2)	44 (69.8)	55 (38.4)	
No	46 (42.2)	82 (57.8)	109 (67.0)	
Willingness to reduce meat consumption due to environmental impact	63 (34.2)	121 (65.8)	184 (100)	<0.001 *
Yes	32 [a] (25.6)	93 [b] (74.4)	125 (67.9)	
No	31 [a] (52.5)	28 [b] (47.5)	59 (32.1)	

The results are expressed as the number of individuals (percentage). * Statistically significant ($p < 0.05$). Frequencies in the same row marked with different letters (a,b) are statistically different according to the Z test for proportions ($p < 0.05$).

Table 5 demonstrates the relationship of the availability to lower the frequency of meat eating in participants who consume it more than six times per week. The findings revealed that less frequent consumers, or those who consume meat less than once a day, are substantially ($p < 0.001$) more likely (79.1%) to reduce their consumption owing to health concerns than the most frequent consumers (20.9%).

Table 5. Association of availability to decrease the frequency of meat consumption in participants with consumption greater than six times per week.

| Characteristics | Meat Consumption More than Six Times per Week | | | p | OR | CI (95%) |
	Yes (n = 53)	No (n = 144)	Total (n = 197)			
Availability to reduce the frequency of meat consumption due to health impact	49 (27.2)	131 (72.8)	180 (100)	<0.001 *	3.612	1.73–7.55
Yes	29 [a] (20.9)	110 [b] (79.1)	139 (77.2)			
No	20 [a] (48.8)	21 [b] (51.2)	41 (22.8)			
Availability to reduce the frequency of meat consumption due to environmental impact	51 (27.7)	133 (72.3)	184 (100)	<0.001 *	4.006	2.02–7.93
Yes	23 [a] (18.4)	102 [b] (81.6)	125 (67.9)			
No	28 [a] (47.5)	31 [b] (52.5)	59 (32.1)			

The results are expressed as the number of individuals (percentage). CI, confidence interval; OR, odds ratio. * Statistically significant ($p < 0.05$). Frequencies in the same line marked with different letters (a,b) are statistically different according to the Z test for proportions ($p < 0.05$).

Being a meat consumer less than once a day relates to a 3.6-fold greater readiness to reduce meat eating due to health sensitivity. When it comes to the willingness to reduce meat consumption due to environmental concerns, less frequent consumers (consumption one time per day) are more willing to do so (81.6%) than the most frequent consumers (daily consumption), who only have 18.4% of affirmative answers. Due to environmental sensitivity, being a less frequent consumer than daily relates to a 4.0 times greater desire to cut meat intake.

Table 6 shows the results of the association by sex of availability to reduce the frequency of meat consumption in the most frequent consumers (more than six times per week). This difference was statistically significant ($p < 0.001$). Being a meat consumer daily and being a female seem to be associated with an eight times greater willingness to reduce meat consumption due to sensitivity to the impact on health than being a male and a frequent meat consumer (one time per day). Regarding availability to reduce meat consumption due to sensitivity to environmental impact, it was found that females more frequently reported being available to reduce meat consumption (69.6%) compared with males (30.4%). Being a meat consumer daily and being a female seem to be associated with a 6.4 times greater availability to reduce meat consumption due to sensitivity to the impact on health than being a male and a frequent meat consumer (one time per day).

Table 6. Association by sex of availability to reduce the frequency of meat consumption in participants with a frequency of meat consumption greater than six times per week.

Characteristics	Meat Consumption More than Six Times per Week											
	M (n = 19)	p	OR	CI (95%)	F (n = 34)	p	OR	CI (95%)	Total (n = 53)	p	OR	CI (95%)
Availability to reduce the frequency of meat consumption due to health impact	19 (38.8)	0.388	1.620	0.534–4.865	30 (61.2)	<0.001 *	8.009	2.632–24.36	49 (100)	<0.001 *	3.612	1.73–7.55
Yes	10 (34.5)				19 (65.5)				29 (77.2)			
No	09 (45.0)				11 (55.0)				20 (22.8)			
Availability to reduce the frequency of meat consumption due to environmental impact	19 (37.3)	0.146	2.256	0.746–6.822	32 (62.7)	<0.001 *	6.417	2.55–16.13	51 (100)	<0.001 *	4.006	2.02–7.93
Yes	07 (30.4)				16 (69.6)				23 (45.1)			
No	12 (42.9)				16 (57.1)				28 (54.9)			

The results are expressed as the number of individuals (percentage). F, female; CI, confidence interval; M, male; OR, odds ratio. * Statistically significant ($p < 0.05$).

4. Discussion

According to current knowledge, this is the first study in Portugal to examine the frequency of meat intake and sensitivity to the impact on health and the environment in residents of the Lisbon metropolitan region. Food sustainability and healthy eating are widely disseminated through various media to influence habits and, as a result, lessen the impact on health and the environment with more aware choices [19]. Excessive meat consumption has negative health repercussions as well as a significant ecological imprint, and dietary modifications are becoming increasingly important [9,20].

The findings revealed no differences in sensitivity to the ecological footprint between groups I and II, which were formed based on various age ranges. It was expected to find differences between the studied groups, and our findings were consistent with those presented in a study conducted in several European Union countries [21] in which the goal was to evaluate the possible presence of differences in sensitivity to the ecological footprint and meat consumption in two well-differentiated age ranges (GI: 20–29 years and GII: 40–64 years old).

We anticipated that the younger group would have better environmental awareness and sensitivity to lowering meat intake due to the negative environmental and health implications than GII. GI has different cultural, political, and gastronomic influences than GII because it is made up of younger elements. Because they were older, the persons in GII may have been more exposed to more unpredictability in food availability throughout their lives than the subjects in GI, who were from a younger generation. Participants in GII were most likely subject to food policies in Portugal that were based on assuring food accessibility until they reached maturity. GI individuals, on the other hand, were from an age in which food regulations began to prioritize nutritional status and health promotion [22].

The current study found no significant differences between the two groups evaluated in Portugal regarding their knowledge of the ecological footprint of meat. A high percentage of participants, regardless of age or sex, indicated that they did not have this knowledge. Despite the different influence of food policies in Portugal on the two evaluated groups, the present study found no significant differences concerning this knowledge. This fact was somewhat unsettling because it showed the need for improvements in communication and the perception of information on the part of the customers whose responses were analyzed, as well as maybe additional consumers from the Portuguese population. There were no discernible differences regarding knowledge regarding the ecological footprint of meat among age groups or between the sexes, and there are no comparative studies on this topic that have been conducted in Portugal. It is also important to note that the evaluated sample had a large representation of participants with secondary or higher education. Although it was anticipated that participants with more educational qualifications would have a greater knowledge about the ecological footprint of meat, the results did not show any differences between the groups based on this variable [6,23,24].

It was also observed that those who consumed meat one to three times per week were more frequently in GII, whereas participants who consumed meat more than six times per week daily were more frequently in GI. The fact that the differences identified were not statistically significant demonstrates that the age range does not appear to have any bearing on the number of times that people consume meat. These results were not what was expected because there has been a growing trend among young people to become aware of the ecological footprint of meat. This information has been widely disseminated on the internet [25] and in other media, as well as the promotion of the Mediterranean dietary pattern [26], which is based on promoting the consumption of vegetable protein to the detriment of animal protein. Arnaudova et al. (2022) [27], who analyzed the frequency of meat intake in university students, did not find any significant differences by age or sex in their findings. The findings of the current study agreed with the findings of the research work by Arnaudova et al. (2022) [27]. The research conducted by Verain and Dagevos (2022) [24], which described and compared people who consume meat, lends support to the notion that the primary motive of people who do not consume meat is concern for the welfare of animals, with health and sustainability coming in a distant second and third place, respectively. Another study was carried out in countries of the European Union [21], which investigated whether reducing meat consumption would be associated with the concept of "eating a healthy and sustainable diet." The authors concluded that in southern Europe, the respondents do not associate reducing meat consumption as an active positive behavior toward healthy eating and/or a contribution to the sustainability of the planet.

In the current analysis, there were not found any statistically significant variations between age groups regarding the desire to limit the amount of meat consumed. On the other hand, when looking at the complete sample, it was discovered that a greater number of participants ($n = 139$) indicated that they were willing to cut their consumption of meat due to concerns regarding its influence on health as opposed to concerns regarding its impact on the environment ($n = 63$). When the examination of availability to reduce meat consumption was carried out by sex, disparities were discovered. It was found that females were more likely to be available to reduce this consumption due to their sensitivity to the influence that it had on both their health and the environment. On the other hand, it was discovered that this availability was greater for reasons related to health (OR = 8.0; $p < 0.001$) than it was for reasons related to the environment (OR = 6.4; $p < 0.001$). A study that was conducted out on 713 German adults with diverse patterns of meat consumption, published by Verain and Dagevos (2022) [24], reveals that males have more resistance to reducing their meat intake, possibly due to a lack of awareness, a lack of interest, or cultural reasons. According to the findings of other studies [23,28], females are more aware of the effects of human activity on the environment, whereas males are less worried about environmental issues. Carvalho and Li (2009) [29] conducted a research study on the lack of desire by males to reduce their intake of meat. The authors concluded that this lack of motivation may be related to males having a weaker view of their own health status in comparison with females.

In the current study, it was shown that individuals who ate meat less frequently (less than once per day) reported being more open to reducing their consumption of meat when compared with individuals who ate meat more frequently. These results were observed for sensitivity to both the impact on health and the environment. However, less frequent consumers were 3.6 times more likely ($p < 0.001$) to reduce their consumption of meat due to their awareness of the negative impact it had on their health and 4.0 times more likely ($p < 0.001$) to do so for environmental reasons. There are several studies that can be found in the scientific literature that discuss a variety of arguments in favor of lowering one's consumption of meat. Others refer to sensitivity to health impacts as the primary cause [24,30], and the price of meat has also been seen as one of the key reasons for reducing its consumption [30]. Some of the reasons have to do with animal welfare [12,31], while others point to sensitivity to health impacts as the main reason [24,30].

In a study that was conducted [32] in Canada, the impact of community interventions on changing eating habits was analyzed, and the conclusion reached was that an individual's level of knowledge alters the tendency to internalize the message and subsequent action in reducing meat intake. The study was carried out to evaluate the impact of community interventions on changing eating habits. This research also focused on the significance of making alternative food selections after reducing the amount of meat consumed, and it implied that these shifts did not necessarily have positive effects on the environment. It is of the utmost importance that community actions be suited to the target audience that is intended to be affected, and to do this, it is vital to know the population and differentiate between the groups within it. It is also important to educate people so that they may make informed decisions about the dietary alternatives that will help them reduce their meat consumption while also benefiting the environment. Because eating meat has such a significant negative effect on both human health and the natural world, adopting new eating patterns and making more conscientious and environmentally friendly decisions is more important than ever. One of the first stages toward accomplishing this objective is being familiar enough with the people to be able to intervene in a forceful manner [1,9,12,20,31,32].

It will also be important to consider the possible effects of seasonality on meat consumption in Portugal. Although the study was conducted from November 2022 to March 2023, the questionnaire was applied from the end of January until March. Thus, the influence of the holiday season was not confirmed. In Portugal, the availability of some foods may be influenced by seasonality, as with fruit, vegetables, and fish, but the tables of seasonality and food availability in the national market do not include meat [33]. It is also important to point out that based on the latest results of the Food Balance Sheet for the five-year period (2016–2020), its availability has increased by 8.7% (+6.7 kg/inhabitant) in relation to the homologous previous period, currently being the group of the food wheel with the greatest deviation of availability for consumption in relation to the recommended daily consumption [1]. Thus, since 2012, meat consumption in Portugal has been three times higher (16.4%) than recommended (5%) on the food wheel and with little seasonal variation.

The price of meat is also a possible factor contributing to its lower daily consumption. Food price inflation between November 2022 and March 2023 was quite high [34]. The foods that had the most significant increases between February and March 2023 were (1) dairy products (+27.3%), (2) fish (+27%), (3) grocery products (+25%), (4) fruits and vegetables (+24.7%), and meat (+22.8%) [35]. The increase in the price of meat and other foods described is a factor that may have contributed to a lower consumption of meat due to a decrease in the consumer's purchasing power. However, the results of the III Great National Sustainability Survey [36], presented in October 2022, had already shown a significant reduction in meat consumption (−32%) compared with 2018 (pre-pandemic). Thus, the effect of the pandemic seems to have had a greater impact on reducing meat consumption than the price increase since several foods that can be protein alternatives to meat had an even greater increase (e.g., fish, dairy products, and grocery stores). Furthermore, during periods of greater financial trouble, consumers also change their meat buying patterns, favoring types of meat with lower prices per kilogram (e.g., pork meat).

Study Limitations

The current study had a few flaws and restrictions. The validated questionnaires on this topic referred to consumption frequencies and/or eating habits; however, no validated questionnaire on the subject being studied was found in the scientific literature. Consequently, it was necessary to create a new questionnaire. Although the sample size was representative of the population in the sense that it was larger than the minimum sample size associated with a confidence level of 95% and a margin of error of 10%, the authors intend to continue this work in the future and increase the number of participants to decrease the error to 5%, which would require 385 participants in each group. Although the questionnaire was administered without any kind of personal identity record, there was still a possibility that there was a bias related to social desirability and participation. This was another drawback of the study. Very few of the participants in this study had even completed their primary or secondary education, which meant that the work did not adequately reflect people with lower levels of literary qualifications. It will be necessary in the future to carry out an evaluation that also includes a greater number of participants with characteristics that are inadequately reflected in the work that has already been performed on the research. Another aspect that was not considered was related to the amount of meat consumed since only the frequency of consumption was evaluated. It will be necessary to incorporate a methodology for assessing the food portion of meat consumed in combination with the frequency of consumption into the work that will be performed in the future.

5. Conclusions

This study contributed to the evaluation of the frequency of meat consumption, the knowledge of the ecological footprint, and the availability of participants to reduce their meat consumption because of sensitivity to the impact on health and the environment, among residents of the metropolitan region of Lisbon. Regardless of age or sex, most participants said that they lacked understanding regarding the ecological footprint of meat consumption. There was no discernible difference in the frequency of meat eating based on age or sex. Less frequent meat consumers (consumption of less than once per day) were more available to minimize their meat consumption than more frequent meat consumers (consumption of more than six times per week) because they were more sensitive to the influence that their behavior may have on their health or the environment. When it came to people who ate meat more than six times a week, females were more available than males to cut their consumption of meat if doing so would have a positive effect on their health or the environment.

Additional research is required to properly analyze the prevalence of meat intake and the options available to lessen that prevalence. In the future, it is planned to continue the inquiry into this topic, with the goals of increasing the sample size, expanding the analyzed geographic area, including additional potential variables that may motivate people to consume less meat, and quantifying the food portion that was consumed.

Author Contributions: Conceptualization, A.T. and A.V.; methodology, A.T. and A.V.; software, A.T. and A.V.; validation, A.T., P.P., H.C., and A.V.; formal analysis, A.T.; investigation, A.T.; resources, A.T.; writing—original draft preparation, A.T.; writing—review and editing, P.P., H.C. and A.V.; visualization, A.T.; supervision, P.P., H.C. and A.V.; project administration, A.V. All authors have read and agreed to the published version of the manuscript.

Funding: This research received no external funding.

Institutional Review Board Statement: The study was conducted in accordance with the Declaration of Helsinki and approved by the Ethics Committee of Atlantic—University Higher Institution (23/01/2023).

Informed Consent Statement: Informed consent was obtained from all subjects involved in the study.

Data Availability Statement: Not applicable.

Conflicts of Interest: The authors declare no conflict of interest.

References

1. Balança Alimentar Portuguesa 2016–2020. Available online: file:///C:/Users/valen/Downloads/BAP_2016_2020%20(3).pdf (accessed on 8 May 2023).
2. Bento, A.; Gonçalves, C.; Cordeiro, T.; Vaz de Almeida, M.D. Portugal nutritional transition during the last 4 decades: 1974–2011. *Porto Biomed. J.* **2018**, *3*, e25. [CrossRef] [PubMed]
3. Monteiro, M.; Fontes, T.; Ferreira-Pêgo, C. Nutrition literacy of portuguese adults—A pilot study. *Int. J. Environ. Res. Public Health* **2021**, *18*, 3177. [CrossRef] [PubMed]
4. Inquérito Alimentar Nacional Relatório Resultados 2015–2016. Available online: https://ian-af.up.pt/sites/default/files/IAN-AF%20Relat%C3%B3rio%20Resultados_0.pdf (accessed on 8 May 2023).
5. National Food, Nutrition and Physical Activity Survey of the Portuguese General Population. Available online: https://www.ian-af.up.pt/sites/default/files/IAN-AF%20Summary%20of%20Results_1.pdf (accessed on 8 May 2023).
6. Estudo de Adesão ao Estudo de Adesão ao Padrão Alimentar Mediterrânico. Available online: https://nutrimento.pt/activeapp/wp-content/uploads/2020/10/Estudo-de-adesa%CC%83o-ao-padra%CC%83o-alimentar-mediterra%CC%82nico.pdf (accessed on 8 May 2023).
7. Papier, K.; Fensom, G.K.; Knuppel, A.; Appleby, P.N.; Tong, T.Y.N.; Schmidt, J.A.; Travis, R.C.; Key, T.J.; Perez-Cornago, A. Meat consumption and risk of 25 common conditions: Outcome-wide analyses in 475,000 men and women in the UK Biobank study. *BMC Med.* **2021**, *19*, 53. [CrossRef] [PubMed]
8. Giromini, C.; Givens, D.I. Benefits and Risks Associated with Meat Consumption during Key Life Processes and in Relation to the Risk of Chronic Diseases. *Foods* **2022**, *11*, 2063. [CrossRef] [PubMed]
9. González, N.; Marquès, M.; Nadal, M.; Domingo, J.L. Meat consumption: Which are the current global risks? A review of recent (2010–2020) evidences. *Food Res. Int.* **2020**, *137*, 109341. [CrossRef] [PubMed]
10. Salter, A.M. The effects of meat consumption on global health. *Rev. Sci. Tech.* **2018**, *37*, 47–55. [CrossRef] [PubMed]
11. Estado da Saúde na UE, Portugal. Available online: https://health.ec.europa.eu/system/files/2021-12/2021_chp_pt_portuguese.pdf (accessed on 8 May 2023).
12. Sanchez-Sabate, R.; Badilla-Briones, Y.; Sabaté, J. Understanding attitudes towards reducing meat consumption for environmental reasons. A qualitative synthesis review. *Sustainability* **2019**, *11*, 6295. [CrossRef]
13. Food Emissions from Production and the Supply Chain. Available online: https://ourworldindata.org/grapher/food-emissions-supply-chain (accessed on 8 May 2023).
14. Meat Market Review—Emerging Trends and Outlook 2022. Available online: https://www.fao.org/3/cc3164en/cc3164en.pdf (accessed on 9 May 2023).
15. O Estado da Nação e as Políticas Públicas 2022: Recuperação em Tempos de Incerteza. Available online: https://ipps.iscte-iul.pt/divulgacao/estudos-e-publicacoes-3/1117-recuperacao-em-tempos-de-incerteza (accessed on 30 March 2023).
16. Instituto Nacional Estatistica Portugal: População Residente. Available online: https://www.ine.pt/xportal/xmain?xpid=INE&xpgid=ine_main (accessed on 8 May 2023).
17. Calculadora de Tamanho de Amostra SurveyMonkey. Available online: https://pt.surveymonkey.com/mp/sample-size-calculator/ (accessed on 9 January 2023).
18. Google Forms: Online Form Creator. Available online: https://www.google.com/forms/about/ (accessed on 30 March 2023).
19. Wakefield, M.A.; Loken, B.; Hornik, R.C. Use of mass media campaigns to change health behaviour. *Lancet* **2010**, *376*, 1261–1271. [CrossRef] [PubMed]
20. Perignon, M.; Vieux, F.; Soler, L.G.; Masset, G.; Darmon, N. Improving diet sustainability through evolution of food choices: Review of epidemiological studies on the environmental impact of diets. *Nutr. Rev.* **2017**, *75*, 2–17. [CrossRef] [PubMed]
21. Boer, J.; Aiking, H. Do EU consumers think about meat reduction when considering to eat a healthy, sustainable diet and to have a role in food system change? *Appetite* **2022**, *170*, 105880. [CrossRef] [PubMed]
22. Graça, P.; Gregório, M.J. Evolução da política alimentar e de nutrição em Portugal e suas relações com o contexto internacional. *Rev. Ali. Hum.* **2012**, *18*, 3.
23. Allès, B.; Baudry, J.; Méjean, C.; Touvier, M.; Péneau, S.; Hercberg, S.; Kesse-Guyot, E. Comparison of sociodemographic and nutritional characteristics between self-reported vegetarians, vegans, and meat-eaters from the nutrinet-santé study. *Nutrients* **2017**, *9*, 1023. [CrossRef] [PubMed]
24. Verain, M.C.D.; Dagevos, H. Comparing meat abstainers with avid meat eaters and committed meat reducers. *Front. Nutr.* **2022**, *9*, 1016858. [CrossRef] [PubMed]
25. Rótulo da Pegada Ecológica nos Alimentos: Brevemente em Portugal? Available online: https://www.avp.org.pt/rotulo-da-pegada-ecologica-dos-alimentos/ (accessed on 30 March 2023).

26. Padrão Alimentar Mediterrânico: Promotor de Saúde. Available online: https://alimentacaosaudavel.dgs.pt/activeapp2020/wpcontent/uploads/2020/01/Padr%C3%A3o-Alimentar-Mediterr%C3%A2nico-Promotor-de-Sa%C3%BAde-1.pdf (accessed on 8 May 2023).
27. Arnaudova, M.; Brunner, T.A.; Götze, F. Examination of students' willingness to change behaviour regarding meat consumption. *Meat Sci.* **2022**, *184*, 108695. [CrossRef] [PubMed]
28. Barton Laws, M.; Yeh, Y.; Reisner, E.; Stone, K.; Wang, T.; Brugge, D. Gender, Ethnicity and Environmental Risk Perception Revisited: The Importance of Residential Location. *J. Community Health* **2015**, *40*, 948–955. [CrossRef] [PubMed]
29. Carvalho, R.; Ii, F. Chronic diseases, self-perceived health status and health risk behaviors: Gender differences. *Rev. Saude Publica* **2009**, *43*, 38–47.
30. Neff, R.A.; Edwards, D.; Palmer, A.; Ramsing, R.; Righter, A.; Wolfson, J. Reducing meat consumption in the USA: A nationally representative survey of attitudes and behaviours. *Public Health Nutr.* **2018**, *21*, 1835–1844. [CrossRef] [PubMed]
31. Garcez, L.; Padilha, d.O.; Malek, L.; Umberger, W.J. Sustainable Meat: Looking through the Eyes of Australian Consumers. *Sustainability* **2021**, *13*, 5398. [CrossRef]
32. Lacroix, K.; Gifford, R. Targeting interventions to distinct meat-eating groups reduces meat consumption. *Food Qual. Prefer* **2020**, *86*, 103997. [CrossRef]
33. Calendários de Produção Nacional. Available online: https://www.apn.org.pt/documentos/marcadores_e_folhetos/Brochura_calendarios_producao_nacional.pdf (accessed on 28 June 2023).
34. Instituto Nacional de Estatística. Available online: https://www.ine.pt/xportal/xmain?xpgid=ine_tema&xpid=INE&tema_cod=1314&xlang=pt (accessed on 28 June 2023).
35. Deco Proteste—Defesa do Consumidor. Available online: https://www.deco.proteste.pt/familia-consumo/orcamento-familiar/noticias/um-ano-guerra-preco-alimentos-aumentou-mesmo-quando-inflacao-desceu (accessed on 28 June 2023).
36. Grande Consumo—Revista dos Negócios da Distribuição. Available online: https://grandeconsumo.com/portugueses-utilizam-mais-marmita-comem-menos-carne-e-mais-alimentos-biologicos/ (accessed on 28 June 2023).

Disclaimer/Publisher's Note: The statements, opinions and data contained in all publications are solely those of the individual author(s) and contributor(s) and not of MDPI and/or the editor(s). MDPI and/or the editor(s) disclaim responsibility for any injury to people or property resulting from any ideas, methods, instructions or products referred to in the content.

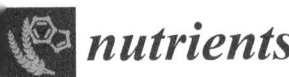

Article

Trends in Beef Intake in the United States: Analysis of the National Health and Nutrition Examination Survey, 2001–2018

Clara S. Lau [1,*], Victor L. Fulgoni III [2], Mary E. Van Elswyk [3] and Shalene H. McNeill [1]

1 National Cattlemen's Beef Association, a contractor to the Beef Checkoff, 9110 East Nichols Ave., Suite 300, Centennial, CO 80112, USA; smcneill@beef.org
2 Nutrition Impact, LLC, Battle Creek, MI 49014, USA; vic3rd@aol.com
3 Van Elswyk Consulting, Inc., Clark, CO 80428, USA; mveconsulting@q.com
* Correspondence: clau@beef.org

Abstract: Evidence-based dietary advice regarding meats (including beef), requires accurate assessment of beef and other red meat intakes across life stages. Beef intake is subject to misclassification due to the use of broad categories such as "red and processed meat". In the current study, intake trends for total beef (i.e., any beef type) and specific beef types (fresh lean, ground, processed) among Americans participating in the National Health and Nutrition Examination Survey (NHANES) 2001–2018 (n = 74,461) were characterized and usual intake was assessed using NHANES 2011–2018 (n = 30,679). The usual intake amounts of beef were compared to those of relevant protein food subgroups modeled in the Healthy U.S.-Style Dietary Pattern (HDP) reported in the 2020–2025 Dietary Guidelines for Americans (DGA). Total per capita beef consumption declined an average of 12 g ($p < 0.0001$) for ages 2–18 years and 5.7 g ($p = 0.0004$) for ages 19–59 years per 2-yr NHANES cycle, over the 18-year timeframe, while remaining unchanged for Americans aged 60+ years. On a per capita basis, Americans aged 2 years and older consumed 42.2 g (1.5 ounces) of total beef per day. Fresh lean beef per capita consumption was 33.4 g (1.2 ounces) per day. Per capita intake was similar across all age groups and below the daily HDP modeled amount of 3.7 ounce equivalents for the "Meats, Poultry, Eggs" (MPE) subgroup, while approximately 75% of beef consumers' intakes of total beef was within HDP modeling. Evidence from intake trends suggests beef is not overconsumed by the majority of Americans but rather within the amounts for MPE and red meat modeled in the HDP of the DGA at the 2000-calorie level.

Keywords: red meat; beef; lean fresh beef; ground beef; processed beef; dietary intake; National Health and Nutrition Examination Survey (NHANES); United States; usual intake; meat products

1. Introduction

Beef is a commonly consumed food and an inherent source of many essential nutrients including high-quality protein, vitamins B6 and B12, zinc, and readily bioavailable heme iron [1,2]. Beef is a red meat, but the commonly used phrases "red meat" and "red and processed meat" encompasses more than just beef, typically referring to the combination of beef, pork, lamb, and game meat, both fresh and processed [3]. The use of broad terminology such as "red and processed meat" increases the risk of misclassification of beef and other red meat intake data [4,5]. Nonetheless, recommendations to eat less "red and processed meat" persist in current dietary guidance in the United States (U.S.) [6,7] based, at least in part, on observational evidence reporting weak associations between "red and processed meat" consumption and risk of chronic disease [8,9]. Interpretation of advice to eat less "red and processed meat" is further complicated by advice that encourages "lean meat" [6,7], as lean beef, red meat, processed meat, and lean meat are not mutually exclusive categories [5]. The Dietary Guidelines for Americans, 2020–2025 (DGA) indicate that protein foods, including lean meats, are core elements in a healthy diet [7]. Although

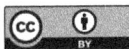

Citation: Lau, C.S.; Fulgoni, V.L., III; Van Elswyk, M.E.; McNeill, S.H. Trends in Beef Intake in the United States: Analysis of the National Health and Nutrition Examination Survey, 2001–2018. *Nutrients* **2023**, *15*, 2475. https://doi.org/10.3390/nu15112475

Academic Editor: Joanna Stadnik

Received: 4 April 2023
Revised: 17 May 2023
Accepted: 22 May 2023
Published: 26 May 2023

Copyright: © 2023 by the authors. Licensee MDPI, Basel, Switzerland. This article is an open access article distributed under the terms and conditions of the Creative Commons Attribution (CC BY) license (https://creativecommons.org/licenses/by/4.0/).

the DGA do not provide beef-specific intake recommendations, the Healthy U.S.-Style Dietary Pattern (HDP), for a 2000-calorie diet, models 3.7 ounces (oz) or 104.9 g of lean meat, poultry and/or eggs per day as part of a healthy dietary pattern [7].

Without a comprehensive and accurate knowledge of intake of individual meat types across all life stages, it is difficult to evaluate the relationships between red and processed meat intake and disease risk to support the development of evidence-based dietary advice [4]. Previous analyses of National Health and Nutrition Examination Survey (NHANES) 1999–2016 reported the consumption of processed meat (including processed red meat and processed poultry meat) remained unchanged, while fresh red meat and fresh beef consumption decreased among adults in the U.S. [10]. During this same time period, fresh poultry, predominantly chicken, significantly increased among U.S. adults [10]. The current study characterizes intake of total beef (i.e., any beef type) and individual beef types (fresh lean, ground, and processed) across life stages using NHANES 2001–2018 data, with the specific objectives to: (1.) Describe intake trends for total beef and individual beef types for the general population across life stages; (2.) Report intake distribution of beef and beef types on both a per capita and per consumer basis; and (3.) Compare per capita and per consumer beef intake to the modeled "Meats, Poultry, Eggs" (MPE) subgroup of the Protein Foods group in the HDP presented in the 2020–2025 DGA.

2. Materials and Methods

2.1. Dietary Intake Assessment

The NHANES is a program of the National Center for Health Statistics which is part of the Centers for Disease Control and Prevention and has the responsibility for producing vital and health statistics for adults and children living across the U.S. The nutrition examination aspect of the survey, What We Eat in America (WWEIA), relies on the U.S. Department of Agriculture (USDA)'s Automated Multiple-Pass Method, a computer-assisted multiple-pass format interview system with standardized probes, developed by the USDA to estimate current dietary intake and to minimize misclassification of dietary intake data of foods [11]. A detailed description of the subject recruitment, survey design, and data collection procedures for NHANES are available online at https://www.cdc.gov/nchs/nhanes/about_nhanes.htm (accessed on 23 April 2021).

NHANES has stringent consent protocols and procedures to ensure confidentiality and protection from identification. The present study was a secondary data analysis of publicly available de-identified data and therefore does not meet the criteria for human subjects research and therefore was exempt from additional approvals by institutional review boards. All participants provided a signed written informed consent. All data obtained from this study are publicly available at: http://www.cdc.gov/nchs/nhanes/ (accessed on 23 April 2021).

2.2. Analytical Sample—Beef Intake Trends

For analyses examining NHANES cycle-to-cycle trends in beef intake, 24-h dietary recall data from the in-person interview (Day 1) from 74,461 subjects aged 2+ years (after exclusions for unreliable or incomplete data n = 10,163, and subjects with no Day 1 dietary intake data n = 5) participating in NHANES 2001–2018 were used. Data were analyzed separately for the following age groups: 2–18 years (children and adolescents), 19–59 years (adults), and 60+ years (older adults), as outlined in the DGA.

2.3. Analytical Sample—Usual Intake of Beef, per Capita and per Consumer

For analyses looking at current beef intake distribution, we used data from NHANES 2011–2018, which provides an updated assessment of previous work [1,12]. The total sample included 30,679 subjects after exclusions. Usual intake was determined using the National Cancer Institute's (NCI) methodology [13] incorporating both days of dietary recall. The two-part model (proportion and amount) was used to determine usual intakes for both per capita (combines consumers and non-consumers of beef) and consumer-only population groups (defined as those with beef consumption on Day 1). Data representing the combination of consumers and non-consumers of beef are referred to as "per capita" in the results and discussed using "average"-related terminology. Data representing consumer-only populations are referred to as "beef consumers" or "consumer-only". Data were analyzed separately for age groups: 2+ years (general population), 2–18 years (children and adolescents), 19–59 years (adults), and 60+ years (older adults), as outlined in the DGA.

2.4. Calculation of Beef-Related Variables

The Food and Nutrient Database for Dietary Studies (FNDDS) is used to code and analyze dietary intakes collected in the WWEIA portion of the NHANES survey (https://www.ars.usda.gov/northeast-area/beltsville-md-bhnrc/beltsville-human-nutrition-research-center/food-surveys-research-group/docs/fndds/; accessed on 23 April 2021). FNDDS food code ingredient data were used to determine the ingredient profile of all food codes consumed. The USDA Food Patterns Equivalent Database (FPED) and the Food Pattern Ingredient Database (FPID) are linked to the food codes and ingredient codes were used to quantify beef content (https://www.ars.usda.gov/northeast-area/beltsville-md-bhnrc/beltsville-human-nutrition-research-center/food-surveys-research-group/docs/fped-overview/; accessed on 23 April 2021). Four types of beef (total beef, ground beef, fresh lean beef, processed beef) were analyzed (Table 1) and calculated separately [3]. A similar approach to reconcile meat sources in multiple meat-ingredient foods was used by O'Connor and colleagues [14]. For beef-related variables determined to be entirely beef, the percentage of beef was assumed to be 100%. For foods/ingredients that contain beef where a second type of meat was indicated by the description, e.g., "bologna, beef and pork", then the percentage used for beef was 50%. Similarly, for foods/ingredients containing beef, where the description suggests that at least two other types of meat were included the percentage contribution by beef was assumed to be 33%. Beef types are not mutually exclusive, so the types will not equal the total, e.g., fresh lean beef includes a portion that is ground, but not all ground beef is lean, and some consumers only consume certain beef types. Furthermore, lean beef is calculated using a USDA-established threshold of 2.63 g solid fat or less per ounce equivalent to qualify as lean beef, with solid fat in excess of 2.63 g allocated to the solid fat component of FPED (Table 1) [3]. Consequently, subject numbers for the total beef category will reflect consumers of both lean and higher fat beef.

Table 1. Beef-related Food Patterns Ingredient Database (FPID) Variables.

Beef Variable	Related FPID Variables	Calculation
Total Beef	pf_meat [1]; pf_cured meat [2]	Descriptions examined to determine the percentage of each variable assumed to be beef. Percentage of beef applied. Total includes solid fat in beef in excess of 2.63 g per ounce (9.28%) [i.e., discretionary fat] and lean beef portion.
Processed Beef	pf_cured meat	Cured meat includes frankfurters, sausages, corned beef, and luncheon meat. Descriptions examined to determine the percentage of each variable assumed to be beef. Percentage of beef applied. Total includes solid fat in beef in excess of 2.63 g per ounce (9.28%) [i.e., discretionary fat] and lean beef portion.
Fresh lean beef	pf_meat	Solid fat in excess of 2.63 g per ounce (9.28%) is subtracted, fresh lean portion remains
Ground beef	pf_meat; the descriptions of ingredients in FPID helped delineate ground beef products (i.e., ground beef or similar term used in food ingredient description)	Total includes solid fat in beef in excess of 2.63 g per ounce (9.28%) [i.e., discretionary fat] and lean beef portion.

[1] pf_meat—FPID variable name "protein food–meat" includes beef, pork, veal, lamb, and game meat, excludes cured and organ meat. [2] pf_curedmeat—FPID variable name "protein-food-cured meat" includes frankfurters, sausages, corned beef, and luncheon meat made from beef, pork, or poultry.

2.5. Comparison of Usual Intake of Beef to "Meats, Poultry, Eggs" Modeled in HDP

In an effort to assess beef intake against dietary advice, data in the current study were compared to the MPE subgroup modeled in the HDP as reported in the DGA [7]. The DGA notes that "Meats include beef, goat, lamb, pork, and game meat (e.g., bison, moose, elk, deer)" and that meats and poultry should be lean or low-fat [7]. Food groups used in the HDP modeling are composed of the most nutrient-dense forms of foods (i.e., prepared with the lowest amounts of sodium, saturated fat and added sugars) [15]. Thus, it is understood that meats in the HDP model represent lean red meat. Supplementary Figure S1 describes the steps used to derive the daily amounts of MPE, collectively, and the amount of lean red meat, individually, as modeled in the HDP and used as comparison points in the current analysis. USDA utilizes food group and subgroup item clusters to complete dietary pattern modeling [15]. Item clusters are groupings of similar foods, in nutrient-dense form, used to calculate the nutrient profile of a food group or subgroup [15]. Proportional intakes of an item cluster based on a composite population-weighted average intake of the general U.S. population and/or varying life stage populations are the benchmarks for USDA dietary pattern models [15,16]. Using this approach, 3.7 ounce equivalents are modeled for the MPE of the HPD at the 2000-calorie level (Supplementary Figure S1). To determine the amount of lean red meat modeled in the 3.7 ounce equivalents of MPE of the HDP, the USDA protein food item cluster was disaggregated on a percent contribution basis into the individual representative foods (Supplementary Figure S1). The amount of lean meat in the protein food item cluster was then totaled and used as the denominator for red meat in the red meat food subgroup, resulting in 1.8 ounce equivalents of lean red meat per day or 12.5 ounce equivalents per week. For the purposes of comparison to the HDP, it is noted that ounce equivalents and ounces are synonymous for lean meat [7]. Further, as noted in Table 1, fresh lean beef data excludes fat contribution in excess of that considered lean (9.28 g fat per 100 g) and is therefore synonymous with lean meat ounce equivalents, as modeled in the HDP. Total beef data will include solid fat in excess of 9.28%.

In the current analysis, we compared both per capita and consumer-only usual intake levels of beef, to that allocated in the modeled amount of MPE in the 2000-calorie level of the HDP, as a way to establish a reference point. Modeling of the HDP involves establishing food groups and food group amounts, in part, based on consumption-weighted nutrient dense food averages over time [15]. Thus, on any given day, consumers might choose only one (e.g., beef) or a few food sources of protein in the MPE group, but over time consumers might end up consuming all the MPE components (such as after a week or so). This also allows allocation of an entire day's MPE modeled allowance to beef, as practically speaking, not everyone includes all components of the MPE subgroup in their daily diet. Additionally, the HDP does not distinguish beef from pork and other red meat, and at the 2000-calorie level of the HDP, 1.8 of the 3.7 oz of MPE is allocated to lean red meat (i.e., both fresh and processed).

2.6. Statistical Analysis

Analyses were performed using SAS 9.4 and data adjusted for the complex sampling (clustered sample) design of NHANES, using appropriate survey weights, strata, and primary sampling units. Least-square means and the standard errors were calculated using regression analyses adjusted for key covariates (age, gender and ethnicity). A *p*-value of <0.05 was deemed significant. To assess intake over time, NHANES cycles were numbered 1–9 for 2001–2002 through 2017–2018, respectively; the regression coefficient generated by these analyses generates a change per NHANES cycle (e.g., every two years). Distribution of usual intakes of beef was also determined using the NCI programs [17,18] on a per capita basis and on a consumer-only basis. Using the distribution of usual intake, we assessed the percentage of the population exceeding certain levels of beef intake. Additionally, we assessed the source-of-food variable to ascertain where subjects were getting ground beef.

3. Results

3.1. Trends in Intake of Beef by Age Group, NHANES 2001–2018

Children and adolescents between 2 and 18 years of age consumed significantly less total beef in 2018 as compared to 2001 ($\beta = -1.66$ g/cycle, $p < 0.0001$), averaging 12 g (0.4 oz) less per day from 2001–2002 (41.9 ± 1.5 g/day (1.5 ± 0.05 oz/day)) compared to 2017–2018 (30.0 ± 2.5 g/day (1.1 ± 0.1 oz/day), Figure 1). Declines in the consumption of each beef type (i.e., fresh lean, processed, ground) contributes to the observed decrease in total beef consumption ($\beta = -1.22$ g/cycle, $p < 0.0001$; $\beta = -0.80$ g/cycle, $p < 0.0001$; $\beta = -0.33$ g/cycle, $p = 0.0005$, respectively).

Compared to 2001, total beef intake in adults aged 19–59 years was an average of 5.7 g (0.2 oz) less per day in 2018 ($\beta = -1.14$ g/cycle, $p = 0.0004$). Of beef types, intakes of fresh lean and processed beef contributed to the significant decline ($\beta = -0.68$ g/cycle, $p = 0.0206$ and $\beta = -0.39$ g/cycle, $p < 0.0001$, respectively) in total beef intake among adults while ground beef intake remained relatively consistent ($\beta = -0.38$ g/cycle, $p = 0.08$).

Older adults aged 60 years and older, on average, maintained their intake of beef over the nine NHANES cycles ($\beta = -0.05$ g/cycle, $p = 0.8866$). Currently, adults aged 60+ years are reported to consume 41.8 ± 3.5 g/day (1.47 ± 0.1 oz/day) of beef compared to 38.3 ± 0.9 g/day (1.35 ± 0.03 oz/day) reported in 2001–2002. Intake of all beef types remained consistent over time.

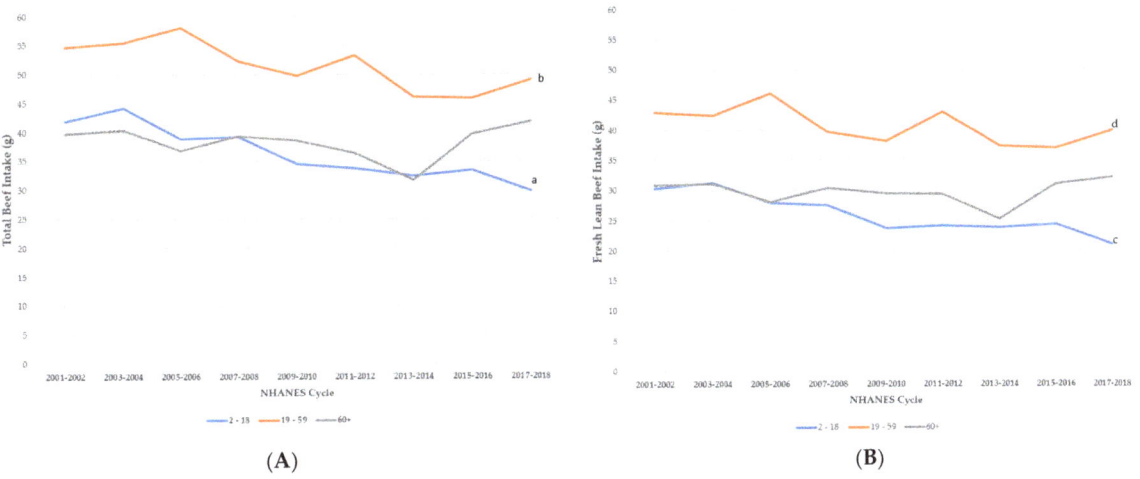

Figure 1. *Cont.*

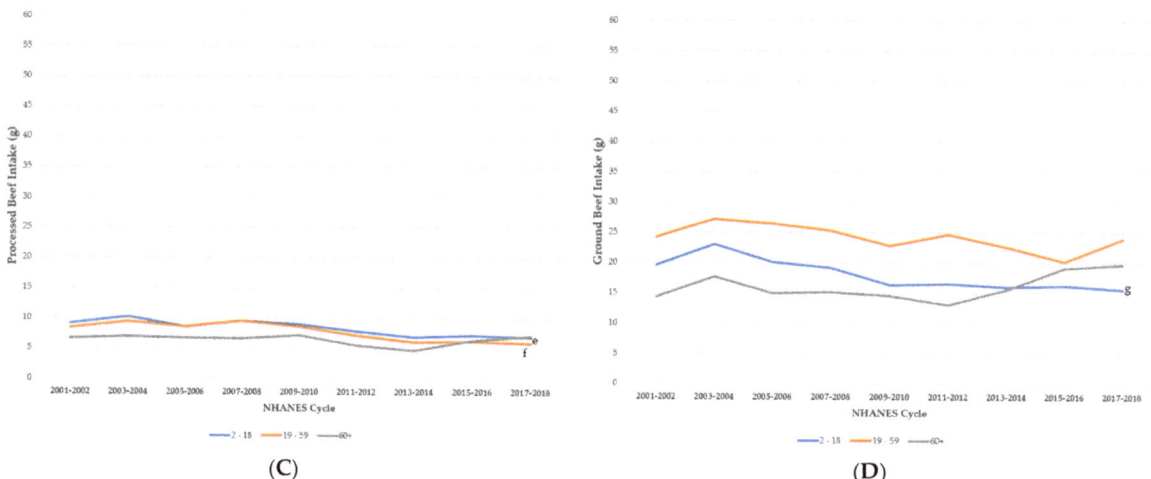

Figure 1. Changes over time in intake of (**A**) total beef; (**B**) fresh lean beef; (**C**) processed beef; and (**D**) ground beef in the United States, by age group. Regression analyses for beef intake over time with age, gender and race/ethnicity as covariates and NHANES survey cycle (2001–2018) as trend variable. Regression coefficient examines amount of change in g/day per cycle; *p*-value assesses whether regression coefficient is different from zero. [a–g] notes significant changes in intake between 2001–2022 and 2017–2018 cycle: [a] β = −1.66 *p* < 0.0001; [b] β = −1.14 *p* = 0.0004; [c] β = −1.22 *p* < 0.0001; [d] β = −0.68 *p* = 0.0206; [e] β = −0.33 *p* = 0.0005; [f] β = −0.39 *p* < 0.0001; [g] β = −0.80 *p* < 0.0001.

3.2. Per Capita Usual Intake of Beef, NHANES 2011–2018

On average, Americans 2 years and older (*n* = 30,679) consumed 42.2 ± 0.9 g (1.5 ± 0.03 oz) of total beef each day. Fresh lean beef intake was reported as 33.4 ± 0.8 g (1.2 ± 0.03 oz) per day (Supplementary Table S1).

Children and adolescents between 2 and 18 years of age (*n* = 10,913) consumed, on average, 31.9 ± 0.9 g (1.1 ± 0.03 oz) of total beef per day. This age group consumed 22.9 ± 0.8 g (0.8 ± 0.03 oz) of fresh lean beef per day (Figure 2, Supplementary Table S1). More specifically, mean usual intake of total beef of males aged 2–18 y was 36.6 ± 1.3 g (1.3 ± 0.04 oz) and of females aged 2–18 y was 27.0 ± 1.0 g (1.0 ± 0.03 oz) per day. Fresh lean beef consumption by these age and gender groups was 26.2 ± 1.1 g (0.9 ± 0.04 oz) and 19.5 ± 0.8 g (0.7 ± 0.03 oz) per day, respectively.

Adults aged 19–59 years (*n* = 13,203) consumed, on average, 47.1 ± 1.1 g (1.7 ± 0.04 oz) of total beef per day. Adults in this age group consumed 38.2 ± 1.0 g (1.4 ± 0.04 oz) of fresh lean beef per day (Figure 2, Supplementary Table S1). More specifically, mean usual intake of total beef of males aged 19–59 years was 60.8 ± 1.7 g (2.1 ± 0.1 oz) and of females aged 19–59 years was 33.1 ± 1.1 g (1.2 ± 0.04 oz) per day. Fresh lean beef consumption by these age and gender groups was 49.0 ± 1.5 g (1.7 ± 0.1 oz) and 27.1 ± 1.0 g (1.0 ± 0.03 oz) per day, respectively.

Older adults aged 60+ years (*n* = 6563) consumed, on average, 40.7 ± 1.2 g (1.4 ± 0.04 oz) of total beef per day. Fresh lean beef consumption by older adults was 32.0 ± 1.2 g (1.1 ± 0.04 oz, Figure 2, Supplementary Table S1). More specifically, mean usual intake of total beef of males aged 60+ years was 51.5 ± 2.1 g (1.8 ± 0.1 oz) per day and of females aged 60+ years it was 31.6 ± 1.3 g (1.1 ± 0.04 oz) per day. Fresh lean beef consumption by males and females 60+ years was reported to be 40.3 ± 2.1 g (1.4 ± 0.1 oz) and 25.1 ± 1.2 g (0.9 ± 0.04 oz) per day, respectively.

Of the beef types reported, processed beef was the least consumed, with mean usual intakes of 7.5 ± 0.4 g (0.3 ± 0.01 oz) per day by 2–18 years, 6.4 ± 0.3 g (0.2 ± 0.01 oz) per day by 19–59 years, and 6.6 ± 0.5 g (0.2 ± 0.02 oz) per day by 60+ years groups (Figure 2, Supplementary Table S1). Between 2001 and 2018, processed beef intake significantly decreased in the total population, specifically in the 2–18 years and 19–59 years age groups, while remaining constant in the 60+ years age group (Figure 1). Mean usual intakes of ground beef were 16.0 ± 0.6 g (0.6 ± 0.02 oz) per day by 2–18 years, 22.7 ± 0.8 g (0.8 ± 0.03 oz) per day by 19–59 years, and 17.1 ± 0.7 g (0.6 ± 0.03 oz) per day by 60+ years groups (Figure 2, Supplementary Table S1). On average, ground beef consumed per capita was from sources other than fast food (Supplementary Table S2).

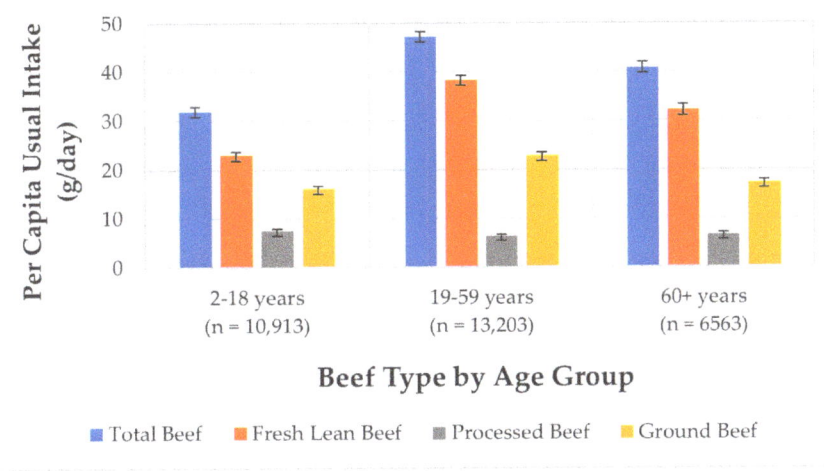

Figure 2. Per capita usual intake of total beef and beef types based on NHANES 2011–2018. Note: Beef types are not mutually exclusive, so the types will not equal the total, (e.g., fresh lean beef includes a portion that is ground, but not all ground beef is lean, and some consumers only consume certain beef types).

3.3. Comparison of Per Capita Usual Intake of Beef to HDP Modeling

Intake distribution of per capita usual intake of total beef and fresh lean beef from NHANES 2011–2018 is reported in Figure 3. All age groups are eating within the 3.7 ounce MPE based on the 2000-calorie level, as modeled in the HDP (Figure 3). On a per capita basis, 82% of the 2–18 years, 62% of the 19–59 years, and 77% of the 60+ years age groups reported intakes of total beef at or below the 1.8 oz of red meat level, as modeled in the HDP at the 2000-calorie level. Additionally, 95% of the 2–18 years, 78% of the 19–59 years, and 92% of the 60+ years age groups are consuming fresh lean beef at levels at or below the 1.8 oz of lean red meat modeled in the HDP at the 2000-calorie level.

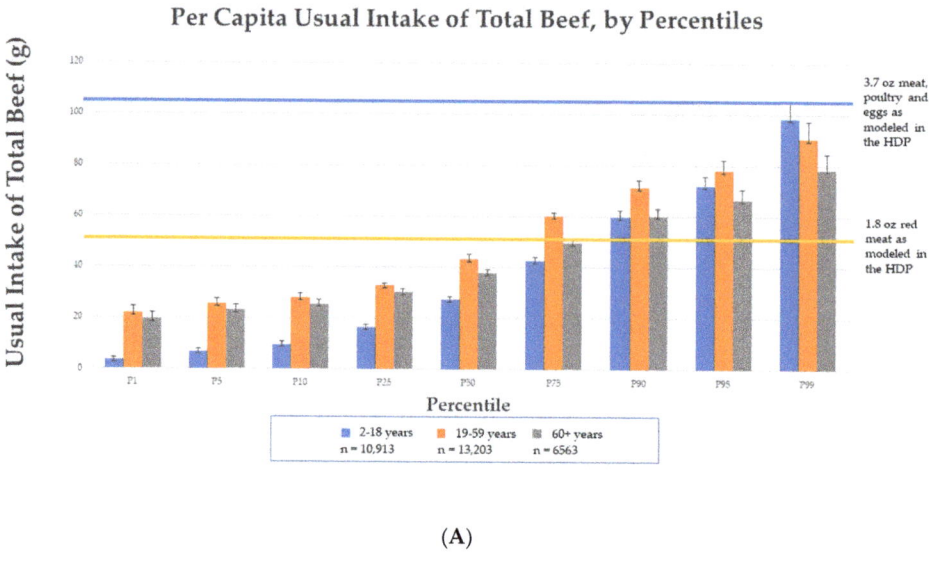

(A)

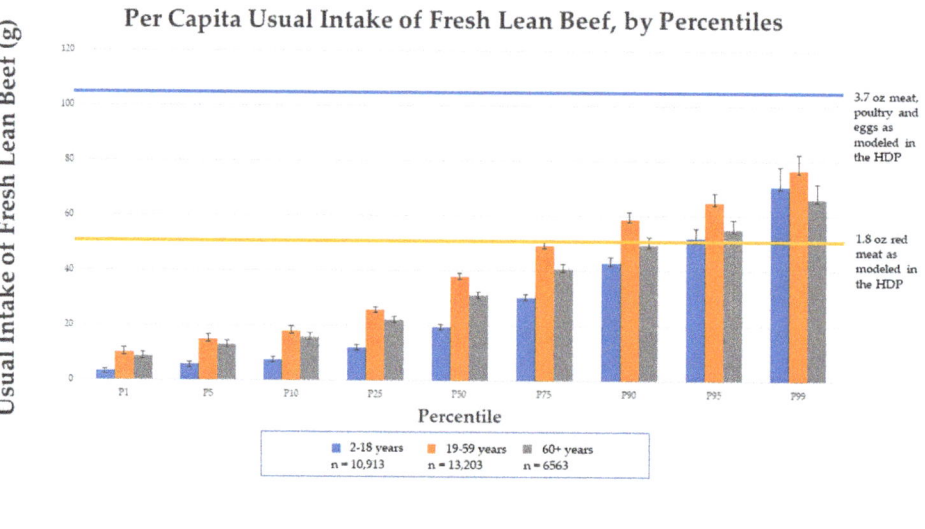

(B)

Figure 3. Percentiles of per capita usual intake of (**A**) total beef and (**B**) fresh lean beef based on NHANES 2011–2018 data by age group and compared to food groups modeled in the Healthy U.S.-Style Dietary Pattern (HDP) at the 2000-calorie level including red meat (i.e., fresh or processed beef, goat, lamb, pork, and game meat).

3.4. Beef Consumer Usual Intake of Beef, NHANES 2011–2018

On the day of recall, approximately half (50.4%) of respondents consumed beef and will be referred to as "beef consumers". Similarly, approximately half of the 2–18 years and 19–59 years subpopulations are beef consumers (52.3% and 51.2%, respectively), while a slightly smaller proportion of the 60+ years subpopulation are beef consumers (45.3%). Data below indicate a higher number of total beef consumers than individual beef types (e.g., not all beef consumers consume all beef types, but all beef consumers consume beef) and because, as noted in the methodology section, total beef intake values are reflective of only the lean portion of beef plus 2.63 g of solid fat per ounce equivalent; therefore, the amounts of total beef and lean beef will be similar. In other words, while the sample sizes reflect the number of consumers of total beef and each beef type, the amount of solid fat in excess of 2.63 g per ounce equivalent found in higher fat beef cuts is allocated to the solid fat component of FPED. The usual intake of beef in beef consumers aged 2 years and older (n = 15,449), was 83.2 ± 0.9 g (2.9 ± 0.03 oz) of total beef each day (Supplementary Table S1). Usual intake of fresh lean beef of beef consumers (n = 11,876) 2 years and older was 83.4 ± 1.0 g (2.9 ± 0.04 oz) per day.

For beef consumers in the 2–18 years age group, the usual intake of total beef was 62.0 ± 1.7 g (2.2 ± 0.1 oz) per day; and the usual intake of fresh lean beef was 64.2 ± 1.8 g (2.3 ± 0.1 oz, Figure 4, Supplementary Table S1) per day. More specifically, usual intake of total beef of males aged 2–18 years was 68.4 ± 2.3 g (2.4 ± 0.1 oz) per day and of females aged 2–18 years it was 54.5 ± 1.6 g (1.9 ± 0.1 oz) per day. Usual intake of fresh lean beef by these age and gender groups was 71.2 ± 2.8 g (2.5 ± 0.1 oz) and 55.9 ± 1.9 g (2.0 ± 0.1 oz) per day, respectively.

For adult beef consumers aged 19–59 years, the usual intake of total beef was 91.8 ± 1.2 g (3.2 ± 0.04 oz) per day. Fresh lean beef consumption by adults under 60 years was reported to be 91.2 ± 1.4 g (3.2 ± 0.1 oz, Figure 4, Supplementary Table S1) per day. More specifically, mean usual intake of total beef of adult males was 109.0 ± 1.9 g (2.4 ± 0.1 oz) per day and of adult females it was 70.2 ± 1.5 g (2.5 ± 0.1 oz) per day. Usual intakes of fresh lean beef by these age and gender groups was 107.4 ± 2.0 g (3.8 ± 0.1 oz) and 70.6 ± 1.5 g (2.5 ± 0.1 oz) per day, respectively.

For older adult beef consumers, aged 60+ years, the usual intake of total beef was 84.1 ± 1.6 g (3.0 ± 0.1 oz) per day. Usual intake of fresh lean beef intake by older adults was 80.9 ± 1.9 g (2.9 ± 0.1 oz, Figure 4, Supplementary Table S1) per day. More specifically, usual intake of total beef of older adult males was 98.3 ± 3.1 g (3.5 ± 0.1 oz) per day and of older adult females was 70.4 ± 1.9 g (2.5 ± 0.1 oz) per day. Usual fresh lean beef intake by these age and gender groups was 95.2 ± 3.2 g (3.4 ± 0.1 oz) per day and 67.3 ± 2.1 g (2.4 ± 0.1 oz) per day, respectively.

Of the beef types reported in beef consumers, processed beef was the least consumed, with mean usual intakes of 30.8 ± 1.4 g (1.1 ± 0.1 oz) per day in 2–18 years, 38.8 ± 1.6 g (1.4 ± 0.1 oz) per day in 19–59 years, and 48.1 ± 2.9 g (1.7 ± 0.1 oz) per day in 60+ years groups (Figure 4, Supplementary Table S1). Ground beef consumers make up approximately a quarter of each age group subpopulation, with mean usual intakes of 57.3 ± 1.5 g (2.0 ± 0.1 oz) per day in 2–18 years, 76.6 ± 2.4 g (2.7 ± 0.1 oz) per day in 19–59 years, and 71.5 ± 3.0 g (2.5 ± 0.1 oz) per day in 60+ years groups (Figure 4, Supplementary Table S1). Among ground beef consumers, 28–39% report consuming ground beef from fast food sources, with mean intakes of 60.5 ± 2.5 g (2.1 ± 0.1 oz) per day in 2–18 years, 74.4 ± 2.0 g (2.6 ± 0.1 oz) per day in 19–59 years, and 65.6 ± 4.2 g (2.3 ± 0.2 oz) per day in 60+ years groups (Supplementary Table S2).

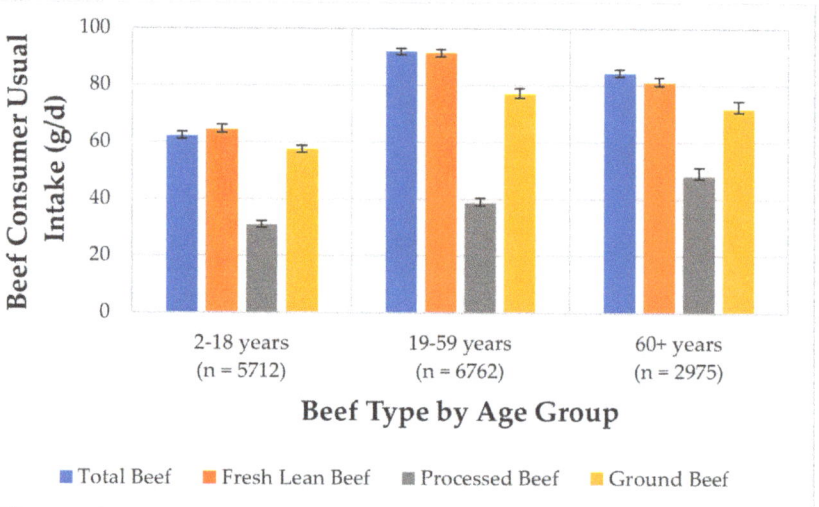

Figure 4. Beef consumer usual intake of beef types, by age group, based on NHANES 2011–2018. Note: Beef types are not mutually exclusive, so the types will not equal the total, (e.g., fresh lean beef includes a portion that is ground, but not all ground beef is lean, and some consumers only consume certain beef types).

3.5. Comparison of Beef Consumer Usual Intakes to HDP Modeling

The distribution of beef consumers' usual intakes of total beef and fresh lean beef are reported in Figure 5, separated by age group (2–18 years, 19–59 years, and 60+ years). If a beef consumer (age 2 years and older) chooses to consume their entire MPE amount in the HDP at the 2000-calorie level, as beef, the mean usual intakes of total beef and fresh lean beef are within the collectively modeled level of 3.7 oz. Most beef consumers included at least 1.8 oz of total beef per day with 38% of the 2–18 years, 5% of the 19–59 years, and 6% of the 60+ years groups reporting intakes at or below the 1.8 oz of red meat level, as modeled in the HDP at the 2000-calorie level. On average, daily intake levels of beef consumers are within the MPE amount, with 7% of the 2–18 years, 31% of the 19–59 years, and 19% of the 60+ years groups reporting intakes at or above the 3.7 oz MPE, as modeled in HDP at the 2000-calorie level. Less than 2% of adults (19–59 years) consume total beef above the 5.5 ounce equivalents for the protein foods group (which includes MPE, seafood, nuts, seeds, and soy products), as modeled in the HDP.

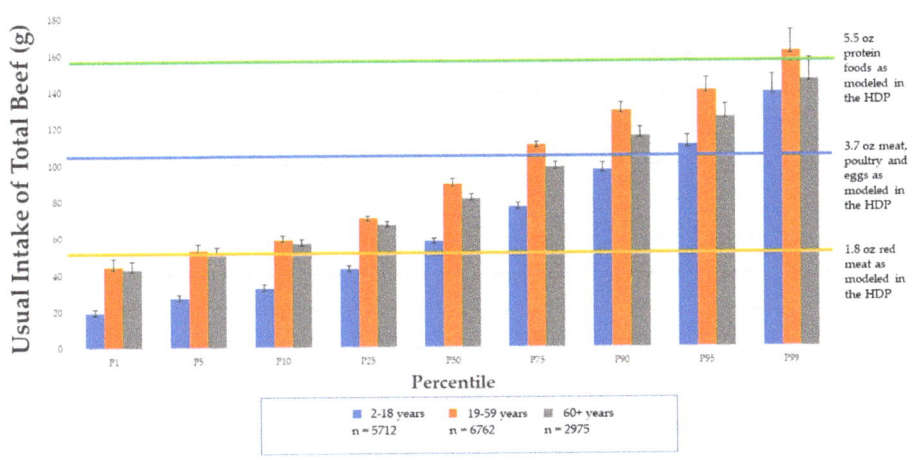

(A)

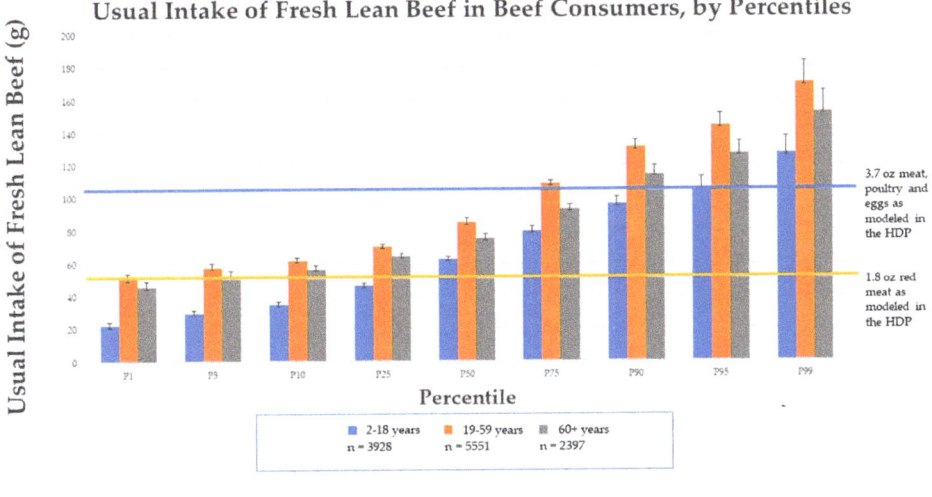

(B)

Figure 5. Percentiles of beef consumer usual intake of (**A**) total beef and (**B**) fresh lean beef based on NHANES 2011–2018 data by age group and compared to food groups modeled in the Healthy U.S.-Style Dietary Pattern (HDP) at the 2000-calorie level including red meat (i.e., fresh or processed beef, goat, lamb, pork, and game meat) and protein foods (i.e., meat, poultry, eggs, seafood, nuts, seeds, and soy products).

4. Discussion

Americans' consumption of beef has significantly declined over the most recent nine cycles (18-year timeframe) of NHANES data. Our findings of declining trends of beef consumption are consistent with Kim et al. [19] and Zeng et al. [10], who reported significant declines in Americans' consumption of total beef in adolescents (age 12–19 years) and of unprocessed beef in adults (20 years and older) based on older NHANES survey data.

The current data analyses indicate that, on average, the majority of Americans consume beef within the amounts for MPE and red meat modeled in the HDP at the 2000-calorie level. Approximately 75% of beef consumers are reported to consume total beef within the modeled amount for MPE in the HDP at the 2000-calorie level, challenging the perception that red meat is "over-consumed" [20–22]. More specifically, beef consumers favor fresh lean beef, typically consuming above the modeled amount of 1.8 oz of red meat but below the modeled amount of 3.7 oz for MPE, in their dietary patterns.

Commonly reported associations between consumption of red and processed meat with increased risk of chronic diseases such as cardiovascular/cardiometabolic disease have raised concerns that beef may be over-consumed [23,24]. However, in recent systematic reviews, authors conclude that red and processed meat consumption is likely not causally related to the development of cardiovascular disease [25] as the magnitude of association is very small and the evidence is of low certainty [26]. Similarly, in another study, researchers noted that the evidence that the association between unprocessed red meat intake with increased risk of disease incidence and mortality was weak and insufficient to make strong or conclusive dietary recommendations [27].

Concerns regarding "over-consumption" of beef may also relate to broader concerns regarding consumption of protein in excess of the minimum level established by the Recommended Dietary Allowance (RDA) [28,29]; however, the consumption of total protein, as a percentage of total energy intake, ranges from 14% to 16% across all age groups, well within the Acceptable Macronutrient Distribution Ranges (AMDR) of 10–35% of total energy intake. Less than 1% of Americans consume protein above the AMDR [30]. The HDP is modeled with protein contributing 18% to the total calories, while the DGA "are designed to meet the RDA and Adequate Intakes for essential nutrients, as well as AMDR, all set by the National Academies," where protein can contribute up to 35% of total calories [7]. Thus, though the modeled amounts in the HDP serve as comparison points for this current analysis, there is flexibility for the individual to consume varying amounts of carbohydrate, protein, and fat, within a healthy eating pattern. Adolescent females (age 14–18 years) were among the most common found to have protein levels below the Estimated Average Requirement (EAR), and adult females aged 19+ years are more likely to fall below the EAR and the RDA for protein compared to adult males of the same age range [30].

The DGA encourages individuals to have the flexibility to choose a healthy dietary pattern within calorie limits that fits their personal preferences and cultural traditions [7]. With the HPD modeled at 18% of calories as protein, there is flexibility to include a higher proportion of total calories as protein (including higher protein as beef), while still within the AMDR, which previous research has demonstrated can support improved health benefits including but not limited to weight management, physical function, and heart health [31–34]. In a recent analysis, researchers demonstrated the feasibility of modifying the amount of protein within the HDP by up to 25% of total calories while meeting all nutrient needs, using the framework implemented by the USDA in developing the HDP [16]. This supports the notion that individuals can have the flexibility to enjoy a variety of protein foods, including beef, and including intake of amounts greater than those modeled in the HDP.

Beef is a commonly consumed whole-food source of high-quality protein that supports healthy aging [35,36]. In the present study, beef consumption of older adults aged 60+ did not decrease over the past 18 years. However, the reported usual intake in older adults is lower than that in the adult group, which suggests beef intake decreases as a person ages, which may lead to a decrease in their intake of high-quality protein and other essential nutrients [30,37]. There is consensus between international expert groups that as people age, there should be an increase in protein intake, as physiological needs change with aging [38,39]. For example, previous research by An and colleagues [40] report that a one ounce equivalent increase in fresh lean beef by older Americans 65+ years was associated with a reduction in the odds of lower extremity mobility limitation by 22% (95% CI: 7%–34%) and any functional limitation by 15% (95% CI: 1%–28%). Similarly, research has suggested that protein and amino acids are positively associated with improved quality of life and well-being [41], and meat (defined by the authors as beef and veal, buffalo meat, pig meat, mutton and lamb, goat meat, horse meat, chicken meat, goose meat, duck meat, turkey meat, rabbit meat, game meat and offal) intake is positively correlated with increased life expectancy [42].

Although approximately 25% of beef consumers exceed the modeled level in the HDP, the excess is less than 2 ounces and does not result in protein consumption that exceeds the AMDR [30]. Based on the available modeled nutrient profiles, an additional 2 ounce equivalent of lean meat would provide an individual aged 19–70 years with an estimated additional 3 g of total fat, 1 g of saturated fat, and 40 mg of cholesterol, as well as 14 g of protein, 1 mg of iron, 2.3 mg of zinc, 52 mg of choline, 0.2 mg vitamin B6, and 1 mcg vitamin B12, if no other adjustments are made to the diet [15].

An et al. [43] previously reported no association between total beef consumption and overall dietary quality measured by the Healthy Eating Index (HEI) 2015 and no association between fresh lean beef consumption and daily intake of saturated fat. Further, fresh, lean beef consumption (2.0 ounce/day) was not associated with daily intake of total energy or sodium but was associated with increased choline, iron, and zinc intake when compared to non-beef consumers [43]. Nicklas et al. [44] reported that lean beef consumers consumed 4.4 ounces of lean beef daily yet consumed more servings of vegetables and fewer servings of milk, oils, grains and fruits than non-beef consumers with no significant difference in diet quality as measured by HEI. Compared to non-beef consumers, lean beef consumers were reported to consume the same amount of total fat with only 0.6% more saturated fat, 0.3% more monounsaturated fat, and 0.8% less polyunsaturated [44]. Therefore, based on these data, it is not expected that consumption of up to 2 ounces more than that modeled in the HDP would be of significant consequence for macronutrient intake and could benefit intake of micronutrients of dietary concern and/or challenge.

Of the individual beef types analyzed, processed beef was consumed the least. Recently, O'Connor and colleagues [45] reported similar findings in their assessment of intake patterns of fresh vs. processed red meat, noting that most of the total red meat consumed by Americans 2+ years was fresh (i.e., unprocessed). The majority of processed red meat consumed by Americans are pork-based with luncheon meat, sausage, ham, bacon, and hot dog representing the top five processed meats consumed [10]. The current data indicate that, on average, the majority of Americans 2+ years consume less than 0.25 ounces of processed beef per day.

Approximately 27% of individuals consumed ground beef on the day of recall. Ground beef is commonly consumed as burgers, as well as an ingredient in mixed dishes such as meatloaf, tacos, burritos, etc. which provide other important nutrients and is an affordable, versatile option for protein, but depending on the recipe, can also lead to increased sodium consumption due to other ingredients [7]. Our analysis concurs with a previous analysis of ground beef consumption patterns in Americans (using data from FoodNet Population Survey, 2006–2007) that noted that ground beef consumption decreases between adults (18–64 years of age) and older adults ($\geq$ 65 years of age) [46]. Additionally, Taylor and colleagues similarly report that less than 40% of ground beef was consumed from fast food establishments [46].

A strength of the current study is the use of a large nationally representative population-based sample of children and adults to assess per capita and consumer-specific usual intakes of beef, using nine cycles (18-years) of NHANES data. Additionally, total beef as well as four individual beef types were separately analyzed to address common types of beef included in habitual diets to provide a fuller picture of beef consumption behaviors of Americans.

While dietary intake data such as NHANES provide direct estimates of intake, there are limitations. For example, NHANES results can be hampered by self-reporting bias [47], though it is expected that a large sample such as NHANES should provide a valid estimate of meat consumption with even a single 24-h recall [10]. On the other hand, national survey data and methods used to estimate meat consumption in the U.S. are varied and designed to meet particular data needs that may or may not meaningfully reflect actual beef intake [10,47–49].

Future NHANES-related research may consider the analysis of the contribution of beef and beef types to nutrient adequacy and/or diet quality of beef consumers and focus on specific vulnerable subpopulations and contribution to nutrient security. This study highlights the importance of the need for more accurate estimations of beef (and beef types) intake, which can increase rigor of future research to quantify the relationship between consumption of beef within broader dietary patterns and various health-related outcomes.

5. Conclusions

Beef is a nutrient-dense commonly consumed food that can contribute a variety of key essential nutrients that Americans may not otherwise consume in sufficient amounts from other foods [1,37]. Nearly every American has room to make improvements in their diet, and evidence-based dietary guidance is needed to support areas in need of improvements and that can benefit people the most. The current study analyzed consumption levels of total beef and beef types (fresh lean beef, ground beef, and processed beef) in Americans 2 years and older over an 18-year period (2001–2018) and found significant declines in beef consumption in children, adolescents, and adults, while consumption remained consistent in older adults. The average amount of total beef consumed increased from children and adolescents to adults but declined in older adults, which can impact aging-related health outcomes. Based on current beef intake data, beef consumers chose fresh lean beef in amounts typically within the MPE guideline, as modeled in the HDP at the 2000-calorie level. Given current beef intake trends, dietary guidance to limit or reduce beef intake could be viewed as lacking nutritional justification and could exacerbate the growing nutrient deficiencies in America. Beef is an inherent whole food source of high-quality dietary protein and several micronutrients including iron, zinc, and B vitamins; thus, a decline in beef intake can lead to unintended consequences of declining contribution of nutrients to the diet, including those identified as shortfall or essential nutrients [22,37,49]. Population-wide recommendations to increase or decrease the intake of any food group require evidence-based justification, given that all food groups provide critical nutrients that may not be readily available in meaningful amounts from other commonly available, popular, and/or affordable alternatives.

Supplementary Materials: The following supporting information can be downloaded at: https://www.mdpi.com/article/10.3390/nu15112475/s1, Figure S1: Determination of Red Meat Contribution to Healthy U.S. Style Eating Pattern (HDP) at the 2000-calorie level; Table S1: Per Capita and Beef Consumer Usual Intakes of Beef Based on NHANES 2001–2018; Table S2: Day 1 Mean Intake of Total Ground Beef and Ground Beef From Fast Food Sources By Americans, Gender Combined–NHANES 2011–2018.

Author Contributions: Conceptualization, C.S.L., M.E.V.E. and V.L.F.III; Methodology, V.L.F.III; Formal Analysis, V.L.F.III; Writing—Original Draft Preparation, C.S.L., V.L.F.III and M.E.V.E.; Writing—Review & Editing, C.S.L., M.E.V.E., V.L.F.III and S.H.M. All authors have approved the submitted version and agree to be personally accountable for their contributions and for ensuring that questions related to the accuracy or integrity of any part of the work, even ones in which the author was not personally involved, are appropriately investigated, resolved, and documented in the literature. All authors have read and agreed to the published version of the manuscript.

Funding: This manuscript is funded by the Beef Checkoff.

Institutional Review Board Statement: Not applicable.

Informed Consent Statement: Not applicable.

Data Availability Statement: NHANES data are publicly available from https://www.cdc.gov/nchs/nhanes/index.htm accessed on 22 June 2021.

Conflicts of Interest: C.L. and S.M. are currently employed by the National Cattlemen's Beef Association (NCBA), a contractor to the Beef Checkoff, as the Senior Director of Nutrition Research and Executive Director, Nutrition Science, Health & Wellness, respectively. M.V.E is an independent consultant and has been paid by NCBA, a contractor to the Beef Checkoff, for work related to this manuscript. V.L.F., as Senior Vice President of Nutrition Impact, LLC performs consulting and database analyses for various food and beverage companies and related entities. V.L.F. received an honorarium from NCBA, a contractor to the Beef Checkoff, for his contributions to this manuscript. Other than that identified in "Conflicts of Interest" above, the Beef Checkoff had no role in the design, execution, interpretation, or writing of the study.

References

1. Zanovec, M.; O'Neil, C.E.; Keast, D.R.; Fulgoni, V.L., 3rd; Nicklas, T.A. Lean beef contributes significant amounts of key nutrients to the diets of US adults: National Health and Nutrition Examination Survey 1999–2004. *Nutr. Res.* **2010**, *30*, 375–381. [CrossRef] [PubMed]
2. Drewnowski, A. The Nutrient Rich Foods Index helps to identify healthy, affordable foods. *Am. J. Clin. Nutr.* **2010**, *91*, 1095S–1101S. [CrossRef] [PubMed]
3. Bowman, S.A.; Clemens, J.C.; Friday, J.E.; Moshfegh, A.J. Food Patterns Equivalents Database 2017–2018: Methodology and User Guide. Available online: http://www.ars.usda.gov/nea/bhnrc/fsrg (accessed on 4 April 2023).
4. Gifford, C.L.; O'Connor, L.E.; Campbell, W.W.; Woerner, D.R.; Belk, K.E. Broad and Inconsistent Muscle Food Classification Is Problematic for Dietary Guidance in the U.S. *Nutrients* **2017**, *9*, 1027. [CrossRef] [PubMed]
5. O'Connor, L.E.; Gifford, C.L.; Woerner, D.R.; Sharp, J.L.; Belk, K.E.; Campbell, W.W. Dietary Meat Categories and Descriptions in Chronic Disease Research Are Substantively Different within and between Experimental and Observational Studies: A Systematic Review and Landscape Analysis. *Adv. Nutr.* **2020**, *11*, 41–51. [CrossRef] [PubMed]
6. Lichtenstein, A.H.; Appel, L.J.; Vadiveloo, M.; Hu, F.B.; Kris-Etherton, P.M.; Rebholz, C.M.; Sacks, F.M.; Thorndike, A.N.; Van Horn, L.; Wylie-Rosett, J. 2021 Dietary Guidance to Improve Cardiovascular Health: A Scientific Statement from the American Heart Association. *Circulation* **2021**, *144*, e472–e487. [CrossRef]
7. U.S. Department of Agriculture and U.S. Department of Health and Human Services. Dietary Guidelines for Americans, 2020–2025. Available online: https://www.dietaryguidelines.gov/sites/default/files/2021-03/Dietary_Guidelines_for_Americans-2020-2025.pdf (accessed on 4 April 2023).
8. O'Connor, L.E.; Campbell, W.W. Red Meat and Health: Getting to the Heart of the Matter. *Nutr. Today* **2017**, *52*, 167–173. [CrossRef]
9. Carroll, A.E.; Doherty, T.S. Meat Consumption and Health: Food for Thought. *Ann. Intern. Med.* **2019**, *171*, 767–768. [CrossRef]
10. Zeng, L.; Ruan, M.; Liu, J.; Wilde, P.; Naumova, E.N.; Mozaffarian, D.; Zhang, F.F. Trends in Processed Meat, Unprocessed Red Meat, Poultry, and Fish Consumption in the United States, 1999–2016. *J. Acad. Nutr. Diet.* **2019**, *119*, 1085–1098. [CrossRef]
11. Ahluwalia, N.; Dwyer, J.; Terry, A.; Moshfegh, A.; Johnson, C. Update on NHANES Dietary Data: Focus on Collection, Release, Analytical Considerations, and Uses to Inform Public Policy. *Adv. Nutr.* **2016**, *7*, 121–134. [CrossRef]
12. O'Neil, C.E.; Zanovec, M.; Keast, D.R.; Fulgoni, V.L., 3rd; Nicklas, T.A. Nutrient contribution of total and lean beef in diets of US children and adolescents: National Health and Nutrition Examination Survey 1999–2004. *Meat Sci.* **2011**, *87*, 250–256. [CrossRef]
13. Tooze, J.A.; Kipnis, V.; Buckman, D.W.; Carroll, R.J.; Freedman, L.S.; Guenther, P.M.; Krebs-Smith, S.M.; Subar, A.F.; Dodd, K.W. A mixed-effects model approach for estimating the distribution of usual intake of nutrients: The NCI method. *Stat. Med.* **2010**, *29*, 2857–2868. [CrossRef]
14. O'Connor, L.E.; Herrick, K.A.; Parsons, R.; Reedy, J. Heterogeneity in Meat Food Groups Can Meaningfully Alter Population-Level Intake Estimates of Red Meat and Poultry. *Front. Nutr.* **2021**, *8*, 778369. [CrossRef]
15. 2020 Dietary Guidelines Advisory Committee and Food Pattern Modeling Team. Food Pattern Modeling: Ages 2 Years and Older. Available online: https://www.dietaryguidelines.gov/sites/default/files/2020-07/FoodPatternModeling_Report_2YearsandOlder.pdf (accessed on 4 April 2023).
16. Murphy, M.M.; Barraj, L.M.; Higgins, K.A. Healthy U.S.-style dietary patterns can be modified to provide increased energy from protein. *Nutr. J.* **2022**, *21*, 39. [CrossRef]
17. Herrick, K.A.; Rossen, L.M.; Parsons, R.; Dodd, K.W. Estimating Usual Dietary in Take from National Health and Nutrition Examination Survey Data Using the National Cancer Institute Method. Available online: https://www.cdc.gov/nchs/data/series/sr_02/sr02_178.pdf (accessed on 4 April 2023).
18. Scientific Report of the 2020 Dietary Guidelines Advisory Committee: Advisory Report to the Secretary of Agriculture and the Secretary of Health and Human Services. Available online: https://www.dietaryguidelines.gov/2020-advisory-committee-report (accessed on 4 April 2023).
19. Kim, H.; Caulfield, L.E.; Rebholz, C.M.; Ramsing, R.; Nachman, K.E. Trends in types of protein in US adolescents and children: Results from the National Health and Nutrition Examination Survey 1999–2010. *PLoS ONE* **2020**, *15*, e0230686. [CrossRef]

20. Frank, S.M.; Jaacks, L.M.; Batis, C.; Vanderlee, L.; Taillie, L.S. Patterns of Red and Processed Meat Consumption across North America: A Nationally Representative Cross-Sectional Comparison of Dietary Recalls from Canada, Mexico, and the United States. *Int. J. Environ. Res. Public Health* **2021**, *18*, 357. [CrossRef]
21. Neff, R.A.; Edwards, D.; Palmer, A.; Ramsing, R.; Righter, A.; Wolfson, J. Reducing meat consumption in the USA: A nationally representative survey of attitudes and behaviours. *Public Health Nutr.* **2018**, *21*, 1835–1844. [CrossRef]
22. Klurfeld, D.M. The whole food beef matrix is more than the sum of its parts. *Crit. Rev. Food Sci. Nutr.* **2022**, 1–9. [CrossRef]
23. Al-Shaar, L.; Satija, A.; Wang, D.D.; Rimm, E.B.; Smith-Warner, S.A.; Stampfer, M.J.; Hu, F.B.; Willett, W.C. Red meat intake and risk of coronary heart disease among US men: Prospective cohort study. *BMJ* **2020**, *371*, m4141. [CrossRef]
24. Papier, K.; Fensom, G.K.; Knuppel, A.; Appleby, P.N.; Tong, T.Y.N.; Schmidt, J.A.; Travis, R.C.; Key, T.J.; Perez-Cornago, A. Meat consumption and risk of 25 common conditions: Outcome-wide analyses in 475,000 men and women in the UK Biobank study. *BMC Med.* **2021**, *19*, 53. [CrossRef]
25. Hill, E.R.; O'Connor, L.E.; Wang, Y.; Clark, C.M.; McGowan, B.S.; Forman, M.R.; Campbell, W.W. Red and processed meat intakes and cardiovascular disease and type 2 diabetes mellitus: An umbrella systematic review and assessment of causal relations using Bradford Hill's criteria. *Crit. Rev. Food Sci. Nutr.* **2022**, 1–18. [CrossRef]
26. Zeraatkar, D.; Han, M.A.; Guyatt, G.H.; Vernooij, R.W.M.; El Dib, R.; Cheung, K.; Milio, K.; Zworth, M.; Bartoszko, J.J.; Valli, C.; et al. Red and Processed Meat Consumption and Risk for All-Cause Mortality and Cardiometabolic Outcomes: A Systematic Review and Meta-analysis of Cohort Studies. *Ann. Intern. Med.* **2019**, *171*, 703–710. [CrossRef] [PubMed]
27. Lescinsky, H.; Afshin, A.; Ashbaugh, C.; Bisignano, C.; Brauer, M.; Ferrara, G.; Hay, S.I.; He, J.; Iannucci, V.; Marczak, L.B.; et al. Health effects associated with consumption of unprocessed red meat: A Burden of Proof study. *Nat. Med.* **2022**, *28*, 2075–2082. [CrossRef] [PubMed]
28. Frank, S.M.; Taillie, L.S.; Jaacks, L.M. How Americans eat red and processed meat: An analysis of the contribution of thirteen different food groups. *Public Health Nutr.* **2022**, *25*, 1406–1415. [CrossRef] [PubMed]
29. Harnack, L.; Mork, S.; Valluri, S.; Weber, C.; Schmitz, K.; Stevenson, J.; Pettit, J. Nutrient Composition of a Selection of Plant-Based Ground Beef Alternative Products Available in the United States. *J. Acad. Nutr. Diet.* **2021**, *121*, 2401–2408.e12. [CrossRef] [PubMed]
30. Berryman, C.E.; Lieberman, H.R.; Fulgoni, V.L., 3rd; Pasiakos, S.M. Protein intake trends and conformity with the Dietary Reference Intakes in the United States: Analysis of the National Health and Nutrition Examination Survey, 2001–2014. *Am. J. Clin. Nutr.* **2018**, *108*, 405–413. [CrossRef]
31. Wolfe, R.R.; Cifelli, A.M.; Kostas, G.; Kim, I.Y. Optimizing Protein Intake in Adults: Interpretation and Application of the Recommended Dietary Allowance Compared with the Acceptable Macronutrient Distribution Range. *Adv. Nutr.* **2017**, *8*, 266–275. [CrossRef]
32. Sayer, R.D.; Speaker, K.J.; Pan, Z.; Peters, J.C.; Wyatt, H.R.; Hill, J.O. Equivalent reductions in body weight during the Beef WISE Study: Beef's role in weight improvement, satisfaction and energy. *Obes. Sci. Pract.* **2017**, *3*, 298–310. [CrossRef]
33. Porter Starr, K.N.; Pieper, C.F.; Orenduff, M.C.; McDonald, S.R.; McClure, L.B.; Zhou, R.; Payne, M.E.; Bales, C.W. Improved Function With Enhanced Protein Intake per Meal: A Pilot Study of Weight Reduction in Frail, Obese Older Adults. *J. Gerontol. A Biol. Sci. Med. Sci.* **2016**, *71*, 1369–1375. [CrossRef]
34. Porter Starr, K.N.; Connelly, M.A.; Orenduff, M.C.; McDonald, S.R.; Sloane, R.; Huffman, K.M.; Kraus, W.E.; Bales, C.W. Impact on cardiometabolic risk of a weight loss intervention with higher protein from lean red meat: Combined results of 2 randomized controlled trials in obese middle-aged and older adults. *J. Clin. Lipidol.* **2019**, *13*, 920–931. [CrossRef]
35. Paddon-Jones, D.; Campbell, W.W.; Jacques, P.F.; Kritchevsky, S.B.; Moore, L.L.; Rodriguez, N.R.; van Loon, L.J. Protein and healthy aging. *Am. J. Clin. Nutr.* **2015**, *101*, 1339S–1345S. [CrossRef]
36. Phillips, S.M.; Fulgoni, V.L., 3rd; Heaney, R.P.; Nicklas, T.A.; Slavin, J.L.; Weaver, C.M. Commonly consumed protein foods contribute to nutrient intake, diet quality, and nutrient adequacy. *Am. J. Clin. Nutr.* **2015**, *101*, 1346S–1352S. [CrossRef] [PubMed]
37. Agarwal, S.; Fulgoni, V.L., 3rd. Contribution of beef to key nutrient intakes in American adults: An updated analysis with NHANES 2011–2018. *Nutr. Res.* **2022**, *105*, 105–112. [CrossRef] [PubMed]
38. Bauer, J.; Biolo, G.; Cederholm, T.; Cesari, M.; Cruz-Jentoft, A.J.; Morley, J.E.; Phillips, S.; Sieber, C.; Stehle, P.; Teta, D.; et al. Evidence-based recommendations for optimal dietary protein intake in older people: A position paper from the PROT-AGE Study Group. *J. Am. Med. Dir. Assoc.* **2013**, *14*, 542–559. [CrossRef] [PubMed]
39. Deutz, N.E.; Bauer, J.M.; Barazzoni, R.; Biolo, G.; Boirie, Y.; Bosy-Westphal, A.; Cederholm, T.; Cruz-Jentoft, A.; Krznaric, Z.; Nair, K.S.; et al. Protein intake and exercise for optimal muscle function with aging: Recommendations from the ESPEN Expert Group. *Clin. Nutr.* **2014**, *33*, 929–936. [CrossRef]
40. An, R.; Nickols-Richardson, S.M.; Alston, R.J.; Shen, S. Fresh and Fresh Lean Beef Intake in Relation to Functional Limitations among US Older Adults, 2005–2016. *Am. J. Health Behav.* **2019**, *43*, 729–738. [CrossRef]
41. Hawley, A.L.; Liang, X.; Børsheim, E.; Wolfe, R.R.; Salisbury, L.; Hendy, E.; Wu, H.; Walker, S.; Tacinelli, A.M.; Baum, J.I. The potential role of beef and nutrients found in beef on outcomes of wellbeing in healthy adults 50 years of age and older: A systematic review of randomized controlled trials. *Meat Sci.* **2022**, *189*, 108830. [CrossRef]
42. You, W.; Henneberg, R.; Saniotis, A.; Ge, Y.; Henneberg, M. Total Meat Intake is Associated with Life Expectancy: A Cross-Sectional Data Analysis of 175 Contemporary Populations. *Int. J. Gen. Med.* **2022**, *15*, 1833–1851. [CrossRef]

43. An, R.; Nickols-Richardson, S.; Alston, R.; Shen, S.; Clarke, C. Total, Fresh, Lean, and Fresh Lean Beef Consumption in Relation to Nutrient Intakes and Diet Quality among U.S. Adults, 2005–2016. *Nutrients* **2019**, *11*, 563. [CrossRef]
44. Nicklas, T.A.; O'Neil, C.E.; Zanovec, M.; Keast, D.R.; Fulgoni, V.L., 3rd. Contribution of beef consumption to nutrient intake, diet quality, and food patterns in the diets of the US population. *Meat Sci.* **2012**, *90*, 152–158. [CrossRef]
45. O'Connor, L.E.; Wambogo, E.A.; Herrick, K.A.; Parsons, R.; Reedy, J. A Standardized Assessment of Processed Red Meat and Processed Poultry Intake in the US Population Aged ≥2 Years Using NHANES. *J. Nutr.* **2022**, *152*, 190–199. [CrossRef]
46. Taylor, E.V.; Holt, K.G.; Mahon, B.E.; Ayers, T.; Norton, D.; Gould, L.H. Ground beef consumption patterns in the United States, FoodNet, 2006 through 2007. *J. Food Prot.* **2012**, *75*, 341–346. [CrossRef] [PubMed]
47. Fehrenbach, K.S.; Righter, A.C.; Santo, R.E. A critical examination of the available data sources for estimating meat and protein consumption in the USA. *Public Health Nutr.* **2016**, *19*, 1358–1367. [CrossRef] [PubMed]
48. Leroy, F.; Cofnas, N. Should dietary guidelines recommend low red meat intake? *Crit. Rev. Food Sci. Nutr.* **2020**, *60*, 2763–2772. [CrossRef] [PubMed]
49. Leme, A.C.; Baranowski, T.; Thompson, D.; Philippi, S.; O'Neil, C.E.; Fulgoni, V.L., 3rd; Nicklas, T.A. Food Sources of Shortfall Nutrients Among US Adolescents: National Health and Nutrition Examination Survey (NHANES) 2011–2014. *Fam. Community Health* **2020**, *43*, 59–73. [CrossRef] [PubMed]

Disclaimer/Publisher's Note: The statements, opinions and data contained in all publications are solely those of the individual author(s) and contributor(s) and not of MDPI and/or the editor(s). MDPI and/or the editor(s) disclaim responsibility for any injury to people or property resulting from any ideas, methods, instructions or products referred to in the content.

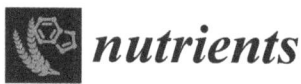 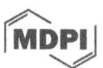

Article

Association of Pork (All Pork, Fresh Pork and Processed Pork) Consumption with Nutrient Intakes and Adequacy in US Children (Age 2–18 Years) and Adults (Age 19+ Years): NHANES 2011–2018 Analysis

Sanjiv Agarwal [1,*] and Victor L. Fulgoni III [2]

1. NutriScience LLC, East Norriton, PA 19403, USA
2. Nutrition Impact, LLC, Battle Creek, MI 49014, USA; vic3rd@aol.com
* Correspondence: agarwal47@yahoo.com; Tel.: +1-630-383-9359

Abstract: Pork is a rich source of high-quality protein and select nutrients. The objective of this work was to assess the intakes of all pork (AP), fresh pork (FP) and processed pork (PP) and their association with nutrient intake and meeting nutrient recommendations using 24 h dietary recall data. Usual intake was determined using the NCI method and the percentage of the population with intakes below the Estimated Average Requirement, or above the Adequate Intake for pork consumers and non-consumers, was estimated. About 52, 15 and 45% of children and 59, 20 and 49% of adults were consumers of AP, FP and PP, respectively, with mean intakes in consumers of 47, 60 and 38 g/day for children and 61, 77 and 48 g/day for adults, respectively. Among consumers of AP, FP and PP, the intakes of copper, potassium, selenium, sodium, zinc, thiamine, niacin, vitamin B_6 and choline were higher ($p < 0.05$) and a higher ($p < 0.05$) proportion met nutrient recommendations for copper, potassium, zinc, thiamin and choline compared to non-consumers. There were additional differences ($p < 0.05$) in intakes and adequacies for other nutrients between consumers and non-consumers depending upon the age group and pork type. In conclusion, pork intake was associated with higher intakes and adequacies in children and adults for certain key nutrients.

Keywords: pork; National Health and Nutrition Examination Survey; vitamins; minerals; usual intakes; nutrient adequacy

Citation: Agarwal, S.; Fulgoni, V.L., III. Association of Pork (All Pork, Fresh Pork and Processed Pork) Consumption with Nutrient Intakes and Adequacy in US Children (Age 2–18 Years) and Adults (Age 19+ Years): NHANES 2011–2018 Analysis. *Nutrients* **2023**, *15*, 2293. https://doi.org/10.3390/nu15102293

Academic Editor: Joanna Stadnik

Received: 27 April 2023
Revised: 10 May 2023
Accepted: 11 May 2023
Published: 13 May 2023

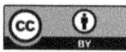

Copyright: © 2023 by the authors. Licensee MDPI, Basel, Switzerland. This article is an open access article distributed under the terms and conditions of the Creative Commons Attribution (CC BY) license (https://creativecommons.org/licenses/by/4.0/).

1. Introduction

Pork is one of the most widely consumed meats in the world, accounting for over one-third of meat production and intake globally, and it is a rich source of high-quality protein and select nutrients [1]. The average annual pork consumption in the US is about 51 pounds per person, which is about one-fourth of overall meat intake and ranks third in annual meat consumption [2]. A 100 g portion of pork (pork, not further specified; FDC ID: 2341267) provides substantial amounts of protein (27.1 g, 54.2% DV), iron (0.79 mg, 4.4% DV), zinc (2.44 mg, 22.2% DV), selenium (44.8 µg, 81.5% DV), magnesium (26 mg; 6.2% DV), phosphorus (245 mg; 19.6% DV), potassium (402 mg, 8.6% DV), thiamin (0.605 mg, 50.4% DV), riboflavin (0.234 mg; 18.0% DV), niacin (7.55 mg; 47.2% DV), choline (81.1 mg, 14.7% DV), and vitamins B_6 (0.615 mg; 36.2% DV) and B_{12} (0.65 µg; 27.1% DV) [3,4]. In cross-sectional analyses, pork consumption has been shown to contribute significantly (more than 10%) to intakes of several nutrients, including protein, phosphorus, potassium, selenium, thiamine, riboflavin, niacin, vitamin B_6, and vitamin B_{12} [5–7], and did not affect diet quality [6]. Limited recent evidence suggests that intake of pork may be associated with cognitive health [8] cardiovascular and metabolic health benefits [9–12] and reduced risk of functional limitations among older adults [13].

Inadequate micronutrient intakes and deficiencies have been identified as major public health problems affecting a large part of the world's population and are important contributors to the global burden of disease and increased risk of morbidity and mortality [14–18]. According to recent estimates, 1.5 to 2 billion people, or one-third of the population, suffer from at least one form of micronutrient deficiency [14–18]. Although continued public health recommendations, including the Dietary Guidelines for Americans, suggest consuming nutrient-dense foods as part of healthy eating pattern, many Americans do not adhere to these recommendations and have inadequate intakes of several essential nutrients [19,20]. Therefore, vitamins A, D, E, and C, and choline, calcium, magnesium, iron (for certain age/gender groups), potassium, and fiber have been identified as "underconsumed nutrients" [20] and of these, vitamin D, calcium, iron, potassium, and fiber have been designated as "nutrients of public health concern" because their low intakes may lead to adverse health outcomes and are potentially associated with increased risk of chronic disease [20]. We hypothesize that intake of pork as a rich source of protein and other nutrients would be associated with improved nutrient adequacy for certain nutrients. Therefore, the objective of the present research was to assess the relationship between intake of pork (including fresh pork as well as processed pork) and meeting nutrient recommendations in US children and adults using the National Health and Nutrition Examination Survey (NHANES) 2011–2018.

2. Materials and Methods

2.1. Database

Dietary intake data from WWEIA component of NHANES 2011–2018 were used in the present analysis. NHANES is an ongoing cross-sectional survey of a nationally representative non-institutionalized civilian population conducted by the National Center for Health Statistics of the Centers for Disease Control and Prevention to monitor food and nutrient intake and the health status of the US population. The data are currently continuously collected using a stratified multistage cluster sampling probability design and are released every 2 years. Participants are interviewed in their homes for demographic, socioeconomic, dietary (24 h dietary recall), and general health information, followed by a comprehensive health examination conducted in a mobile examination center. A detailed description of the subject recruitment, survey design, and data collection procedures is available online [21]. NHANES protocols are approved by the Ethics Review Board of National Center for Health Statistics, and the present study was a secondary data analysis which lacked personal identifiers. Therefore, it was exempt from additional approvals by Institutional Review Boards. All participants provided signed written informed consent. All data obtained from this study are publicly available at: http://www.cdc.gov/nchs/nhanes/, accessed on 12 December 2022.

2.2. Study Population

Data from children age 2–18 years (n = 10,913; population weighted N = 69,849,814) and adults age 19+ years (n = 19,766; population weighted N = 231,605,756) after excluding those with incomplete or unreliable dietary recall as judged by NHANES staff, those with missing day 1 or day 2 dietary data and those pregnant and/or lactating participating in NHANES cycles 2011–2012, 2013–2014, 2015–2016 and 2017–2018 were used.

2.3. Estimates of Dietary Intake

Dietary intake data were obtained from in-person 24 h dietary recall interviews that were administered using an automated, multiple-pass (AMPM) method [22]. Nutrient intakes were obtained from the total nutrient intake files for each NHANES cycle [23]; intakes from dietary supplements were not included. Two dietary recalls were collected for most subjects; the first day dietary recall was collected in person, while the second recall was collected via the telephone. The distributions of usual nutrient intakes were estimated using the National Cancer Institute (NCI) method [24] and the percentage of the population below the Estimated Average Requirement (EAR) or above the Adequate Intake (AI) was determined using the cut-point method, except for iron, for which the probability method was used [25].

2.4. Estimates of Pork Intakes

The Food and Nutrition Database for Dietary Studies (FNDDS) food codes were used to assess pork intakes by determining the amount of pork contained in NHANES survey foods [26]. When pork items were used as "ingredients" of the survey foods, the FNDDS food codes were identified, and recipe calculations were performed using the survey-specific USDA Food Patterns Equivalents database (FPED) which also includes the Food Patterns Equivalents Ingredient Database (FPID) [26]. The FPID descriptions were examined to determine the proportion of pork: 100% if entirely pork; 50% or 33% if the description indicated one or two other meat types, respectively, in addition to pork. For some FNDDS food codes that contained ingredients with missing FPID, the food code ingredient profile was modified either by using a food code from another NHANES cycle or by using another ingredient code with a similar description. Fresh pork (FP) and processed pork (PP) were defined using the pf_meat and pf_cured meat components, respectively [26]. All pork (AP) included all fresh and processed pork. Consumers of AP, FP, and PP were defined as those individuals consuming any amount of AP, FP, or PP on either of the two days of dietary recall.

2.5. Statistics

All analyses were performed using SAS 9.4 (SAS Institute, Cary, NC, USA) software and the data were adjusted for the complex sampling design of NHANES, using appropriate survey weights, strata, and primary sampling units. Day one dietary weights were used in all intake analysis. Data are presented as mean ± standard error; t-tests and z-statistic was used to assess differences between non-consumers and consumers.

3. Results

3.1. Children Age 2–18 Years

About 52, 15, and 45% of children age 2-18 years were consumers of AP, FP, and PP, respectively, with a mean intake of 47, 60 and 38 g/day, respectively, among consumers.

Mean per capita intake of PP, FP and PP were 17, 5 and 12 g/day, respectively. The per capita mean intake of AP has decreased, while intake of FP and PP has not changed over the last 18 years among children age 2-18 years in the US (Figure 1).

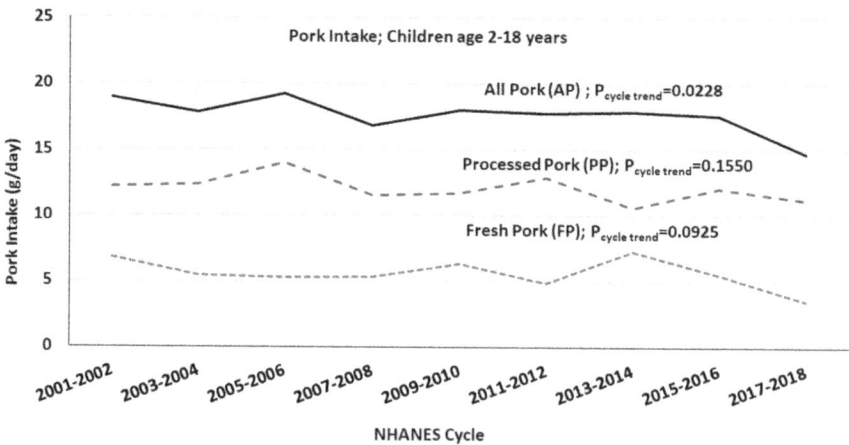

Figure 1. Mean per capita intake of pork among children (age 2–18 years) over NHANES study periods; gender combined data from day one of 24 h dietary recall.

Consumers of different pork types (AP, FP, and PP), compared to respective non-consumers, were more likely to be male (except for FP), obese (only for PP), Asian (only for FP), have a poverty–income ratio (PIR) below 1.35 (except for PP), engage in vigorous physical activity (only for FP) and current smokers (only for AP), and less likely to be of normal weight (only for PP), non-Hispanic White (only for FP), Asian (only for AP and PP), and have a PIR above 1.85 (Table 1).

Table 1. Demographics associated with pork consumption in children (age 2–18 years).

	All Pork (AP)		Fresh Pork (FP)		Processed Pork (PP)	
	Non-Consumers	Consumers	Non-Consumers	Consumers	Non-Consumers	Consumers
Sample N	5156	5757	9077	1836	6103	4810
Population N	33,326,596	36,523,218	59,684,896	10,164,918	38,532,690	31,317,124
Mean Age (Years)	9.94 ± 0.13	10.2 ± 0.1	10.1 ± 0.1	9.95 ± 0.17	9.94 ± 0.11	10.3 ± 0.1
Gender (% Male)	48.9 ± 1.1	52.6 ± 1.0 [#]	50.7 ± 0.9	51.7 ± 1.5	49.2 ± 1.0	52.8 ± 1.1 [#]
Underweight (%)	4.07 ± 0.52	3.32 ± 0.42	3.76 ± 0.38	3.16 ± 0.60	4.00 ± 0.51	3.28 ± 0.47
Normal weight (%)	63.1 ± 1.1	60.8 ± 1.0	62.1 ± 0.8	60.5 ± 1.6	63.1 ± 1.0	60.3 ± 1.1 [#]
Overweight (%)	15.2 ± 0.7	16.4 ± 0.7	15.8 ± 0.5	16.3 ± 1.0	15.3 ± 0.6	16.5 ± 0.7
Obese (%)	17.6 ± 0.9	19.5 ± 0.9	18.4 ± 0.8	20.0 ± 1.2	17.6 ± 0.8	19.9 ± 1.0 [#]
Ethnicity						
Hispanic (%)	22.9 ± 1.9	24.8 ± 2.1	23.8 ± 1.9	24.3 ± 2.7	22.9 ± 1.9	25.2 ± 2.2
n-H White (%)	52.9 ± 2.5	51.0 ± 2.7	53.0 ± 2.5	45.5 ± 3.2 [*]	52.1 ± 2.5	51.6 ± 2.8
n-H Black (%)	13.0 ± 1.3	14.5 ± 1.5	13.4 ± 1.3	16.2 ± 2.1	13.3 ± 1.3	14.4 ± 1.6
Asian (%)	5.33 ± 0.62	4.06 ± 0.43 [#]	3.99 ± 0.43	8.66 ± 1.05 [*]	5.94 ± 0.62	3.11 ± 0.38 [*]
Poverty Income Ratio						
<1.35 (%)	33.7 ± 1.8	36.7 ± 1.8 [#]	34.5 ± 1.7	39.9 ± 2.6 [#]	34.2 ± 1.8	36.5 ± 1.8
1.35 ≤ 1.85 (%)	11.1 ± 0.8	12.0 ± 0.8	11.3 ± 0.7	12.7 ± 1.4	11.3 ± 0.8	11.8 ± 0.9
>1.85 (%)	55.2 ± 2.0	51.4 ± 1.9 [*]	54.2 ± 1.9	47.4 ± 2.2 [*]	54.5 ± 1.9	51.6 ± 2.0 [#]
Education						
<High School (%)	99.3 ± 0.2	99.3 ± 0.2	99.2 ± 0.1	99.7 ± 0.2	99.3 ± 0.2	99.2 ± 0.2
High school (%)	0.73 ± 0.16	0.71 ± 0.18	0.78 ± 0.14	0.32 ± 0.18	0.69 ± 0.15	0.75 ± 0.21
>High School (%)	0.00 ± 0.00	0.00 ± 0.00	0.00 ± 0.00	0.00 ± 0.00	0.00 ± 0.00	0.00 ± 0.000
Physical Activity						
Sedentary (%)	15.6 ± 0.9	14.9 ± 0.8	15.5 ± 0.7	13.9 ± 1.1	15.4 ± 0.9	15.1 ± 0.9
Moderate (%)	24.1 ± 1.0	24.9 ± 0.7	24.9 ± 0.7	22.5 ± 1.6	23.9 ± 0.9	25.3 ± 0.9
Vigorous (%)	60.4 ± 1.2	60.1 ± 1.1	59.7 ± 1.0	63.6 ± 1.8 [#]	60.7 ± 1.2	59.6 ± 1.2
Smoking never (%)	92.8 ± 0.6	91.6 ± 0.6	92.3 ± 0.5	91.3 ± 1.2	92.7 ± 0.6	91.5 ± 0.7
Smoking former (%)	6.04 ± 0.56	6.70 ± 0.53	6.30 ± 0.43	6.90 ± 1.03	6.11 ± 0.54	6.73 ± 0.60
Smoking current (%)	0.80 ± 0.19	1.60 ± 0.31 [#]	1.16 ± 0.22	1.58 ± 0.68	0.86 ± 0.19	1.65 ± 0.38

Two days 24 h dietary recall data from NHANES 2011–2018. Data is presented as Mean ± Standard Error. [#], [*] represent significant differences from non-consumers at $p < 0.05$ and $p < 0.01$, respectively and assessed by t-tests. n-H, non-Hispanic.

Children who consumed AP, FP, and PP had higher intakes of copper (4–9%), magnesium (4–5%), potassium (7–8%), selenium (13–19%), sodium (5–18%), zinc (5–12%), thiamine (11–13%), niacin (6–9%), vitamin B_6 (6–7%), and choline (12–19%) compared to their respective non-consumers. Consumers of AP and PP had higher intakes of calcium (5–8%), iron (5–8%), phosphorus (9–11%), riboflavin (7–8%), vitamin B_{12} (9–10%), and vitamin D (7%) than their respective non-consumers. Consumers of PP had higher intakes of folate (5%) than non-consumers. However, consumers of FP had lower intakes for calcium (6%), iron (3%) and vitamin B_{12} (2%) than non-consumers (Table 2).

Table 2. Usual intakes of nutrients among children (age 2–18 years, gender combined) non-consumers and consumers of different pork types.

	All Pork (AP)		Fresh Pork (FP)		Processed Pork (PP)	
	Non-Consumers	Consumers	Non-Consumers	Consumers	Non-Consumers	Consumers
Sample N	5156	5757	9077	1836	6103	4810
Population N	33,326,596	36,523,218	59,684,896	10,164,918	38,532,690	31,317,124
Calcium (mg)	983 ± 14	1035 ± 11 *	1018 ± 11	954 ± 15 *	976 ± 12	1052 ± 12 *
Copper (mg)	0.89 ± 0.01	0.96 ± 0.01 *	0.92 ± 0.01	0.96 ± 0.02 #	0.89 ± 0.01	0.97 ± 0.01 *
Iron (mg)	13.4 ± 0.2	14.1 ± 0.2 *	13.8 ± 0.1	13.4 ± 0.2	13.3 ± 0.2	14.3 ± 0.2 *
Magnesium (mg)	228 ± 2	238 ± 2 *	232 ± 2	241 ± 4 #	228 ± 2	239 ± 3 *
Phosphorus (mg)	1197 ± 13	1304 ± 13 *	1252 ± 10	1271 ± 19	1198 ± 11	1324 ± 14 *
Potassium (mg)	2055 ± 21	2217 ± 23 *	2116 ± 16	2295 ± 38 *	2073 ± 20	2224 ± 25 *
Selenium (µg)	86 ± 1.0	102 ± 1 *	92.7 ± 0.8	105 ± 2 *	87.7 ± 0.9	103 ± 1 *
Sodium (mg)	2723 ± 29	3185 ± 34 *	2940 ± 26	3095 ± 57 #	2737 ± 26	3240 ± 35 *
Zinc (mg)	9.18 ± 0.12	10.3 ± 0.1 *	9.68 ± 0.10	10.2 ± 0.2 #	9.28 ± 0.12	10.4 ± 0.1 *
Vitamin A, RE (µg)	586 ± 9	604 ± 9	600 ± 8	579 ± 11	585 ± 8	609 ± 10
Thiamin (mg)	1.43 ± 0.02	1.62 ± 0.02 *	1.5 ± 0.01	1.67 ± 0.03 *	1.45 ± 0.02	1.63 ± 0.02 *
Riboflavin (mg)	1.84 ± 0.02	1.97 ± 0.02 *	1.90 ± 0.02	1.94 ± 0.03	1.84 ± 0.02	1.98 ± 0.02 *
Niacin (mg)	20.3 ± 0.3	22.2 ± 0.3 *	21.1 ± 0.2	22.4 ± 0.4 *	20.5 ± 0.2	22.3 ± 0.4 *
Folate, DFE (µg)	495 ± 8	512 ± 8	507 ± 6	487 ± 10	492 ± 7	516 ± 9 #
Vitamin B$_6$ (mg)	1.66 ± 0.02	1.78 ± 0.03 *	1.70 ± 0.02	1.81 ± 0.04 #	1.67 ± 0.02	1.78 ± 0.03 *
Vitamin B$_{12}$ (µg)	4.45 ± 0.08	4.85 ± 0.08 *	4.67 ± 0.06	4.58 ± 0.09	4.46 ± 0.07	4.89 ± 0.09 *
Vitamin C (mg)	71.2 ± 1.7	76 ± 2.1	72.5 ± 1.5	81.5 ± 5.0	71.6 ± 1.6	76.4 ± 2.2
Vitamin D (µg)	5.20 ± 0.12	5.54 ± 0.09 #	5.36 ± 0.09	5.45 ± 0.14	5.23 ± 0.11	5.57 ± 0.10 #
Vitamin E, ATE (mg)	7.08 ± 0.13	7.26 ± 0.10	7.16 ± 0.09	7.20 ± 0.16	7.05 ± 0.11	7.30 ± 0.11
Choline (mg)	226 ± 3	269 ± 3 *	244 ± 2	274 ± 5 *	229 ± 3	273 ± 3 *

Two days 24 h dietary recall data from NHANES 2011–2018. Data presented as mean ± Standard Error; ATE: alpha tocopherol equivalents; DFE: dietary folate equivalents; RE: retinol activity equivalents; #,* represent significant differences from non-consumers at $p < 0.05$ and $p < 0.01$, respectively and assessed by z statistics.

A higher proportion of children met the nutrient recommendations for copper (3–4% units), potassium (6–10% units), zinc (5–8% units), thiamin (2–3% units), and choline (8–9% units) among consumers of AP, FP, and PP compared to non-consumers. Consumers of AP and PP had lower percentages of children below EAR for calcium (5–8% units), iron (2% units), phosphorus (8–9% units), riboflavin (1–2% units), and vitamin B$_{12}$ (2% units) than non-consumers. Consumers of FP had a lower proportion of children below EAR for magnesium (4% units), vitamin B$_6$ (2% units), and vitamin C (11% units) and a higher proportion of children below EAR for calcium (6% units) than non-consumers (Table 3).

Table 3. Nutrient inadequacy/adequacy in children (age 2–18 years, gender combined) non-consumers and consumers of different pork types.

	All Pork (AP)		Fresh Pork (FP)		Processed Pork (PP)	
	Non-Consumers	Consumers	Non-Consumers	Consumers	Non-Consumers	Consumers
Sample N	5156	5757	9077	1836	6103	4810
Population N	33,326,596	36,523,218	59,684,896	10,164,918	38,532,690	31,317,124
	% Children below Estimated Average Requirements (EAR)					
Calcium	48.8 ± 1.5	44.0 ± 1.3 #	45.7 ± 1.4	52.0 ± 1.7 *	49.6 ± 1.4	42.0 ± 1.5 *
Copper	7.05 ± 0.84	3.32 ± 0.59 *	5.52 ± 0.59	2.08 ± 0.59 *	6.73 ± 0.75	3.06 ± 0.66 *
Iron	4.03 ± 0.54	2.15 ± 0.37 *	3.01 ± 0.39	2.54 ± 0.61	4.03 ± 0.49	1.89 ± 0.41 *
Magnesium	36.6 ± 1.3	34.0 ± 1.2	35.6 ± 1.0	31.7 ± 1.6 #	36.1 ± 1.1	34.0 ± 1.3
Phosphorus	19.7 ± 1.4	11.3 ± 1.2 *	15.6 ± 1.1	11.8 ± 1.7	19.4 ± 1.2	10.1 ± 1.3 *
Selenium	0.16 ± 0.08	0.02 ± 0.02	0.11 ± 0.05	0.0004 ± 0.01 #	0.10 ± 0.06	0.02 ± 0.03

Table 3. Cont.

	All Pork (AP)		Fresh Pork (FP)		Processed Pork (PP)	
	Non-Consumers	Consumers	Non-Consumers	Consumers	Non-Consumers	Consumers
Zinc	15.1 ± 1.6	7.58 ± 1.22 *	11.7 ± 1.2	6.4 ± 1.5 *	14.6 ± 1.4	6.82 ± 1.43 *
Vitamin A	26.0 ± 1.5	23.8 ± 1.7	24.8 ± 1.3	25.2 ± 2.1	26.2 ± 1.3	23.31 ± 1.95
Thiamin	3.14 ± 0.58	0.62 ± 0.29 *	2.02 ± 0.41	0.12 ± 0.12 *	2.78 ± 0.50	0.62 ± 0.34 *
Riboflavin	2.06 ± 0.45	0.68 ± 0.27 *	1.28 ± 0.35	0.73 ± 0.26	2.10 ± 0.43	0.54 ± 0.27 *
Niacin	0.65 ± 0.23	0.17 ± 0.11	0.42 ± 0.15	0.05 ± 0.06 #	0.53 ± 0.19	0.16 ± 0.13
Folate	5.39 ± 0.84	3.81 ± 0.88	4.47 ± 0.83	4.26 ± 1.23	5.44 ± 0.77	3.53 ± 1.04
Vitamin B_6	3.33 ± 0.74	1.66 ± 0.60	2.74 ± 0.61	0.76 ± 0.48 #	3.16 ± 0.69	1.61 ± 0.66
Vitamin B_{12}	2.41 ± 0.46	0.87 ± 0.33 *	1.65 ± 0.36	0.81 ± 0.37	2.31 ± 0.42	0.78 ± 0.34 *
Vitamin C	23.1 ± 1.3	21.3 ± 1.8	23.7 ± 1.1	13.0 ± 4.2 #	22.5 ± 1.3	21.8 ± 1.9
Vitamin D	93.1 ± 0.8	93.9 ± 0.7	93.3 ± 0.6	94.2 ± 1.2	93.0 ± 0.8	94.1 ± 0.8
Vitamin E	66.1 ± 1.7	65.9 ± 1.1	66.1 ± 1.2	64.6 ± 2.1	66.2 ± 1.5	65.8 ± 1.3
% Children above Adequate Intake (AI)						
Potassium	27.3 ± 1.5	34.4 ± 1.4 *	29.6 ± 1.1	39.8 ± 2.6 *	28.2 ± 1.3	34.4 ± 1.6 *
Sodium	99.7 ± 0.1	100 ± 0.02 #	99.8 ± 0.1	100 ± 0.02 #	99.7 ± 0.1	100 ± 0.02 #
Choline	16.1 ± 1.2	25.3 ± 0.9 *	19.7 ± 0.8	27.6 ± 1.7 *	16.7 ± 1.0	26.1 ± 1.0 *

Two days 24 h dietary recall data from NHANES 2011–2018. Data presented as mean ± Standard Error; #,* represent significant differences from non-consumers at $p < 0.05$ and $p < 0.01$, respectively and assessed using z statistics.

3.2. Adults Age 19+ Years

About 59, 20, and 49% of adults age 19+ years were consumers of AP, FP, and PP, respectively, with a mean intake of 61, 77, and 48 g/day, respectively, among consumers.

The mean per capita intake of PP, FP and PP was 25, 10, and 16 g/day, respectively. The per capita mean intake of AP and PP has decreased, while the intake of FP has not changed over the last 18 years among those age 19+ years in the US (Figure 2).

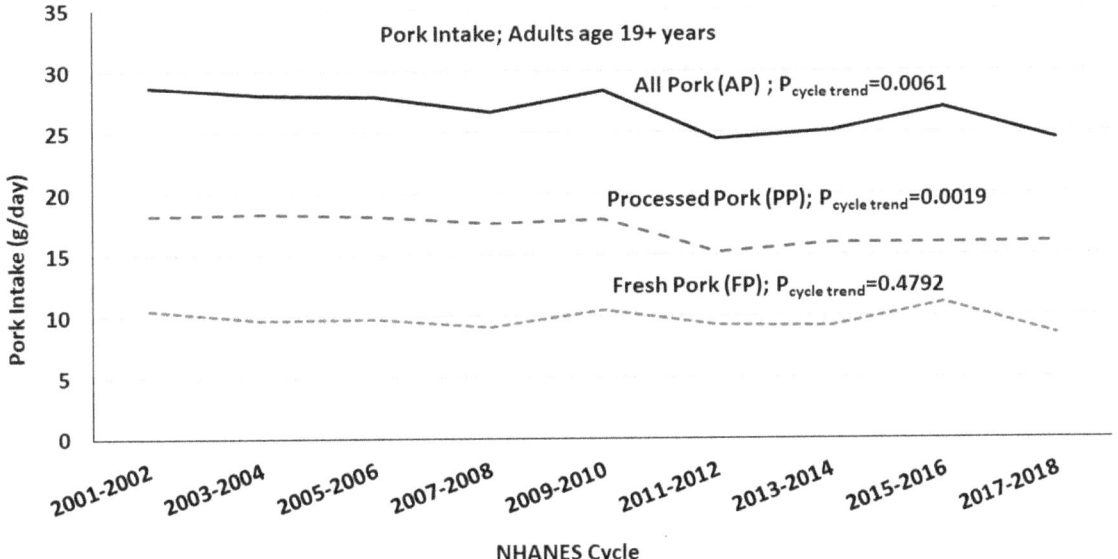

Figure 2. Mean per capita intake of pork among adults (age 19+ years) over NHANES study periods; gender combined data from day one of 24 h dietary recall.

Consumers (aged 19+ years) of different pork types (AP, FP, and PP), compared to their respective non-consumers, were more likely to be older, male, obese, non-Hispanic White (only for PP), non-Hispanic Black, Asian (only for FP), have education below High School, High School (except for FP), be sedentary, be a former smoker (only for AP), be current smokers (except for FP), and be less likely to be of normal weight (except for FP), overweight (only for FP), non-Hispanic White (only for FP), Asian (except for FP), have education above High School, engage in vigorous activity (except for PP), and be never smokers (Table 4).

Table 4. Demographics associated with pork consumption in adults (age 19+ years).

	All Pork (AP)		Fresh Pork (FP)		Processed Pork (PP)	
	Non-Consumers	Consumers	Non-Consumers	Consumers	Non-Consumers	Consumers
Sample N	8211	11,555	15,367	4399	10,340	9426
Population N	95,898,484	135,707,272	184,749,722	46,856,034	118,070,955	113,534,800
Mean Age (Years)	46.5 ± 0.4	48.5 ± 0.4 *	47.4 ± 0.3	48.6 ± 0.6 *	47.0 ± 0.4	48.3 ± 0.4 *
Gender (% Male)	44.8 ± 0.8	52.6 ± 0.6 *	48.4 ± 0.6	53.2 ± 1.0 *	45.8 ± 0.7	53.1 ± 0.7 *
Underweight (%)	1.61 ± 0.23	1.48 ± 0.16	1.54 ± 0.15	1.51 ± 0.24	1.69 ± 0.22	1.37 ± 0.17
Normal weight (%)	30.6 ± 1.0	25.3 ± 0.8 *	27.6 ± 0.7	27.0 ± 1.0	30.2 ± 0.9	24.7 ± 0.9 *
Overweight (%)	32.4 ± 0.9	32.2 ± 0.8	33.0 ± 0.6	29.2 ± 1.1 *	31.5 ± 0.8	33.0 ± 0.9
Obese (%)	35.4 ± 1.0	41.1 ± 0.8 *	37.8 ± 0.8	42.3 ± 1.0 *	36.7 ± 0.9	40.9 ± 0.9 *
Ethnicity						
Hispanic (%)	15.4 ± 1.2	14.8 ± 1.2	15.0 ± 1.2	15.3 ± 1.4	15.3 ± 1.2	14.8 ± 1.3
n-H White (%)	63.4 ± 1.7	65.4 ± 1.9	65.7 ± 1.6	59.8 ± 2.3 *	62.4 ± 1.8	66.8 ± 1.8 *
n-H Black (%)	10.6 ± 0.9	12.0 ± 1.1 #	11.0 ± 0.9	13.1 ± 1.4 #	10.7 ± 0.9	12.1 ± 1.1 #
Asian (%)	6.75 ± 0.62	4.67 ± 0.48 *	4.61 ± 0.42	9.17 ± 0.98 *	7.97 ± 0.71	3.00 ± 0.31 *
Poverty Income Ratio						
<1.35 (%)	24.4 ± 1.0	24.2 ± 1.0	24.1 ± 1.0	24.9 ± 1.5	24.4 ± 1.0	24.1 ± 1.1
1.35 ≤ 1.85 (%)	10.3 ± 0.7	9.71 ± 0.48	9.84 ± 0.46	10.3 ± 0.8	10.4 ± 0.6	9.45 ± 0.50
>1.85 (%)	65.4 ± 1.4	66.1 ± 1.3	66.1 ± 1.2	64.8 ± 1.9	65.2 ± 1.4	66.4 ± 1.3
Education						
<High School (%)	34.9 ± 1.4	38.9 ± 1.1 *	36.4 ± 1.2	40.5 ± 1.4 *	35.9 ± 1.2	38.6 ± 1.2 *
High School (%)	31.7 ± 1.0	33.4 ± 0.7 #	32.8 ± 0.7	32.5 ± 1.1	31.4 ± 0.8	34.0 ± 0.8 *
>High School (%)	33.4 ± 1.4	27.7 ± 1.3 *	30.8 ± 1.3	27.1 ± 1.6 *	32.6 ± 1.3	27.4 ± 1.3 *
Physical Activity						
Sedentary (%)	19.7 ± 0.6	22.6 ± 0.8 *	20.9 ± 0.6	23.3 ± 1.0 #	20.4 ± 0.6	22.3 ± 0.8 #
Moderate (%)	35.8 ± 0.9	35.7 ± 0.8	35.4 ± 0.7	37.1 ± 1.2	36.0 ± 0.8	35.5 ± 0.9
Vigorous (%)	44.5 ± 0.9	41.7 ± 1.0 #	43.7 ± 0.8	39.6 ± 1.2 *	43.6 ± 0.9	42.1 ± 1.0
Smoking never (%)	57.2 ± 0.9	52.4 ± 0.8 *	55.1 ± 0.7	51.7 ± 1.2 *	56.5 ± 0.9	52.2 ± 0.8 *
Smoking former (%)	25.3 ± 0.9	27.5 ± 0.6 #	26.1 ± 0.6	28.3 ± 1.1	25.7 ± 0.8	27.5 ± 0.7
Smoking current (%)	17.3 ± 0.8	19.9 ± 0.7 *	18.5 ± 0.7	19.8 ± 1.1	17.6 ± 0.8	20.0 ± 0.8 *

Two days 24 h dietary recall data from NHANES 2011–2018. Data are presented as Mean ± Standard Error. #,* represent significant differences from non-consumers at $p < 0.05$ and $p < 0.01$, respectively, and assessed using t-tests. n-H: non-Hispanic.

Adult consumers of AP, FP, and PP had higher intakes of iron (3–6%), phosphorus (3–12%), potassium (6–8%), selenium (15–19%), sodium (7–20%), zinc (8–11%), thiamine (14–20%), riboflavin (1–10%), niacin (9–11%), vitamin B_6 (4–6%), and choline (13–21%) compared to their respective non-consumers. Consumers of AP and PP had higher intakes of calcium (5–11%) and vitamin B_{12} (6–8%) than their respective non-consumers. Consumers of PP had higher intakes of vitamin D (6%). However, consumers of AP had lower intakes of vitamin C (5%), and consumers of FP had lower intakes of calcium (9%), vitamin A (9%) and vitamin E (4%) compared to their respective non-consumers (Table 5).

Table 5. Usual intakes of nutrients among adults (age 19+ years, gender combined) non-consumers and consumers of different pork types.

	All Pork (AP)		Fresh Pork (FP)		Processed Pork (PP)	
	Non-Consumers	Consumers	Non-Consumers	Consumers	Non-Consumers	Consumers
Sample N	8211	11,555	15,367	4399	10,340	9426
Population N	95,898,484	135,707,272	184,749,722	46,856,034	118,070,955	113,534,800
Calcium (mg)	944 ± 10	987 ± 8 *	987 ± 6	902 ± 11 *	922 ± 8	1019 ± 9 *
Copper (mg)	1.24 ± 0.02	1.27 ± 0.01	1.25 ± 0.01	1.28 ± 0.01	1.24 ± 0.01	1.27 ± 0.01
Iron (mg)	14.2 ± 0.2	15 ± 0.1 *	14.6 ± 0.1	15 ± 0.2 #	14.3 ± 0.1	15.0 ± 0.1 *
Magnesium (mg)	306 ± 3	309 ± 2	307 ± 2	312 ± 3	306 ± 3	309 ± 2
Phosphorus (mg)	1317 ± 13	1457 ± 8 *	1391 ± 7	1432 ± 13 *	1320 ± 11	1481 ± 9 *
Potassium (mg)	2558 ± 25	2756 ± 19 *	2643 ± 17	2803 ± 33 *	2591 ± 21	2769 ± 21 *
Selenium (μg)	104 ± 1	124 ± 1 *	112 ± 1	130 ± 1 *	108 ± 1	124 ± 1 *
Sodium (mg)	3171 ± 25	3812 ± 23 *	3495 ± 17	3757 ± 34 *	3221 ± 22	3881 ± 24 *
Zinc (mg)	10.6 ± 0.1	11.8 ± 0.1 *	11.1 ± 0.1	12.0 ± 0.1 *	10.7 ± 0.1	11.8 ± 0.1 *
Vitamin A, RE (μg)	652 ± 13	637 ± 10	656 ± 9	595 ± 16 *	636 ± 11	652 ± 10
Thiamin (mg)	1.46 ± 0.01	1.73 ± 0.01 *	1.55 ± 0.01	1.86 ± 0.02 *	1.51 ± 0.01	1.72 ± 0.01 *
Riboflavin (mg)	2.05 ± 0.02	2.23 ± 0.02 *	2.15 ± 0.02	2.18 ± 0.02 *	2.06 ± 0.02	2.26 ± 0.02 *
Niacin (mg)	24.7 ± 0.3	27.4 ± 0.2 *	25.8 ± 0.2	28.0 ± 0.3 *	25.1 ± 0.2	27.5 ± 0.2 *
Folate, DFE (μg)	523 ± 7	533 ± 4	529 ± 4	534 ± 7	524 ± 6	534 ± 5
Vitamin B_6 (mg)	2.10 ± 0.03	2.21 ± 0.02 *	2.14 ± 0.02	2.27 ± 0.03 *	2.12 ± 0.02	2.21 ± 0.02 *
Vitamin B_{12} (μg)	4.85 ± 0.08	5.16 ± 0.07 *	5.05 ± 0.06	4.95 ± 0.11	4.83 ± 0.07	5.23 ± 0.08 *
Vitamin C (mg)	82.2 ± 1.6	78.0 ± 1.3 #	79.7 ± 1.2	79.9 ± 1.9	81.6 ± 1.5	77.7 ± 1.3
Vitamin D (μg)	4.48 ± 0.09	4.64 ± 0.07	4.56 ± 0.06	4.58 ± 0.13	4.45 ± 0.09	4.71 ± 0.8 #
Vitamin E, ATE (mg)	9.32 ± 0.15	9.21 ± 0.10	9.35 ± 0.11	8.94 ± 0.12 #	9.15 ± 0.13	9.37 ± 0.11
Choline (mg)	299 ± 3	362 ± 3 *	328 ± 2	369 ± 5 *	307 ± 3	366 ± 3 *

Two days 24 h dietary recall data from NHANES 2011–2018. Data presented as mean ± Standard Error; ATE: alpha tocopherol equivalents; DFE: dietary folate equivalents; RE: retinol activity equivalents; #,* represent significant differences from non-consumers at $p < 0.05$ and $p < 0.01$, respectively, and assessed using z statistics.

A higher proportion of adults met the nutrients recommendations for copper (2–5% units), iron (2–4% units), phosphorus (~1% unit), potassium (4–5% units), selenium (1% units), sodium (1–2% units), zinc (5–12% units), thiamin (8–12% units), riboflavin (1–4% units), niacin (1–3% units), vitamin B_6 (5–6% units), and choline (5–6% units) among consumers of AP, FP, and PP compared to their respective non-consumers. Consumers of AP and PP had lower proportion of adults below EAR for calcium (6–11% units), folate (3–4% units), and vitamin B_{12} (5% units) than their respective non-consumers. Consumers of PP had lower proportion of adults below EAR vitamin A (5% units) than non-consumers. However, consumers of AP and PP had a higher proportion of adults below EAR for vitamin D (2–3% units); consumers of AP and FP had a higher proportion of adults below EAR for vitamin E (4–5% units), and consumers of FP had a higher proportion of adults below EAR for calcium (8% units) and vitamin A (8% units) compared to their respective non-consumers (Table 6).

Table 6. Nutrient inadequacy/adequacy in adult (age 19+ years, gender combined) non-consumers and consumers of different pork types.

	All Pork (AP)		Fresh Pork (FP)		Processed Pork (PP)	
	Non-Consumers	Consumers	Non-Consumers	Consumers	Non-Consumers	Consumers
Sample N	8211	11,555	15,367	4399	10,340	9426
Population N	95,898,484	135,707,272	184,749,722	46,856,034	118,070,955	113,534,800
	% Adults below Estimated Average Requirements (EAR)					
Calcium	46.9 ± 1.1	41.1 ± 1.0 *	41.9 ± 0.7	49.9 ± 1.2 *	49.0 ± 0.9	37.6 ± 1.0 *
Copper	10.7 ± 0.6	5.58 ± 0.46 *	8.12 ± 0.48	6.11 ± 0.75 #	10.1 ± 0.5	5.20 ± 0.47 *

Table 6. Cont.

	All Pork (AP)		Fresh Pork (FP)		Processed Pork (PP)	
	Non-Consumers	Consumers	Non-Consumers	Consumers	Non-Consumers	Consumers
Iron	7.58 ± 0.40	4.03 ± 0.22 *	5.75 ± 0.26	4.00 ± 0.43 *	7.01 ± 0.34	3.91 ± 0.25 *
Magnesium	52.2 ± 1.3	53.1 ± 0.9	52.6 ± 0.9	52.4 ± 1.3	52.4 ± 1.0	53.1 ± 1.0
Phosphorus	1.77 ± 0.25	0.32 ± 0.05 *	0.87 ± 0.11	0.52 ± 0.12 #	1.68 ± 0.23	0.23 ± 0.06 *
Selenium	1.46 ± 0.30	0.13 ± 0.04 *	0.75 ± 0.11	0.09 ± 0.05 *	1.28 ± 0.24	0.12 ± 0.04 *
Zinc	24.6 ± 1.2	12.6 ± 1.0 *	18.9 ± 0.9	13.6 ± 1.4 *	23.4 ± 1.1	11.7 ± 1.2 *
Vitamin A	44.9 ± 1.3	44.7 ± 1.5	43.1 ± 1.1	51.2 ± 2.5 *	46.6 ± 1.2	42.0 ± 1.6 #
Thiamin	14.6 ± 0.9	2.98 ± 0.38 *	9.42 ± 0.54	1.04 ± 0.36 *	12.0 ± 0.8	3.06 ± 0.44 *
Riboflavin	5.66 ± 0.56	2.23 ± 0.23 *	3.83 ± 0.29	2.50 ± 0.42 *	5.38 ± 0.50	1.86 ± 0.23 *
Niacin	3.25 ± 0.48	0.73 ± 0.13 *	1.93 ± 0.22	0.65 ± 0.22 *	2.71 ± 0.38	0.65 ± 0.15 *
Folate	15.6 ± 1.0	12.4 ± 0.9 #	14.0 ± 0.7	13.2 ± 1.5	15.5 ± 1.0	11.9 ± 1.0 *
Vitamin B_6	15.1 ± 1.1	9.45 ± 0.73 *	13.0 ± 0.8	8.08 ± 1.08 *	14.2 ± 0.9	9.48 ± 0.87 *
Vitamin B_{12}	8.34 ± 0.96	3.26 ± 0.47 *	5.88 ± 0.55	3.93 ± 0.83	8.16 ± 0.75	2.74 ± 0.47 *
Vitamin C	47.2 ± 1.3	49.5 ± 1.1	48.6 ± 1.1	47.8 ± 1.7	47.1 ± 1.2	49.8 ± 1.2
Vitamin D	93.8 ± 0.5	96.5 ± 0.4 *	95.0 ± 0.4	96.2 ± 0.7	94.3 ± 0.5	96.4 ± 0.4 *
Vitamin E	76.8 ± 1.3	81.0 ± 0.8 *	78.0 ± 1.0	83.2 ± 1.1 *	78.5 ± 1.0	79.9 ± 1.0
	% Adults above Adequate Intake (AI)					
Potassium	29.2 ± 1.2	33.4 ± 1.0 *	30.8 ± 0.9	35.8 ± 1.7 #	30.1 ± 1.1	33.9 ± 1.1 #
Sodium	98.2 ± 0.4	99.8 ± 0.07 *	99.1 ± 0.1	99.6 ± 0.13 *	98.4 ± 0.3	99.8 ± 0.1 *
Choline	4.43 ± 0.53	10.6 ± 0.9 *	7.33 ± 0.54	12.1 ± 1.3 *	5.15 ± 0.55	11.0 ± 1.0 *

Two days 24 h dietary recall data from NHANES 2011–2018. Data presented as mean ± Standard Error; #,* represent significant differences from non-consumers at $p < 0.05$ and $p < 0.01$, respectively and assessed using z statistics.

4. Discussion

The results of this analysis of cross-sectional data from NHANES indicate that children and adult consumers of pork have higher intakes and lower prevalence of inadequacies of several key micronutrients, including many under-consumed nutrients and nutrients of concern, compared to those who did not consume pork. Interestingly, the results for most nutrients are similar for fresh pork and processed pork consumers.

To date, only a limited number of studies have evaluated the impact of pork intake on micronutrient intakes, and even fewer have assessed the association of pork intake with meting nutrient recommendations. In an earlier cross-sectional analysis of NHANES 2003–2006, Murphy et al. [5] reported that fresh pork and fresh lean pork contributed more than 10% of daily intake of protein, phosphorus, potassium, zinc, selenium, thiamine, riboflavin, niacin, vitamin B_6, and vitamin B_{12} in the diets of consumers. Increased fresh and lean pork intakes were related to small but significantly ($p < 0.01$) improved daily nutritional intakes of protein (4 g), magnesium (4 mg), phosphorus (30 mg), potassium (83–85 mg), selenium (7 µg), zinc (0.3 mg), thiamine (0.2 mg), riboflavin (0.04 mg), niacin (0.8 mg), and vitamin B_6 (0.1 mg) compared to non-consumers in another cross-sectional analysis of NHANES 2005–2016 [6]. In a secondary analysis of the 2007 Australian National Children's Nutrition and Physical Activity Survey [7], fresh pork contributed substantially to the total intakes of thiamin (15%), protein (13%), niacin (10%), zinc (9%), phosphorous (7%), and potassium (6%); while processed pork contributed protein (6.3%), zinc (5.4%), and niacin (5.2%), in the diets of children. In the present analysis of NHANES 2011–2018, we find that both children and adult consumers of different pork types had consistently significantly higher intakes of several micronutrients, including potassium, selenium, zinc, thiamine, niacin, vitamin B_6, and choline, compared to their respective non-consumers. Consumers of one or the other pork types also had significantly higher intakes of several other micronutrients. Interestingly, calcium intakes were higher among consumers of both AP and PP but lower among consumers of FP. The reasons for this anomaly are not immediately apparent and require further investigation, but we hypothesize that consumers of pork may also consume more calcium-rich dairy products.

In addition to higher intakes, consumers of different pork types also had a lower prevalence of % population below EAR and higher prevalence of % population above AI compared to non-consumers for several nutrients. To the best of our knowledge, ours is this first investigation on different types of pork intakes and meeting nutrient recommendations. However, many of the observed differences in the prevalence of nutritional inadequacies (% population below EAR) or % population above AI between consumers and non-consumers of different types of pork were in mid-single digits for both children and adults (see Tables 3 and 5). To put these results into perspective, since we used population weighted nationally representative data, a sample size of 5757 children and 11,555 adult consumers of AP represented 36,523,218 children and 135,707,272 adult consumers of AP; a 1% unit change in prevalence of meeting nutritional requirement among consumers would translate to 365,232 children and 1,357,072 adults. For example, based on our results 7.09% more children and 4.25% more adult consumers of AP being above the AI for potassium, we estimate that pork (AP) intake was associated with over 2.5 million more children and over 5.7 million more adults meeting the adequate intake level of potassium.

There is a consistent ongoing global debate on the climate and other environmental effects of animal agriculture and animal sourced food production while ensuring food security for the growing populations. Many scientists and policy makers are increasingly concerned with the environmental consequences in addition to the potential health consequences of meat (especially red meat) consumption and have advocated to limit or eliminate animal-sourced food from the diet [27–30]. However, such recommendations that primarily account for the environmental impact of animal sourced foods do not necessarily account for their potential effect on food availability and nutrient intake and could have potential unintended consequences [31–33]. However, pork production has been shown to be associated with greenhouse gas emission to a lesser extent compared to ruminant meat [34], and therefore would have less environmental impact.

The major strengths of our study included the use of a large nationally representative, population-based sample achieved through combining several sets of NHANES data releases and the use of the NCI method to assess usual intake to assess the percentage of the population below the EAR or above the AI. A major limitation of the current study, as with any cross-sectional study, is the inability to determine the cause-and-effect relationship. Additionally, there is the potential for bias in the use of self-reported dietary recalls relying on memory [35].

Finally, our findings suggest several future research opportunities: (1) while we looked at broad age groups to determine the overall impact of pork, there may be value in further evaluation of the association of pork intake in diverse groups based on age, socioeconomic status, and race/ethnicity; (2) if possible, an evaluation of the impact of specific pork cuts/parts of the pig may be worthwhile; (3) given the different base diets around the world, it may be worthwhile to evaluate the impact of pork in different parts of the world based on geography/cultural background; and (4) modeling to help define what foods would need to be consumed in greater quantities to replace nutrients from pork if removed from the diet.

5. Conclusions

The results show that pork intake was associated with improved nutrient intake and meeting nutrient recommendations in US children (age 2–18 years) and adults (age 19+ years) for certain key nutrients. It is therefore likely that pork may play a critical role in reducing the incidence of under-nutrition. At a minimum, those that advocate removal of meat and, in particular, pork from dietary guidelines need to ensure the nutrients provided by pork are replaced with other dietary changes. Future studies are needed to examine the long-term impact of pork consumption on diet quality, nutrient intake, and health promotion.

Author Contributions: The authors' responsibilities were as follows—S.A.: project conception, research design, development of overall research plan, interpretation of the data, preparation of the first draft of the manuscript, and revision of the manuscript; V.L.F.III: project conception, research design, development of overall research plan, NHANES database analysis and statistical analysis, interpretation of the data, and revision of the manuscript. All authors have read and agreed to the published version of the manuscript.

Funding: This research was funded by the Pork Checkoff. Pork Checkoff had no role in the analyses/interpretation of results and did not review the manuscript prior to submission.

Institutional Review Board Statement: The data used for this manuscript were from the National Health and Nutrition Examination Survey (NHANES) 2001–2018; data collection for NHANES was approved by the Research Ethics Review Board of the National Center for Health Statistics. NHANES has stringent consent protocols and procedures to ensure confidentiality and protection from identification. This study was a secondary data analysis, which lacked personal identifiers, and therefore did not require Institutional Review Board review.

Informed Consent Statement: The data used for this manuscript were from the National Health and Nutrition Examination Survey (NHANES) 2001–2018 and all participants or proxies provided written informed consent.

Data Availability Statement: The datasets analyzed in this study are available in the Center for Disease Control and Prevention repository; available online: http://www.cdc.gov/nchs/nhanes/ (accessed on 12 December 2022).

Acknowledgments: The study and the writing of the manuscript were supported by the Pork Checkoff.

Conflicts of Interest: S.A. as Principal of NutriScience LLC performs nutrition science consulting for various food and beverage companies and related entities. V.L.F.III as Senior Vice President of Nutrition Impact, LLC performs consulting and database analyses for various food and beverage companies and related entities.

References

1. Ritchie, H.; Rosado, P.; Roser, M. Meat and Dairy Production. Published online at OurWorldInData.org. 2017. Available online: https://ourworldindata.org/meat-production (accessed on 15 February 2023).
2. Davis, C.G.; Lin, B.-H. Factors Affecting US Pork Consumption: USDA/ERS report LDP-M-130-01. Available online: https://www.ers.usda.gov/webdocs/outlooks/37377/15778_ldpm13001_1_.pdf?v=5569.5 (accessed on 17 February 2023).
3. USDA; ARS. FoodData Central: ID 2341267, 2022. Available online: https://fdc.nal.usda.gov/ (accessed on 24 March 2023).
4. US FDA. Daily Value on the New Nutrition and Supplement Facts Labels. Available online: https://www.fda.gov/food/new-nutrition-facts-label/daily-value-new-nutrition-and-supplement-facts-labels (accessed on 24 March 2023).
5. Murphy, M.M.; Spungen, J.H.; Bi, X.; Barraj, L.M. Fresh and fresh lean pork are substantial sources of key nutrients when these products are consumed by adults in the United States. *Nutr. Res.* **2011**, *31*, 776–783. [CrossRef] [PubMed]
6. An, R.; Nickols-Richardson, S.M.; Alston, R.; Clarke, C. Fresh and lean pork consumption in relation to nutrient intakes and diet quality among US adults, NHANES 2005–2016. *Health Behav. Policy Rev.* **2019**, *6*, 570–581. [CrossRef]
7. Nolan-Clark, D.J.; Neale, E.P.; Charlton, K.E. Processed pork is the most frequently consumed type of pork in a survey of Australian children. *Nutr. Res.* **2013**, *33*, 913–921. [CrossRef] [PubMed]
8. Wade, A.T.; Davis, C.R.; Dyer, K.A.; Hodgson, J.M.; Woodman, R.J.; Keage, H.A.D.; Murphy, K.J. A Mediterranean Diet with Fresh, Lean Pork Improves Processing Speed and Mood: Cognitive Findings from the MedPork Randomised Controlled Trial. *Nutrients* **2019**, *11*, 1521. [CrossRef]
9. Murphy, K.J.; Thomson, R.L.; Coates, A.M.; Buckley, J.D.; Howe, P.R. Effects of eating fresh lean pork on cardiometabolic health parameters. *Nutrients* **2012**, *4*, 711–723. [CrossRef] [PubMed]
10. Murphy, K.J.; Parker, B.; Dyer, K.A.; Davis, C.R.; Coates, A.M.; Buckley, J.D.; Howe, P.R. A comparison of regular consumption of fresh lean pork, beef and chicken on body composition: A randomized cross-over trial. *Nutrients* **2014**, *6*, 682–696. [CrossRef]
11. An, R.; Liu, J.; Liu, R. Pork Consumption in Relation to Body Weight and Composition: A Systematic Review and Meta-analysis. *Am. J. Health Behav.* **2020**, *44*, 513–525. [CrossRef]
12. Stettler, N.; Murphy, M.M.; Barraj, L.M.; Smith, K.M.; Ahima, R.S. Systematic review of clinical studies related to pork intake and metabolic syndrome or its components. *Diabetes Metab. Syndr. Obes.* **2013**, *6*, 347–357. [CrossRef]
13. An, R.; Nickols-Richardson, S.M.; Alston, R.J.; Shen, S.; Clarke, C. Fresh- and lean-pork intake in relation to functional limitations among US older adults, 2005–2016. *Nutr. Health* **2020**, *26*, 295–301. [CrossRef]
14. HLPE. *Nutrition and Food Systems. A Report by the High Level Panel of Experts on Food Security and Nutrition of the Committee on World Food Security*; FAO: Rome, Italy, 2017.

15. Bailey, R.L.; West, K.P.; Black, R.E. The epidemiology of global micronutrient deficiencies. *Ann. Nutr. Metab.* **2015**, *66*, S22–S33. [CrossRef]
16. Beal, T.; Massiot, E.; Arsenault, J.E.; Smith, M.R.; Hijmans, R.J. Global trends in dietary micronutrient supplies and estimated prevalence of inadequate intakes. *PLoS ONE* **2017**, *12*, e0175554. [CrossRef] [PubMed]
17. Han, X.; Ding, S.; Lu, J.; Li, Y. Global, regional, and national burdens of common micronutrient deficiencies from 1990 to 2019: A secondary trend analysis based on the Global Burden of Disease 2019 study. *EClinicalMedicine* **2022**, *12*, 101299. [CrossRef]
18. Kumssa, D.B.; Joy, E.J.M.; Ander, E.L.; Watts, M.J.; Young, S.D.; Walker, S.; Broadley, M.R. Dietary calcium and zinc deficiency risks are decreasing but remain prevalent. *Sci. Rep.* **2015**, *5*, 10974. [CrossRef]
19. U.S. Department of Health and Human Services; U.S. Department of Agriculture. *2015–2020 Dietary Guidelines for Americans*, 8th ed.; December 2015. Available online: http://health.gov/dietaryguidelines/2015/guidelines/ (accessed on 24 March 2022).
20. U.S. Department of Agriculture; U.S. Department of Health and Human Services. *Dietary Guidelines for Americans, 2020–2025*, 9th ed.; December 2020. Available online: https://DietaryGuidelines.gov (accessed on 24 March 2023).
21. Centers for Disease Control and Prevention; National Center for Health Statistics. *National Health and Nutrition Examination Survey*; National Center for Health Statistics: Hyattsville, MD, USA, 2021. Available online: https://www.cdc.gov/nchs/nhanes/index.htm (accessed on 12 December 2022).
22. Raper, N.; Perloff, B.; Ingwersen, L.; Steinfeldt, L.; Anand, J. An overview of USDA's dietary intake data system. *J. Food Comp. Anal.* **2004**, *17*, 545–555. [CrossRef]
23. USDA/ARS. USDA Food and Nutrient Database for Dietary Studies. Food Surveys Research Group Home Page. Available online: http://www.ars.usda.gov/nea/bhnrc/fsrg (accessed on 12 December 2022).
24. Tooze, J.A.; Kipnis, V.; Buckman, D.W.; Carroll, R.J.; Freedman, L.S.; Guenther, P.M.; Krebs-Smith, S.M.; Subar, A.F.; Dodd, K.W. A mixed-effects model approach for estimating the distribution of usual intake of nutrients: The NCI method. *Stat. Med.* **2010**, *29*, 2857–2868. [CrossRef]
25. Institute of Medicine. *DRIs: Applications in Dietary Assessment*; National Academies Press: Washington, DC, USA, 2000.
26. USDA/ARS. USDA Food Patterns Equivalents Database. Food Surveys Research Group. Available online: https://www.ars.usda.gov/northeast?area/beltsville?md?bhnrc/beltsville?human?nutrition?research?center/food?surveys?research?group/docs/fped?overview? (accessed on 12 December 2022).
27. Institute of Medicine. *Sustainable Diets: Food for Healthy People and a Healthy Planet; Workshop Summary*; The National Academies Press: Washington, DC, USA, 2014.
28. Willett, W.; Rockström, J.; Loken, B.; Springmann, M.; Lang, T.; Vermeulen, S.; Garnett, T.; Tilman, D.; DeClerck, F.; Wood, A.; et al. Food in the Anthropocene: The EAT-Lancet Commission on healthy diets from sustainable food systems. *Lancet* **2019**, *393*, 447–492. [CrossRef] [PubMed]
29. Westhoek, H.; Lesschen, J.P.; Rood, T.; Wagner, S.; De Marco, A.; Murphy-Bokern, D.; Leip, A.; van Grinsven, H.; Sutton, M.A.; Oenema, O. Food choices, health and environment: Effects of cutting Europe's meat and dairy intake. *Glob. Environ. Chang.* **2014**, *26*, 196–205. [CrossRef]
30. Hedenus, F.; Wirsenius, S.; Johansson, D.J.A. The importance of reduced meat and dairy consumption for meeting stringent climate change targets. *Clim. Chang.* **2014**, *124*, 79–91. [CrossRef]
31. Springmann, M.; Wiebe, K.; Mason-D'Croz, D.; Sulser, T.B.; Rayner, M.; Scarborough, P. Health and nutritional aspects of sustainable diet strategies and their association with environmental impacts: A global modelling analysis with country-level detail. *Lancet Planet. Health* **2018**, *2*, e451–e461. [CrossRef]
32. Tso, R.; Forde, C.G. Unintended Consequences: Nutritional Impact and Potential Pitfalls of Switching from Animal- to Plant-Based Foods. *Nutrients* **2021**, *13*, 2527. [CrossRef]
33. Salomé, M.; Huneau, J.F.; Le Baron, C.; Kesse-Guyot, E.; Fouillet, H.; Mariotti, F. Substituting Meat or Dairy Products with Plant-Based Substitutes Has Small and Heterogeneous Effects on Diet Quality and Nutrient Security: A Simulation Study in French Adults (INCA3). *J. Nutr.* **2021**, *151*, 2435–2445. [CrossRef] [PubMed]
34. Tilman, D.; Clark, M. Global diets link environmental sustainability and human health. *Nature* **2014**, *515*, 518–522. [CrossRef] [PubMed]
35. Subar, A.F.; Freedman, L.S.; Tooze, J.A.; Kirkpatrick, S.I.; Boushey, C.; Neuhouser, M.L.; Thompson, F.E.; Potischman, N.; Guenther, P.M.; Tarasuk, V.; et al. Addressing Current Criticism Regarding the Value of Self-Report Dietary Data. *J. Nutr.* **2015**, *145*, 2639–2645. [CrossRef] [PubMed]

Disclaimer/Publisher's Note: The statements, opinions and data contained in all publications are solely those of the individual author(s) and contributor(s) and not of MDPI and/or the editor(s). MDPI and/or the editor(s) disclaim responsibility for any injury to people or property resulting from any ideas, methods, instructions or products referred to in the content.

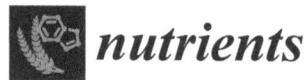 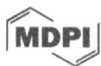

Review

Risk Assessment of Micronutrients Deficiency in Vegetarian or Vegan Children: Not So Obvious

Jean-Pierre Chouraqui

Paediatric Nutrition and Gastroenterology, Paediatrics Department, University Hospital of Grenoble-Alpes (CHUGA), Quai Yermoloff, 38700 La Tronche, France; chouraquijp@wanadoo.fr

Abstract: Vegetarian diets have gained in popularity worldwide and therefore an increasing number of children may be exposed to the resulting nutritional consequences. Among them, the risk of micronutrient shortfall is particularly of concern. This narrative review aims to assess and discuss the relevance of micronutrient deficiency risk based on the available data. It mainly draws attention to iron, zinc, iodine, and vitamins B12 and D intake. Diets that are more restrictive in animal source foods, such as vegan diets, have a greater likelihood of nutritional deficiencies. However, the actual risk of micronutrient deficiency in vegetarian children is relatively difficult to assert based on the limitations of evidence due to the lack of well-designed studies. The risk of vitamin B12 deficiency must be considered in newborns from vegan or macrobiotic mothers and children with the most restrictive diet, as well as the risk of iron, zinc, and iodine deficiency, possibly by performing the appropriate tests. A lacto-ovo-vegetarian diet exposes a low risk if it uses a very varied diet with a sufficient intake of dairy products. Vegan and macrobiotic diets should be avoided during pregnancy and childhood. There is a need for education and nutrition guidance and the need for supplementation should be assessed individually.

Keywords: infants; children; vegetarian; vegan; macrobiotic

1. Introduction

Micronutrients are vitamins and minerals that are needed in very small amounts for health (mg or μg/day), and that enable the body to produce enzymes, hormones, and other substances which are essential for proper growth and development [1]. Micronutrients are therefore even more crucial during the phases of rapid growth and development in childhood, i.e., the 1000 first days and first years of life and adolescence [2–5]. Micronutrient deficiencies may lead to deleterious health conditions, and less clinically noticeable disorders such as lower academic performance and an increased risk of diseases [2,3,6,7]. On the other hand, there is increasing evidence that diets during childhood and adolescence can impact health in later adulthood [8]. The World Health Organization's (WHO) Ambition and Action in Nutrition 2016–2025 aimed to provide a fit-for-purpose nutrition strategy and recalled the resolution WHA 37.18 on prevention and management of micronutrient malnutrition [9].

Micronutrients can only be provided in the diet and their deficiencies in children without underlying disease are food-borne. In general, micronutrients content tends to be denser, more varied, and more bioavailable in animal-source foods (ASF, including meat, fish, eggs, dairy products, and animal-derived ingredients) than in foods of plant origin (FPO) [6,10,11]. ASF are the almost exclusive dietary sources of vitamin B12 and vitamin D, apart from the possible contributions by certain mushrooms and yeasts. ASF is also the source of highly bioavailable vitamin A (retinol), iron, and zinc. Moreover, they provide a daily intake of riboflavin, choline, and vitamin E. Otherwise, vegetable oil and nuts may represent the most prominent sources of vitamin E. Dietary iodine intake depends mainly on that of iodized salt or otherwise from ASF and to a lesser extent from FPO depending then on the iodine content of the local soil and water.

Citation: Chouraqui, J.-P. Risk Assessment of Micronutrients Deficiency in Vegetarian or Vegan Children: Not So Obvious. *Nutrients* 2023, 15, 2129. https://doi.org/10.3390/nu15092129

Academic Editor: Diana H. Taft

Received: 20 March 2023
Revised: 16 April 2023
Accepted: 22 April 2023
Published: 28 April 2023

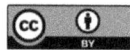

Copyright: © 2023 by the author. Licensee MDPI, Basel, Switzerland. This article is an open access article distributed under the terms and conditions of the Creative Commons Attribution (CC BY) license (https://creativecommons.org/licenses/by/4.0/).

Populations consuming little or no ASF, i.e., a vegetarian diet, are therefore exposed to the risk of deficiency in some or all these nutrients depending on their level of ASF intake [12]. The degree of ASF restriction as well as that of the permitted foods define the different vegetarian patterns [13–15]. All patterns include prolonged breastfeeding as much as possible. The lacto-ovo-vegetarian diet (LOV), very often assimilated to a vegetarian diet, is most often practiced, and excludes meat (all types and derived processed products), fish, and seafood but includes dairy products, eggs, and honey, together with a wide variety of plant foods. In addition, lacto-vegetarians also exclude eggs, while pollotarians consume poultry, pescatarians consume fish and seafood, and ovo-vegetarians may consume eggs but not milk. Occasionally and variably flexitarians will eat meat or fish. Veganism is much more restrictive and excludes all ASF, as well as products containing ingredients derived from ASF and all items of animal origin (e.g., wool, silk, leather). A macrobiotic diet is based on cereals, pulses, vegetables, seaweed, and soy products and may include fish.

As a benchmark, it should be acknowledged that in some parts of the world, mainly in Asia, human beings have been able for millennia not only to survive but also to maintain long and healthy lives on diets free from flesh [16–18]. Such diet remains part of the cultural and religious tradition in these countries essentially out of respect for all living beings [19]. Furthermore, avoidance of ASF is increasingly popular in industrialized countries due to a growing concern for animal welfare, sustainable development, and health, not to mention the socioeconomic impact of animal product consumption [15,20–28]. In households, children's eating behavior depends on parents purchasing family food, setting an example, and wanting their children to share their beliefs and eating habits [27,29,30]. On the other hand, more and more establishments such as kindergartens, schools, colleges, restaurants, and hospitals are providing vegetarian options at least one or two days a week for educational and environmental reasons. As a result, the question of the risks and benefits of vegetarian diets in childhood arises. Among the risks, those linked to an insufficient intake of micronutrients constitute a particularly important issue. This narrative review aims to assess and discuss the relevance of micronutrient deficiency risk based on the available data.

2. Search Strategy

A comprehensive search of the literature using PubMed, EMBASE, Google Scholar, and the Cochrane Library was conducted from 1980 up to January 2023. The keywords (words or MeSH terms) used were: 'micronutrients', 'vitamin', 'mineral', 'vegetarian', or 'vegan', 'pregnancy', 'lactation', 'breastfeeding', 'newborn', 'infant', 'toddler', 'child', 'adolescent', 'dietary intake', or 'deficiencies'. Moreover, a search was undertaken to identify relevant papers referred to in previously identified articles. Original papers, reviews, meta-analyses, position papers, and guidelines published by expert scientific groups or societies were included. Articles in English or with relevant English abstracts and in French were selected. When relevant data were identified in another language, an online translator was used so as not to overlook that information. After reading the title and abstract of the identified articles, duplicate references were removed. Thus, of the 332 publications first selected, 122 are finally cited.

3. Vitamins

3.1. Vitamin Supply from Foods from Plant Origin

FPO may be a significant source of antioxidant vitamins such as vitamin C (ascorbic acid), E (tocopherol), and provitamin A carotenoids, as well as vitamin K (phylloquinone), but also vitamin B1 (thiamine), B2 (riboflavin), B3 (niacin, PP), B5 (pantothenic acid), B6 (pyridoxine), B7 (biotin), B9 (folates) [31–34]. However, the impact of cooking (heating and leaching) and processing on the available vitamin content should not be neglected [34]. Compared to intakes of these vitamins in omnivorous children, those in vegetarians and vegans have been shown either identical or even higher in most studies, especially in vegans [35–49]. Lower intake of vitamin B2 has been reported in children following a macrobiotic diet compared to omnivores [35]. No studies assessed the vitamin K or vitamin B5 intake.

On the other hand, the dietary intake of vitamin D is very limited and can only come from infant's and young child's formulas and to a lesser extent from some fatty fishes or even less from some mushrooms [50–54]. Compared to the intake in omnivorous children, no study found a difference in vegetarian children [45–47], but one found a lower intake in vegan children [41].

The major issue in vegetarian diets is related to the total lack of vitamin B12 in FPO [55]. The only possible plant source of vitamin B12 could be some algae but with a low bioavailability [56,57].

3.2. Vitamin B12 Concern

Vitamin B12 is essential for human metabolism acting as a coenzyme in the conversion of methylmalonyl-CoA to succinyl-CoA in propionate metabolism and the transmethylation of homocysteine to methionine [58]. After reviewing published dietary reference values, the European Food Safety Authority (EFSA) sets an adequate dietary intake of cobalamin of 4.5 µg/d for pregnant women, 5 µg/d for lactating women, 0.5 µg/d for infants under 7 months of age, 1.5 µg/d for infants 7–11 months and children aged 1–6 years, 2.5 µg/d for children 7–10 years old, 3.5 µg/d for teenagers 11–14 years old and 4 µg/d for adolescent 15–17 years old. Symptoms and the long-term prognosis of cobalamin deficiency in children depend on the severity and duration of the deficiency [56]. The diagnosis may be difficult in the mild case and in the absence of specific signs which may lead to a substantial diagnosis delay that can be pejorative in terms of prognosis. Practitioners should be aware of this possibility in infants from vegetarian mothers and children on a vegetarian diet who do not take supplements.

3.2.1. Newborns and Infants

The need for vitamin B12 is increased during pregnancy and lactation in relation to the expansion of tissues and supply to the fetus and the newborn [58,59]. When adhering to vegetarian diets for at least 3 years without supplementation, 22% of pregnant women have been shown to be vitamin B12 deficient [60]. Maternal vitamin B12 deficiency is associated with low birth weight in addition to an increased risk of pregnancy complications [61]. Cobalamin status in the first six months of life depends on maternal cobalamin status during pregnancy [55,62]. The offspring of vitamin B12-deficient mothers are usually asymptomatic at birth but may develop clinical signs at the age of 4–6 months [63]. Symptoms may include megaloblastic anemia, feeding difficulties, failure to thrive, irritability, muscular hypotonia, tremors and seizures, and impaired neurodevelopment which may be irreversible [61,63].

The cobalamin concentration of breast milk reflects maternal cobalamin concentration in blood [56]. The main nutritional deficit of breast milk from vegetarian and vegan mothers is that of vitamin B12 [64,65]. A vegetarian diet in the mother is the main cause (64% of cases) of vitamin B12 deficiency in breastfed infants [66]. In India, the country with the highest prevalence of vegetarians [67], 63.7% of 149 exclusively breastfed infants (3.1 ± 1 mo) had low levels of serum vitamin B12 (<200 pg/mL), but only 21% of them had a vegetarian mother [68]. Symptoms of cobalamin deficiency in breastfed infants are usually manifested between 4 to 8 months of age [56,69,70]. Numerous breastfed infants of vegetarian or vegan mothers have been reported to develop severe vitamin B12 deficiency with anemia, failure to thrive, hypotonia, developmental delay, microcephaly, and cerebral atrophy [69–73].

3.2.2. Children and Adolescents

The reported intakes of vitamin B12 in children are depicted in Figure 1. The more the diet restricts ASF intake and the longer the compliance with this restriction, the lower the intake [35,36,39–41,43,46–49,74,75].

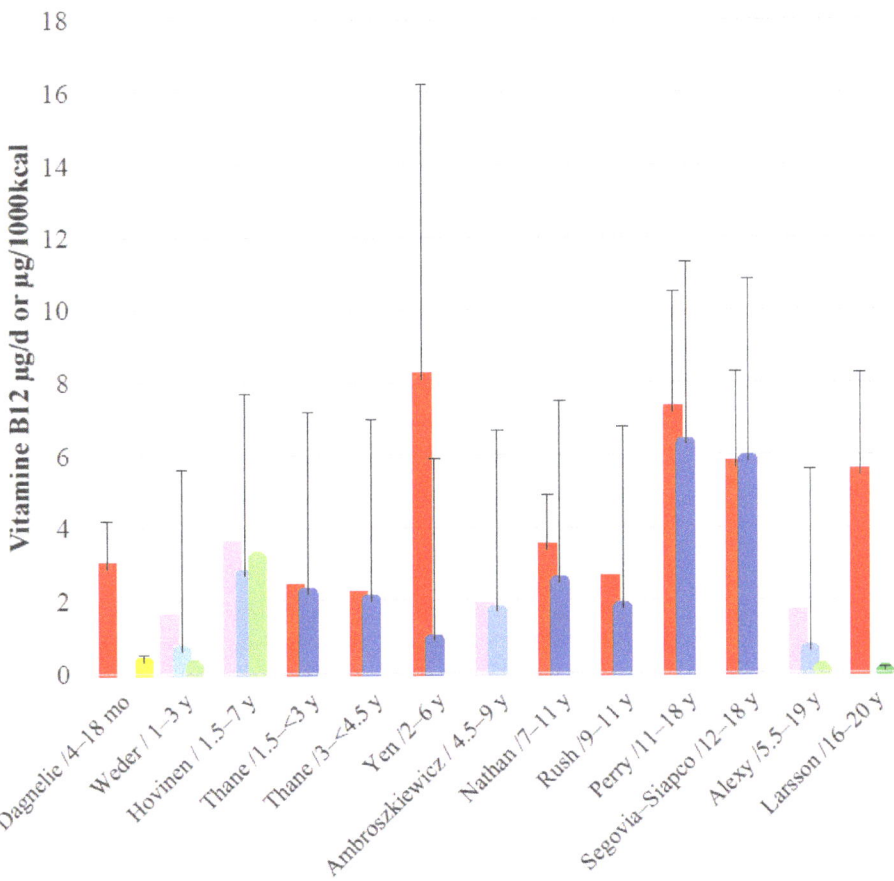

Figure 1. Bar chart to present the reported vitamin B12 intake in lacto-ovo-vegetarian (LOV), vegan or macrobiotic children compared to omnivorous counterparts [35,36,39–41,43,46–49,74,75]. The dark-colored bars display the mean with SD, when available, whereas the light-colored bars display the median value.

Many studies have confirmed the existence of a vitamin status deficiency in children by showing a low level of serum cobalamin, and/or an increase in plasma methylmalonic acid or homocysteine [35,74–78]. However, others failed to get the same results, probably due to not taking into account possible supplements, or a short duration of the restrictive diet [39,43,63,74,78,79]. Vitamin B12 deficiency develops slowly given that vitamin B12 may be stored in the liver [76]. Overall, the reported prevalence of vitamin B12 deficiency was 62% in pregnant vegetarians, 25–85% in vegetarian children, and 21–41% in vegetarian adolescents [80]. The greater prevalence of deficiency was in vegans and those who had adhered to a vegetarian diet since birth. Nearly 40% of 210 apparently healthy Indian children aged 6–23 months have been shown to be deficient in vitamin B12 (<210 pg/mL), especially since they had not consumed cow's milk for at least 6 months (OR 2.6, 95% CI 1.4–4.6) [81]. Severe vitamin B12 deficiency in children on a vegan diet and requiring hospitalization was reported in Italy [82]. In a macrobiotic community, 55% of children were vitamin B12-deficient according to their urinary methylmalonic acid [83]. Overall, deficiency symptoms are the same as those described above in infants [69,84]. In the Indian study enrolling 27 young children (6–27 months), anemia was found in 83%, developmental delay or regression in all, and cerebral atrophy was found in the 9 children who underwent neuroimaging [84]. Usually, an appropriate diagnosis of vitamin B12 deficiency is based on the coexistence of megaloblastic anemia with neurological disorders. However, given that folate intake is most of the time high in vegetarians, the pathognomonic haematologic characteristics of vitamin B12 deficiency may be masked [76,85].

4. Minerals

FPO are relatively rich in certain minerals such as potassium and magnesium but have variable content in zinc, copper, and selenium and only contain non-haeme iron with poor bioavailability [10,31,32,86]. Absorption of iron, zinc, and calcium is reduced by phytates and/or oxalates which are quite abundant in unrefined cereals, whole grains, and legumes [76,86–89]. However, due to its abundance in the human body, calcium is not considered a micronutrient [90–94]. Inadequate intake and/or poor bioavailability of these microminerals are the main cause of deficiency [90].

4.1. Iron

The main role of iron in the body is to ensure the oxygen-carrying capacity of hemoglobin and tissue oxygenation. Current knowledge on iron homeostasis, dietary intake, and prevention of iron deficiency has been recently addressed in this journal [86]. Inadequate intake of bioavailable iron may lead to depletion in body stores and iron deficiency which can be assessed by the measurement of serum ferritin in the absence of inflammation. Children are at particular risk of iron deficiency due to their rapid growth. Iron deficiency will precede the onset of iron deficiency anemia which can lead to poor neurodevelopment. Dietary iron intake and absorption are the main factors driving body iron status alongside blood losses. Most FPO have low iron content which is inorganic iron with low bioavailability (1–12%), without counting the possible iron leaching during cooking [86,88]. Iron bioavailability is moreover hampered by dietary fiber, and phytate but increased by vitamin C. Reported intakes, shown in Figure 2, were generally comparable or even higher in children following a vegetarian, a vegan, or a macrobiotic diet than in those omnivorous [35–37,39–42,44,46–49,74,95].

However, none of these studies considered iron bioavailability. As a consequence, when assessed, the iron store was shown reduced [35,36,38,39,42,44,48,74]. This is even though it is acknowledged that iron absorption is increased when iron status is deficient which leads to hepcidin suppression [86]. Few studies reported lower hemoglobin concentration [36,38]. Rare cases of iron deficiency anemia due to a vegetarian diet have been reported [41,44,96]. The risk of iron deficiency is increased in the event of an unfavorable socio-economic situation [86].

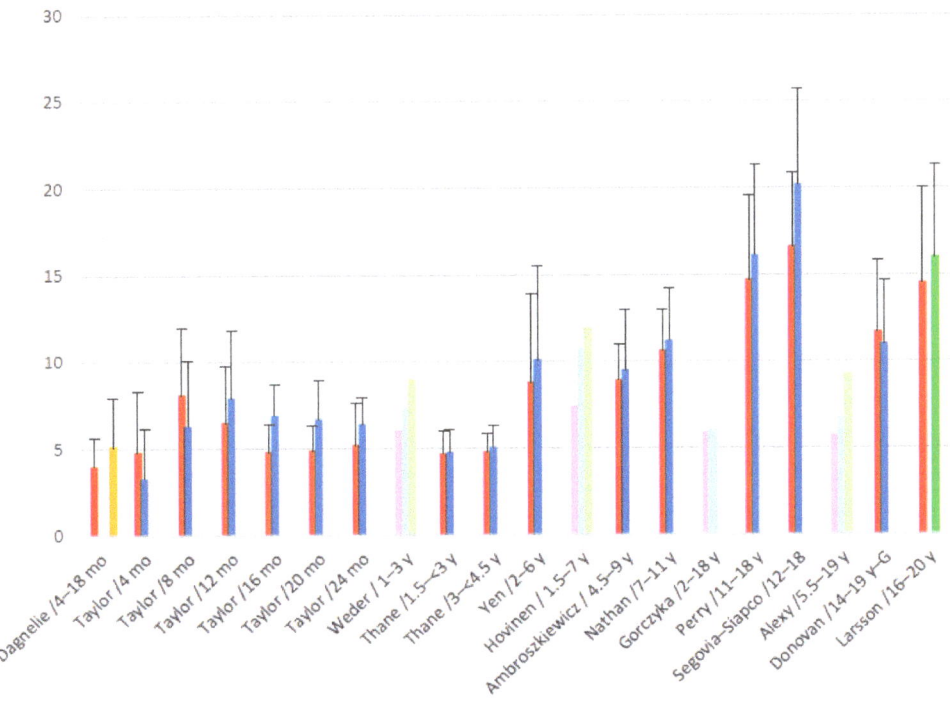

Figure 2. Bar chart presenting the reported iron intake in lacto-ovo-vegetarian (LOV) and vegan children compared to omnivorous counterparts [35–37,39–42,44,46–49,74,95]. The dark-colored bars display the mean with SD, when available, whereas the light-colored bars display the median value.

4.2. Zinc

Zinc provides the prosthetic group of several enzymes to assist in the most major metabolic pathways and is involved in the receptor proteins for vitamins A and D, as well as for thyroid and steroid hormones [87,97]. Worldwide, it has been estimated that 17% of the population may have inadequate zinc intake with a lower percentage in high-income countries than in low-income regions [98]. In this survey, on average 34.8 ± 20% of zinc intake was from ASF. The highest zinc content is found in oysters, shellfish, and red meat, whereas FPO providing the most zinc are whole grains, fortified cereals, pulses, nuts, and seeds [76,97]. However, as for iron, the rich content of phytate, oxalate, or fiber in FPO may interfere with zinc absorption [87,97]. Total dietary phytate and the phytate/zinc molar ratio were shown positively correlated with the risk of inadequate zinc intake (r = 0.62 and 0.92, respectively; $p < 0.01$) [98]. These considerations were not considered in the studies reported in Figure 3.

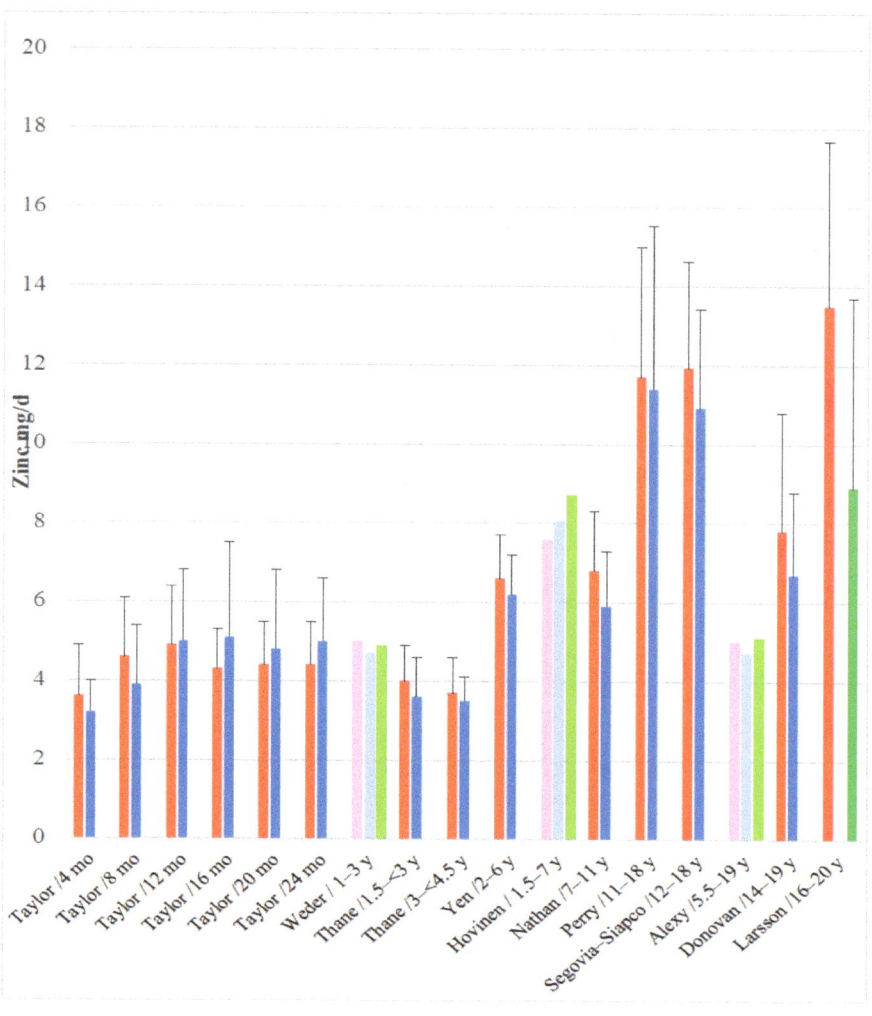

Figure 3. Bar chart to present the reported zinc intake in lacto-ovo-vegetarian (LOV) and vegan children compared to omnivorous counterparts [36,37,39–42,46–49,95]. The dark-colored bars display the mean with SD, when available, whereas the light-colored bars display the median value.

The reported intakes of vegetarian or vegan children were similar to that of omnivorous counterparts in most of these studies [37,39,40,42,47,49,95], with similar plasma zinc concentrations [39,47]. However, in three studies, the intake was lower in vegetarian children than in omnivores [36,41,46]. None of these studies reported clinical features of zinc deficiency but some case reports in young vegan children fed with plant milk [96]. The clinical setting of zinc deficiency may range from poor appetite and anorexia, decreased growth velocity, increased susceptibility to infection, diarrhea, depressed mood, and skin rashes at orifices [90].

4.3. Iodine

Iodine is a mandatory structural and functional element of thyroid hormones and, subsequently, has an important role in the growth, development of neurological, and cognitive functions [99,100]. The iodine concentration, as iodide, in water and foods is highly variable.

The main iodine sources are marine products, eggs, milk, and iodized salt. In meats as well as in FPO the iodine content depends on the richness of the soil of the food production region [90,94]. Adults who consume diets excluding iodine-rich foods have been shown to have an increased risk of iodine deficiency [100,101]. Studies assessing iodine intake in vegetarian children are scarce. A German study found that LOV children had lower intake than omnivores [49]. This was not found in a few Finnish young vegan children who also had similar iodine urine concentration to that of omnivores [47].

4.4. Other Microminerals

Although variably provided by plants, these micromineral intakes have very rarely been evaluated in vegetarian children. Apart from ASF, they may be mainly provided by grains legumes and seeds depending on the soil content [32,102]. Copper intake has been found to be similar or higher in vegetarian children in two studies [37,95]. Canadian LOV adolescents had higher manganese intake than their omnivorous counterparts [37]. Selenium intake in Swedish vegan adolescents were lower than that of omnivorous adolescents [41]. Apart from these few studies, no other study was found in particular regarding the intake of chromium or molybdenum.

5. Discussion and Recommendations

This review emphasizes that the more children are subjected to a diet restricted in ASF (vegan or macrobiotic), the more they are at risk of developing a deficiency in certain micronutrients. All micronutrients, especially vitamin B12 cannot be obtained in an adequate amount from non-ASF. Moreover, some such as carotenoids which can be found as precursors in FPO have a poor conversion to their active form (retinol) and others (e.g., iron and zinc) display low bioavailability. However available data from the studies carried out so far do not formally allow us to find a clear relationship between the diet, which can have diverse patterns, and the intake or the status of micronutrients. There are several reasons for this, some of which represent the limitations of this review, which should be acknowledged.

5.1. Limitations

Many of the reported studies are relatively old, with 53% of them conducted more than 25 years ago [35–41,77,95], and only a third less than 10 years ago [45–49,74,78]. All are observational studies, frequently enrolling a quite small number of children based on the voluntary participation of the parents. Parents who are likely to be concerned about their own health and that of their child and who are better able to practice a balanced diet and give supplements. The use of such supplements is rarely specified in the calculation of intake. Little information is provided about the duration of a vegetarian or a vegan diet in the various population groups, whereas there is inconsistency in the definition of vegetarianism, leading to a great heterogeneity in the vegetarian spectrum and a great dispersion in the results as shown in the figures. The heterogeneity of the results may also be linked to the use of different modes of assessment of intakes, which may use a food frequency questionnaire or a dietary record on one or three days. Moreover, most of the studies have been conducted in industrialized and high-income countries and neither socioeconomic status nor the environment was considered. Last but not least, very few studies have set the evidence of micronutrient shortfall by performing the appropriate tests in blood or urine samples and thus assessing the child's micronutrient status.

The nutritional adequacy of a vegetarian diet must be judged individually, given that a vegetarian diet can be composed in many different ways. On the other hand, in addition to the concern about micronutrients, other disadvantages, and risks must be analyzed. Of additional concern are energy, protein, n-3 long chain-polyunsaturated fatty acids, and calcium intake as well as protein quality and bone health.

5.2. Recommendations

From an ethical point of view, the food choice of parents must be respected, whatever the reason. Health professionals must inform parents of the possible risks of an ill-conceived vegetarian diet, but also of the possible benefits in terms of the health of a well-balanced diet. The diet and physical status of pregnant and nursing women and of children or adolescents following a restrictive diet must be carefully monitored and the help of a trained nutritionist may be needed. The main challenge for practitioners is to assess the risk of nutritional deficiency and to determine the need for laboratory tests.

In descending order, the most inappropriate ASF-restrictive diets are the macrobiotic, the vegan, the pescatarian, the lacto-vegetarian, the ovo-vegetarian, the LOV, and the flexitarian diets. A well-balanced LOV diet may be a healthy choice if the potential nutrient deficits are recognized and acted upon. Several dietary guidelines on vegetarian and vegan diets have been developed in this regard [103–107].

Vegan mothers, infants, and children may require supplementation with vitamin B12, iron, and zinc [76,107–111]. Exclusive breastfeeding is recommended for the 1st 4–6 months provided that the mother is supplemented with vitamin B12. Otherwise, an infant formula must be given, followed after the introduction of complementary food by a follow-on-formula, then a young child formula, which should be used as long as possible up to three years of age [112,113]. In cases of refusal of cow milk-based formulae, an alternative is a soya or hydrolyzed rice infant formula [114]. However, industrial or home-made preparations incorrectly named "plant-based milk", i.e., non-dairy beverages made from a water-based plant extract such as rice, soya, almond, coconut, grains, or other extracts must be strictly avoided because they are not suitable for feeding young children [96].

Complementary feeding should be carefully planned to ensure all critical nutrients are provided in agreement with current nutritional recommendations, and this is quite challenging [26,76,107,108,110,112,115–119]. It should include a wide variety of foods (grains, legumes, pulses, vegetables, fruit, nuts, and seeds). The use of iron- or bio-fortified food should be encouraged [76,86,110]. Apart from taking supplements, it is much more difficult or even impossible for vegans to ensure an adequate intake of vitamin B12 and iron. On the other hand, vitamin D supplementation should be recommended in all children, especially infants and adolescents, whatever their diet [51,53,54].

Parents and adolescents knowledge of nutrition, with which habits and beliefs interfere, determine their food choices according to the availability of certain foods and the subsequent nutrition adequacy of any one particular plant-based diet. This highlights the importance for health professionals to inform and advise families who follow a restrictive diet. Pregnant women, newborns, children, and adolescents with a vegetarian dietary pattern need medical supervision. The underlying problem is the frequent ignorance of the ins and outs of such diets and the solutions to be provided. This is the result of a lack of nutritional education and training in medical schools and postgraduate courses [118–122].

6. Conclusions

Since children's diets are largely driven by their parents, the prevalence of vegetarian diets during childhood is certainly on the rise parallel in industrialized countries. Maintenance of a vegetarian diet can be challenging. The risk of micronutrient deficiency in vegetarian children is relatively difficult to assert based on the current limitations of evidence due to the lack of well-designed studies. This means the need for more adequately powered trials to better identify any problems, which are not easy to conduct.

However, the risk of vitamin B12 deficiency must be considered in newborns from vegan or macrobiotic mothers and children with severe restrictions of ASF. Iron deficiency needs to be assessed individually in vegan children, as well as that of iodine and zinc. For this, some appropriate tests can be carried out, bearing in mind that the more restrictive the diet in ASF, the greater the risk. A LOV diet exposure is a low risk as long as it uses a very varied diet with a sufficient intake of dairy products and especially specific formula in infants and young children. Most of the deficiencies may be preventable through nutrition guidance and the consumption of a well-planned diet containing diverse foods, as well as food fortification and supplementation, where needed. On the other hand, it would be better to avoid vegan and macrobiotic diets during pregnancy and childhood. However, when it comes to micronutrients, special attention should be paid to vitamin B12, iron, zinc, iodine, and vitamin D.

Parents and teenagers must be informed of the serious consequences of failing to follow the advice and prescriptions regarding supplementation of the diet and the need for medical and dietic regular supervision.

Funding: This research received no external funding.

Institutional Review Board Statement: Not applicable.

Informed Consent Statement: Not applicable.

Data Availability Statement: Not applicable.

Conflicts of Interest: The author declares no conflict of interest.

Abbreviations

ASF   animal food sources
FPO   foods of plant origin
LOV   lacto-ovo-vegetarian

References

1. World Health Organization. Micronutrients. Geneva. 2022. Available online: https://www.who.int/health-topics/micronutrients#tab=tab_1 (accessed on 6 December 2022).
2. Black, R.E.; Victora, C.G.; Walker, S.P.; Bhutta, Z.A.; Christian, P.; de Onis, M.; Ezzati, M.; Grantham-McGregor, S.; Katz, J.; Martorell, R.; et al. Maternal and Child Nutrition Study Group. Maternal and child undernutrition and overweight in low-income and middle-income countries. *Lancet* **2013**, *382*, 427–451, Erratum in *Lancet* **2013**, *382*, 396. [CrossRef] [PubMed]
3. Christian, P.; Mullany, L.C.; Hurley, K.M.; Katz, J.; Black, R.E. Nutrition and maternal, neonatal, and child health. *Semin. Perinatol.* **2015**, *39*, 361–372, Erratum in *Semin. Perinatol* **2015**, *39*, 505. [CrossRef] [PubMed]
4. Mattei, D.; Pietrobelli, A. Micronutrients and Brain Development. *Curr. Nutr. Rep.* **2019**, *8*, 99–107. [CrossRef]
5. Inzaghi, E.; Pampanini, V.; Deodati, A.; Cianfarani, S. The Effects of Nutrition on Linear Growth. *Nutrients* **2022**, *14*, 1752. [CrossRef]
6. Murphy, S.P.; Allen, L.H. Nutritional importance of animal source foods. *J. Nutr.* **2003**, *133* (Suppl. S2), 3932S–3935S. [CrossRef] [PubMed]
7. Das, J.K.; Salam, R.A.; Mahmood, S.B.; Moin, A.; Kumar, R.; Mukhtar, K.; Lassi, Z.S.; Bhutta, Z.A. Food fortification with multiple micronutrients: Impact on health outcomes in general population. *Cochrane Database Syst. Rev* **2019**, *12*, CD011400. [CrossRef]
8. Koletzko, B.; Godfrey, K.M.; Poston, L.; Szajewska, H.; van Goudoever, J.B.; de Waard, M.; Brands, B.; Grivell, R.M.; Deussen, A.R.; Dodd, J.M.; et al. Nutrition During Pregnancy, Lactation and Early Childhood and its Implications for Maternal and Long-Term Child Health: The Early Nutrition Project Recommendations. *Ann. Nutr. Metab.* **2019**, *74*, 93–106. [CrossRef]
9. World Health Organization. Ambition and Action in Nutrition 2016–2025. Geneva. 2017. Licence: CC BY-NC-SA 3.0 IGO. Available online: https://apps.who.int/iris/bitstream/handle/10665/255485/9789241512435-eng.pdf?ua=1 (accessed on 6 December 2022).
10. Allen, L.H. To what extent can food-based approaches improve micronutrient status? *Asia. Pac. J. Clin. Nutr.* **2008**, *17* (Suppl. S1), 103–105.
11. Consalez, F.; Ahern, M.; Andersen, P.; Kjellevold, M. The Effect of the Meat Factor in Animal-Source Foods on Micronutrient Absorption: A Scoping Review. *Adv. Nutr.* **2022**, *13*, 2305–2315. [CrossRef]
12. Rudloff, S.; Bührer, C.; Jochum, F.; Kauth, T.; Kersting, M.; Körner, A.; Koletzko, B.; Mihatsch, W.; Prell, C.; Reinehr, T.; et al. Vegetarian diets in childhood and adolescence: Position paper of the nutrition committee, German Society for Paediatric and Adolescent Medicine (DGKJ). *Mol. Cell. Pediatr.* **2019**, *6*, 4. [CrossRef]

13. Bettinelli, M.E.; Bezze, E.; Morasca, L.; Plevani, L.; Sorrentino, G.; Morniroli, D.; Giannì, M.; Mosca, F. Knowledge of Health Professionals Regarding Vegetarian Diets from Pregnancy to Adolescence: An Observational Study. *Nutrients* **2019**, *11*, 1149. [CrossRef]
14. Kiely, M.E. Risks and benefits of vegan and vegetarian diets in children. *Proc. Nutr. Soc.* **2021**, *80*, 159–164. [CrossRef]
15. Bakaloudi, D.R.; Halloran, A.; Rippin, H.L.; Oikonomidou, A.C.; Dardavesis, T.I.; Williams, J.; Wickramasinghe, K.; Breda, J.; Chourdakis, M. Intake and adequacy of the vegan diet. A systematic review of the evidence. *Clin. Nutr.* **2021**, *40*, 3503–3521. [CrossRef] [PubMed]
16. Leitzmann, C. Vegetarian nutrition: Past, present, future. *Am. J. Clin. Nutr.* **2014**, *100* (Suppl. S1), 496S–502S. [CrossRef] [PubMed]
17. Appleby, P.N.; Key, T.J. The long-term health of vegetarians and vegans. *Proc. Nutr. Soc.* **2016**, *75*, 287–293. [CrossRef] [PubMed]
18. Mann, N.J. A brief history of meat in the human diet and current health implications. *Meat. Sci.* **2018**, *144*, 169–179. [CrossRef] [PubMed]
19. Chouraqui, J.P.; Turck, D.; Briend, A.; Darmaun, D.; Bocquet, A.; Feillet, F.; Frelut, M.L.; Girardet, J.P.; Guimber, D.; Hankard, R.; et al. Committee on Nutrition of the French Society of Pediatrics. Religious dietary rules and their potential nutritional and health consequences. *Int. J. Epidemiol.* **2021**, *50*, 12–26. [CrossRef]
20. Rosenfeld, D.L.; Burrow, A.L. Vegetarian on purpose: Understanding the motivations of plant-based dieters. *Appetite* **2017**, *116*, 456–463. [CrossRef]
21. IPSOS Mori. An Exploration into Diets around the World. 2018. Available online: https://www.ipsos.com/sites/default/files/ct/news/documents/2018-09/an_exploration_into_diets_around_the_world.pdf (accessed on 13 September 2022).
22. Godfray, H.C.J.; Aveyard, P.; Garnett, T.; Hall, J.W.; Key, T.J.; Lorimer, J.; Pierrehumbert, R.T.; Scarborough, P.; Springmann, M.; Jebb, S.A. Meat consumption, health, and the environment. *Science* **2018**, *361*, eaam5324. [CrossRef]
23. Milford, A.B.; Le Mouël, C.; Bodirsky, B.L.; Rolinski, S. Drivers of meat consumption. *Appetite* **2019**, *141*, 104313. [CrossRef]
24. Dorard, G.; Mathieu, S. Vegetarian and omnivorous diets: A cross-sectional study of motivation, eating disorders, and body shape perception. *Appetite* **2021**, *156*, 104972. [CrossRef] [PubMed]
25. Salter, A.M. The effects of meat consumption on global health. *Rev. Sci. Tech.* **2018**, *37*, 47–55. [CrossRef] [PubMed]
26. Baldassarre, M.E.; Panza, R.; Farella, I.; Posa, D.; Capozza, M.; Mauro, A.D.; Laforgia, N. Vegetarian and Vegan Weaning of the Infant: How Common and How Evidence-Based? A Population-Based Survey and Narrative Review. *Int. J. Environ. Res. Public Health* **2020**, *17*, 4835. [CrossRef]
27. Bivi, D.; Di Chio, T.; Geri, F.; Morganti, R.; Goggi, S.; Baroni, L.; Mumolo, M.G.; de Bortoli, N.; Peroni, D.G.; Marchi, S.; et al. Raising Children on a Vegan Diet: Parents' Opinion on Problems in Everyday Life. *Nutrients* **2021**, *13*, 1796. [CrossRef] [PubMed]
28. Kim, G.; Oh, J.; Cho, M. Differences between Vegetarians and Omnivores in Food Choice Motivation and Dietarian Identity. *Foods* **2022**, *11*, 539. [CrossRef]
29. Larsen, J.K.; Hermans, R.C.; Sleddens, E.F.; Engels, R.C.; Fisher, J.O.; Kremers, S.P. How parental dietary behavior and food parenting practices affect children's dietary behavior. Interacting sources of influence? *Appetite* **2015**, *89*, 246–257. [CrossRef]
30. Eurispes. Quanti Sono i Vegani in Italia? 2022. Available online: https://www.veganok.com/vegani-in-italia/ (accessed on 13 September 2022).
31. Clarys, P.; Deliens, T.; Huybrechts, I.; Deriemaeker, P.; Vanaelst, B.; De Keyzer, W.; Hebbelinck, M.; Mullie, P. Comparison of nutritional quality of the vegan, vegetarian, semi-vegetarian, pesco-vegetarian and omnivorous diet. *Nutrients* **2014**, *6*, 1318–1332. [CrossRef]
32. Rauma, A.L.; Mykkänen, H. Antioxidant status in vegetarians versus omnivores. *Nutrition* **2000**, *16*, 111–119. [CrossRef] [PubMed]
33. Meléndez-Martínez, A.J. An Overview of Carotenoids, Apocarotenoids, and Vitamin A in Agro-Food, Nutrition, Health, and Disease. *Mol. Nutr. Food. Res.* **2019**, *63*, e1801045; Erratum in: *Mol. Nutr. Food Res.* **2020**, *64*, e2070024. [CrossRef]
34. Hrubša, M.; Siatka, T.; Nejmanová, I.; Vopršalová, M.; Kujovská Krčmová, L.; Matoušová, K.; Javorská, L.; Macáková, K.; Mercolini, L.; Remião, F.; et al. Biological Properties of Vitamins of the B-Complex, Part 1: Vitamins B1, B2, B3, and B5. *Nutrients* **2022**, *14*, 484. [CrossRef]
35. Dagnelie, P.C.; van Staveren, W.A. Macrobiotic nutrition and child health: Results of a population-based, mixed-longitudinal cohort study in The Netherlands. *Am. J. Clin. Nutr.* **1994**, *59* (Suppl. S5), 1187S–1196S. [CrossRef]
36. Nathan, I.; Hackett, A.F.; Kirby, S. The dietary intake of a group of vegetarian children aged 7–11 years compared with matched omnivores. *Br. J. Nutr.* **1996**, *75*, 533–544. [CrossRef] [PubMed]
37. Donovan, U.M.; Gibson, R.S. Dietary intakes of adolescent females consuming vegetarian, semi–vegetarian, and omnivorous diets. *J. Adolesc. Health* **1996**, *18*, 292–300. [CrossRef]
38. Krajcovicová-Kudláčková, M.; Simoncic, R.; Béderová, A.; Grancicová, E.; Magálová, T. Influence of vegetarian and mixed nutrition on selected haematological and biochemical parameters in children. *Nahrung* **1997**, *41*, 311–314. [CrossRef] [PubMed]
39. Thane, C.W.; Bates, C.J. Dietary intakes and nutrient status of vegetarian preschool children from a British national survey. *J. Hum. Nutr. Diet.* **2000**, *13*, 149–162. [CrossRef]
40. Perry, C.L.; McGuire, M.T.; Neumark-Sztainer, D.; Story, M. Adolescent vegetarians: How well do their dietary patterns meet the healthy people 2010 objectives? *Arch. Pediatr. Adolesc. Med.* **2002**, *156*, 431–437. [CrossRef]
41. Larsson, C.L.; Johansson, G.K. Dietary intake and nutritional status of young vegans and omnivores in Sweden. *Am. J. Clin. Nutr.* **2002**, *76*, 100–106. [CrossRef] [PubMed]

42. Yen, C.E.; Yen, C.H.; Huang, M.C.; Cheng, C.H.; Huang, Y.C. Dietary intake and nutritional status of vegetarian and omnivorous preschool children and their parents in Taiwan. *Nutr. Res.* **2008**, *28*, 430–436. [CrossRef] [PubMed]
43. Yen, C.E.; Yen, C.H.; Cheng, C.H.; Huang, Y.C. Vitamin B-12 status is not associated with plasma homocysteine in parents and their preschool children: Lacto-ovo, lacto, and ovo vegetarians and omnivores. *J. Am. Coll. Nutr.* **2010**, *29*, 7–13. [CrossRef]
44. Gorczyca, D.; Prescha, A.; Szeremeta, K.; Jankowski, A. Iron status and dietary iron intake of vegetarian children from Poland. *Ann. Nutr. Metab.* **2013**, *62*, 291–297. [CrossRef]
45. Ambroszkiewicz, J.; Chełchowska, M.; Szamotulska, K.; Rowicka, G.; Klemarczyk, W.; Strucińska, M.; Gajewska, J. Bone status and adipokine levels in children on vegetarian and omnivorous diets. *Clin. Nutr.* **2019**, *38*, 730–737. [CrossRef] [PubMed]
46. Segovia-Siapco, G.; Sabaté, J. Health and sustainability outcomes of vegetarian dietary patterns: A revisit of the EPIC-Oxford and the Adventist Health Study-2 cohorts. *Eur. J. Clin. Nutr.* **2019**, *72* (Suppl. S1), 60–70; Erratum in *Eur. J. Clin. Nutr* **2019**, *73*, 968. [CrossRef] [PubMed]
47. Hovinen, T.; Korkalo, L.; Freese, R.; Skaffari, E.; Isohanni, P.; Niemi, M.; Nevalainen, J.; Gylling, H.; Zamboni, N.; Erkkola, M.; et al. Vegan diet in young children remodels metabolism and challenges the statuses of essential nutrients. *EMBO. Mol. Med.* **2021**, *13*, e13492. [CrossRef]
48. Alexy, U.; Fischer, M.; Weder, S.; Längler, A.; Michalsen, A.; Sputtek, A.; Keller, M. Nutrient Intake and Status of German Children and Adolescents Consuming Vegetarian, Vegan or Omnivore Diets: Results of the VeChi Youth Study. *Nutrients* **2021**, *13*, 1707. [CrossRef] [PubMed]
49. Weder, S.; Keller, M.; Fischer, M.; Becker, K.; Alexy, U. Intake of micronutrients and fatty acids of vegetarian, vegan, and omnivorous children (1–3 years) in Germany (VeChi Diet Study). *Eur. J. Nutr.* **2022**, *61*, 1507–1520. [CrossRef]
50. Braegger, C.; Campoy, C.; Colomb, V.; Decsi, T.; Domellof, M.; Fewtrell, M.; Hojsak, I.; Mihatsch, W.; Molgaard, C.; Shamir, R.; et al. ESPGHAN Committee on Nutrition. Vitamin D in the healthy European paediatric population. *J. Pediatr. Gastroenterol. Nutr.* **2013**, *56*, 692–701. [CrossRef] [PubMed]
51. Saggese, G.; Vierucci, F.; Prodam, F.; Cardinale, F.; Cetin, I.; Chiappini, E.; De' Angelis, G.L.; Massari, M.; Miraglia Del Giudice, E.; Miraglia Del Giudice, M.; et al. Vitamin D in pediatric age: Consensus of the Italian Pediatric Society and the Italian Society of Preventive and Social Pediatrics, jointly with the Italian Federation of Pediatricians. *Ital. J. Pediatr.* **2018**, *44*, 51. [CrossRef] [PubMed]
52. Liu, Z.; Huang, S.; Yuan, X.; Wang, Y.; Liu, Y.; Zhou, J. The role of vitamin D deficiency in the development of paediatric diseases. *Ann. Med.* **2023**, *55*, 127–135. [CrossRef]
53. Jullien, S. Vitamin D prophylaxis in infancy. *BMC Pediatr.* **2021**, *21* (Suppl. S1), 319. [CrossRef]
54. Bacchetta, J.; Edouard, T.; Laverny, G.; Bernardor, J.; Bertholet-Thomas, A.; Castanet, M.; Garnier, C.; Gennero, I.; Harambat, J.; Lapillonne, A.; et al. Vitamin D and calcium intakes in general pediatric populations: A French expert consensus paper. *Arch. Pediatr.* **2022**, *29*, 312–325. [CrossRef]
55. Chittaranjan, Y. Vitamin B12: An intergenerational story. *Nestle. Nutr. Inst. Workshop Ser.* **2020**, *93*, 91–102. [CrossRef] [PubMed]
56. Bjørke-Monsen, A.L.; Ueland, P.M. Cobalamin status in children. *J. Inherit. Metab. Dis.* **2011**, *34*, 111–119. [CrossRef] [PubMed]
57. Watanabe, F.; Yabuta, Y.; Tanioka, Y.; Bito, T. Biologically active vitamin B12 compounds in foods for preventing deficiency among vegetarians and elderly subjects. *J. Agric. Food Chem.* **2013**, *61*, 6769–6775. [CrossRef] [PubMed]
58. EFSA NDA Panel (EFSA Panel on Dietetic Products, Nutrition and Allergies). Scientific Opinion on Dietary Reference Values for cobalamin (vitamin B12). *EFSA J.* **2015**, *13*, 4150. [CrossRef]
59. Rizzo, G.; Laganà, A.S.; Rapisarda, A.M.; La Ferrera, G.M.; Buscema, M.; Rossetti, P.; Nigro, A.; Muscia, V.; Valenti, G.; Sapia, F.; et al. Vitamin B12 among vegetarians: Status, assessment and supplementation. *Nutrients* **2016**, *8*, 767. [CrossRef]
60. Koebnick, C.; Hoffmann, I.; Dagnelie, P.C.; Heins, U.A.; Wickramasinghe, S.N.; Ratnayaka, I.D.; Gruendel, S.; Lindemans, J.; Leitzmann, C. Long-term ovo-lacto vegetarian diet impairs vitamin B-12 status in pregnant women. *J. Nutr.* **2004**, *134*, 3319–3326. [CrossRef]
61. Finkelstein, J.L.; Layden, A.J.; Stover, P.J. Vitamin B-12 and Perinatal Health. *Adv. Nutr.* **2015**, *6*, 552–563. [CrossRef]
62. Varsi, K.; Ueland, P.M.; Torsvik, I.K.; Bjørke-Monsen, A.L. Maternal Serum Cobalamin at 18 Weeks of Pregnancy Predicts Infant Cobalamin Status at 6 Months-A Prospective, Observational Study. *J. Nutr.* **2018**, *148*, 738–745. [CrossRef]
63. Reischl-Hajiabadi, A.T.; Garbade, S.F.; Feyh, P.; Weiss, K.H.; Mütze, U.; Kölker, S.; Hoffmann, G.F.; Gramer, G. Maternal vitamin B12 deficiency detected by newborn screening—Evaluation of causes and characteristics. *Nutrients* **2022**, *14*, 3767. [CrossRef]
64. Perrin, M.T.; Pawlak, R.; Dean, L.L.; Christis, A.; Friend, L. A cross-sectional study of fatty acids and brain-derived neurotrophic factor (BDNF) in human milk from lactating women following vegan, vegetarian, and omnivore diets. *Eur. J. Nutr.* **2019**, *58*, 2401–2410. [CrossRef]
65. Karcz, K.; Królak-Olejnik, B. Vegan or vegetarian diet and breast milk composition—A systematic review. *Crit. Rev. Food Sci. Nutr.* **2021**, *61*, 1081–1098. [CrossRef]
66. Mathey, C.; Di Marco, J.N.; Poujol, A.; Cournelle, M.A.; Brevaut, V.; Livet, M.O.; Chabrol, B.; Michel, G. Stagnation pondérale et régression psychomotrice révélant une carence en vitamine B12 chez 3 nourrissons [Failure to thrive and psychomotor regression revealing vitamin B12 deficiency in 3 infants]. *Arch. Pediatr.* **2007**, *14*, 467–471. [CrossRef]
67. Sahgal, N.; Evans, J.; Salazar, A.M.; Starr, K.J.; Corichi, M. Religion in India: Tolerance and Segregation. 10: Religion and Food. Pew Research Center 2021. Available online: https://www.pewresearch.org/religion/2021/06/29/religion-and-food/ (accessed on 13 February 2023).

68. Kadiyala, A.; Palani, A.; Rajendraprasath, S.; Venkatramanan, P. Prevalence of vitamin B12 deficiency among exclusively breast fed term infants in South India. *J. Trop. Pediatr.* **2021**, *67*, fmaa114. [CrossRef]
69. Dubaj, C.; Czyż, K.; Furmaga-Jabłońska, W. Vitamin B12 deficiency as a cause of severe neurological symptoms in breast fed infant—A case report. *Ital. J. Pediatr.* **2020**, *46*, 40. [CrossRef]
70. Honzik, T.; Adamovicova, M.; Smolka, V.; Magner, M.; Hruba, E.; Zeman, J. Clinical presentation and metabolic consequences in 40 breastfed infants with nutritional vitamin B12 deficiency–what have we learned? *Eur. J. Paediatr. Neurol.* **2010**, *14*, 488–495. [CrossRef] [PubMed]
71. Kocaoglu, C.; Akin, F.; Caksen, H.; Böke, S.B.; Arslan, S.; Aygün, S. Cerebral atrophy in a vitamin B12-deficient infant of a vegetarian mother. *J. Health Popul. Nutr.* **2014**, *32*, 367–371. [PubMed]
72. Reghu, A.; Hosdurga, S.; Sandhu, B.; Spray, C. Vitamin B12 deficiency presenting as oedema in infants of vegetarian mothers. *Eur. J. Pediatr.* **2005**, *164*, 257–258. [CrossRef]
73. von Schenck, U.; Bender-Götze, C.; Koletzko, B. Persistence of neurological damage induced by dietary vitamin B-12 deficiency in infancy. *Arch. Dis. Child.* **1997**, *77*, 137–139. [CrossRef] [PubMed]
74. Ambroszkiewicz, J.; Klemarczyk, W.; Mazur, J.; Gajewska, J.; Rowicka, G.; Strucińska, M.; Chełchowska, M. Serum Hepcidin and Soluble Transferrin Receptor in the Assessment of Iron Metabolism in Children on a Vegetarian Diet. *Biol. Trace. Elem. Res.* **2017**, *180*, 182–190. [CrossRef] [PubMed]
75. Rush, E.C.; Chhichhia, P.; Hinckson, E.; Nabiryo, C. Dietary patterns and vitamin B(12) status of migrant Indian preadolescent girls. *Eur. J. Clin. Nutr* **2009**, *63*, 585–587. [CrossRef]
76. Agnoli, C.; Baroni, L.; Bertini, I.; Ciappellano, S.; Fabbri, A.; Papa, M.; Pellegrini, N.; Sbarbati, R.; Scarino, M.L.; Siani, V.; et al. Position paper on vegetarian diets from the working group of the Italian Society of Human Nutrition. *Nutr. Metab. Cardiovasc. Dis.* **2017**, *27*, 1037–1052. [CrossRef] [PubMed]
77. Schneede, J.; Dagnelie, P.C.; van Staveren, W.A.; Vollset, S.E.; Refsum, H.; Ueland, P.M. Methylmalonic acid and homocysteine in plasma as indicators of functional cobalamin deficiency in infants on macrobiotic diets. *Pediatr. Res.* **1994**, *36*, 194–201. [CrossRef] [PubMed]
78. Světnička, M.; Sigal, A.; Selinger, E.; Heniková, M.; El-Lababidi, E.; Gojda, J. Cross-Sectional Study of the Prevalence of Cobalamin Deficiency and Vitamin B12 Supplementation Habits among Vegetarian and Vegan Children in the Czech Republic. *Nutrients* **2022**, *14*, 535. [CrossRef] [PubMed]
79. Leung, S.S.; Lee, R.H.; Sung, R.Y.; Luo, H.Y.; Kam, C.W.; Yuen, M.P.; Hjelm, M.; Lee, S.H. Growth and nutrition of Chinese vegetarian children in Hong Kong. *J. Paediatr. Child. Health* **2001**, *37*, 247–253. [CrossRef]
80. Pawlak, R.; Parrott, S.J.; Raj, S.; Cullum-Dugan, D.; Lucus, D. How prevalent is vitamin B(12) deficiency among vegetarians? *Nutr. Rev.* **2013**, *71*, 110–117. [CrossRef]
81. Kalyan, G.B.; Mittal, M.; Jain, R. Compromised vitamin B12 status of Indian infants and toddlers. *Food. Nutr. Bull.* **2020**, *41*, 430–437. [CrossRef]
82. Ferrara, P.; Corsello, G.; Quattrocchi, E.; Dell'Aquila, L.; Ehrich, J.; Giardino, I.; Pettoello-Mantovani, M. Caring for Infants and Children Following Alternative Dietary Patterns. *J. Pediatr.* **2017**, *187*, 339–340.e1. [CrossRef]
83. Miller, D.R.; Specker, B.L.; Ho, M.L.; Norman, E.J. Vitamin B-12 status in a macrobiotic community. *Am. J. Clin. Nutr.* **1991**, *53*, 524–529. [CrossRef]
84. Goraya, J.S.; Kaur, S.; Mehra, B. Neurology of Nutritional Vitamin B12 Deficiency in Infants: Case Series from India and Literature Review. *J. Child. Neurol.* **2015**, *30*, 1387–1831. [CrossRef]
85. Johnson, M.A. If high folic acid aggravates vitamin B12 deficiency what should be done about it? *Nutr. Rev.* **2007**, *65*, 451–458. [CrossRef]
86. Chouraqui, J.P. Dietary Approaches to Iron Deficiency Prevention in Childhood-A Critical Public Health Issue. *Nutrients* **2022**, *14*, 1604. [CrossRef]
87. Willoughby, J.L.; Bowen, C.N. Zinc deficiency and toxicity in pediatric practice. *Curr. Opin. Pediatr.* **2014**, *26*, 579–584. [CrossRef]
88. Platel, K.; Srinivasan, K. Bioavailability of Micronutrients from Plant Foods: An Update. *Crit. Rev. Food Sci. Nutr.* **2016**, *56*, 1608–1619. [CrossRef] [PubMed]
89. Craig, W.J.; Mangels, A.R.; Fresán, U.; Marsh, K.; Miles, F.L.; Saunders, A.V.; Haddad, E.H.; Heskey, C.E.; Johnston, P.; Larson-Meyer, E.; et al. The Safe and Effective Use of Plant-Based Diets with Guidelines for Health Professionals. *Nutrients* **2021**, *13*, 4144. [CrossRef]
90. Krebs, N.F.; Hambidge, K.M. Trace elements. In *Nutrition in Pediatrics*, 5th ed.; Duggan, C., Watkins, J.B., Koletzko, B., Walker, W.A., Eds.; Peoples Medical Publishing House: Shelton, CT, USA, 2016; Volume 1, pp. 95–116.
91. Institute of Medicine. *Dietary Reference Intakes for Vitamin A, Vitamin K, Arsenic, Boron, Chromium, Copper, Iodine, Iron, Manganese, Molybdenum, Nickel, Silicon, Vanadium, and Zinc*; The National Academies Press: Washington, DC, USA, 2001. [CrossRef]
92. Mensink, G.B.; Fletcher, R.; Gurinovic, M.; Huybrechts, I.; Lafay, L.; Serra-Majem, L.; Szponar, L.; Tetens, I.; Verkaik-Kloosterman, J.; Baka, A.; et al. Mapping low intake of micronutrients across Europe. *Br. J. Nutr.* **2013**, *110*, 755–773. [CrossRef]
93. Weikert, C.; Trefflich, I.; Menzel, J.; Obeid, R.; Longree, A.; Dierkes, J.; Meyer, K.; Herter-Aeberli, I.; Mai, K.; Stangl, G.I.; et al. Vitamin and Mineral Status in a Vegan Diet. *Dtsch. Arztebl. Int.* **2020**, *117*, 575–582. [CrossRef]
94. Morris, A.L.; Mohiuddin, S.S. Biochemistry, *Nutrients*; StatPearls Publishing: Treasure Island, FL, USA, 2022. Available online: https://www.ncbi.nlm.nih.gov/books/NBK554545/ (accessed on 8 March 2023).

95. Taylor, A.; Redworth, E.W.; Morgan, J.B. Influence of diet on iron, copper, and zinc status in children under 24 months of age. *Biol. Trace. Elem. Res.* **2004**, *97*, 197–214. [CrossRef] [PubMed]
96. Le Louer, B.; Lemale, J.; Garcette, K.; Orzechowski, C.; Chalvon, A.; Girardet, J.P.; Tounian, P. Conséquences nutritionnelles de l'utilisation de boissons végétales inadaptées chez les nourrissons de moins d'un an [Severe nutritional deficiencies in young infants with inappropriate plant milk consumption]. *Arch. Pediatr.* **2014**, *21*, 483–488. [CrossRef]
97. Maywald, M.; Rink, L. Zinc in Human Health and Infectious Diseases. *Biomolecules* **2022**, *12*, 1748. [CrossRef]
98. Wessells, K.R.; Brown, K.H. Estimating the global prevalence of zinc deficiency: Results based on zinc availability in national food supplies and the prevalence of stunting. *PLoS ONE* **2012**, *7*, e50568. [CrossRef] [PubMed]
99. EFSA NDA Panel (EFSA Panel on Panel on Dietetic Products Nutrition and Allergies). Scientific Opinion on Dietary Reference Values for iodine. *EFSA J.* **2014**, *12*, 3660. [CrossRef]
100. Eveleigh, E.R.; Coneyworth, L.J.; Avery, A.; Welham, S.J.M. Vegans, Vegetarians, and Omnivores: How Does Dietary Choice Influence Iodine Intake? A Systematic Review. *Nutrients* **2020**, *12*, 1606. [CrossRef]
101. Groufh-Jacobsen, S.; Hess, S.Y.; Aakre, I.; Folven Gjengedal, E.L.; Blandhoel Pettersen, K.; Henjum, S. Vegans, Vegetarians and Pescatarians Are at Risk of Iodine Deficiency in Norway. *Nutrients* **2020**, *12*, 3555. [CrossRef] [PubMed]
102. Comerford, K.B.; Miller, G.D.; Reinhardt Kapsak, W.; Brown, K.A. The Complementary Roles for Plant-Source and Animal-Source Foods in Sustainable Healthy Diets. *Nutrients* **2021**, *13*, 3469. [CrossRef] [PubMed]
103. Messina, V.; Mangels, A.R. Considerations in planning vegan diets: Children. *J. Am. Diet. Assoc.* **2001**, *101*, 661–669. [CrossRef] [PubMed]
104. Richter, M.; Boeing, H.; Grünewald-Funk, D.; Heseker, H.; Kroke, A.; Leschik-Bonnet, E.; Oberritter, H.; Strohm, D.; Watzl, B. Vegan diet. Position of the German Nutrition Society (DGE). *Ernähr. Umsch.* **2016**, *63*, 92–102, Erratum in *Ernähr. Umsch.* **2016**, *63*, M262. [CrossRef]
105. Menal-Puey, S.; Marques-Lopes, I. Development of a food guide for the vegetarians of Spain. *J. Acad. Nutr. Diet.* **2017**, *117*, 1509–1516. [CrossRef]
106. Federal Commission for Nutrition (FCN). Vegan Diets: Review of Nutritional Benefits and Risks. Expert Report of the FCN. Bern: Federal Food Safety and Veterinary Office. 2018. Available online: https://www.blv.admin.ch/blv/en/home/das-blv/organisation/kommissionen/eek/vor-und-nachteile-vegane-ernaehrung.html (accessed on 13 February 2023).
107. Dietary Guidelines Advisory Committee. *Scientific Report of the 2020 Dietary Guidelines Advisory Committee: Advisory Report to the Secretary of Agriculture and the Secretary of Health and Human Services*; U.S. Department of Agriculture, Agricultural Research Service: Washington, DC, USA, 2020. Available online: https://www.dietaryguidelines.gov/sites/default/files/2020-07/ScientificReport_of_the_2020DietaryGuidelinesAdvisoryCommittee_first-print.pdf (accessed on 13 February 2023).
108. Van Winckel, M.; Vande Velde, S.; De Bruyne, R.; Van Biervliet, S. Clinical practice: Vegetarian infant and child nutrition. *Eur. J. Pediatr.* **2011**, *170*, 1489–1494. [CrossRef]
109. Melina, V.; Craig, W.; Levin, S. Position of the Academy of Nutrition and Dietetics: Vegetarian Diets. *J. Acad. Nutr. Diet.* **2016**, *116*, 1970–1980. [CrossRef]
110. Baroni, L.; Goggi, S.; Battaglino, R.; Berveglieri, M.; Fasan, I.; Filippin, D.; Griffith, P.; Rizzo, G.; Tomasini, C.; Tosatti, M.A.; et al. Vegan Nutrition for Mothers and Children: Practical Tools for Healthcare Providers. *Nutrients* **2018**, *11*, 5. [CrossRef]
111. Müller, P. Vegan diet in young children. *Nestle. Nutr. Inst. Workshop Ser.* **2020**, *93*, 103–110. [CrossRef] [PubMed]
112. Fewtrell, M.; Bronsky, J.; Campoy, C.; Domellöf, M.; Embleton, N.; Fidler Mis, N.; Hojsak, I.; Hulst, J.M.; Indrio, F.; Lapillonne, A.; et al. Complementary Feeding: A Position Paper by the European Society for Paediatric Gastroenterology, Hepatology, and Nutrition (ESPGHAN) Committee on Nutrition. *J. Pediatr. Gastroenterol. Nutr* **2017**, *64*, 119–132. [CrossRef] [PubMed]
113. Chouraqui, J.P.; Turck, D.; Tavoularis, G.; Ferry, C.; Dupont, C. The Role of Young Child Formula in Ensuring a Balanced Diet in Young Children (1–3 Years Old). *Nutrients* **2019**, *11*, 2213. [CrossRef]
114. Bocquet, A.; Dupont, C.; Chouraqui, J.P.; Darmaun, D.; Feillet, F.; Frelut, M.L.; Girardet, J.P.; Hankard, R.; Lapillonne, A.; Rozé, J.C.; et al. Committee on Nutrition of the French Society of Pediatrics (CNSFP). Efficacy and safety of hydrolyzed rice-protein formulas for the treatment of cow's milk protein allergy. *Arch. Pediatr.* **2019**, *26*, 238–246. [CrossRef]
115. Amit, M. Vegetarian diets in children and adolescents. *Paediatr. Child Health* **2010**, *15*, 303–314.
116. National Health and Medical Research Council. Eat for health—Australian dietary guidelines. 2013; 212p. Available online: https://www.eatforhealth.gov.au/sites/default/files/content/n55_australian_dietary_guidelines.pdf (accessed on 13 February 2023).
117. Gomes Silva, S.C.; Pinho, J.P.; Borges, C.; Teixeira Santos, C.; Santos, A.; Graça, A. Guidelines for a healthy vegetarian diet. In *National Programme for the Promotion of a Healthy Diet*; Direção-Geral da Saúde: Lisbon, Portugal, 2015; 45p. Available online: https://nutrimento.pt/activeapp/wp--content/uploads/2015/12/Guidelines-for-a-healthy-vegetarian-diet.pdf (accessed on 13 February 2023).
118. Patel, P.; Kassam, S. Evaluating nutrition education interventions for medical students: A rapid review. *J. Hum. Nutr. Diet.* **2022**, *35*, 861–871. [CrossRef] [PubMed]
119. STAGE (Strategic Technical Advisory Group of Experts); Duke, T.; AlBuhairan, F.S.; Agarwal, K.; Arora, N.K.; Arulkumaran, S.; Bhutta, Z.A.; Binka, F.; Castro, A.; Claeson, M.; et al. World Health Organization and knowledge translation in maternal, newborn, child and adolescent health and nutrition. *Arch. Dis. Child.* **2022**, *107*, 644–649. [CrossRef]

120. Kushner, R.F.; Van Horn, L.; Rock, C.L.; Edwards, M.S.; Bales, C.W.; Kohlmeier, M.; Akabas, S.R. Nutrition education in medical school: A time of opportunity. *Am. J. Clin. Nutr.* **2014**, *99* (Suppl. S5), 1167S–1173S. [CrossRef]
121. Bassin, S.R.; Al-Nimr, R.I.; Allen, K.; Ogrinc, G. The state of nutrition in medical education in the United States. *Nutr. Rev.* **2020**, *78*, 764–780. [CrossRef]
122. Villette, C.; Vasseur, P.; Lapidus, N.; Debin, M.; Hanslik, T.; Blanchon, T.; Steichen, O.; Rossignol, L. Vegetarian and Vegan Diets: Beliefs and Attitudes of General Practitioners and Pediatricians in France. *Nutrients* **2022**, *14*, 3101. [CrossRef]

Disclaimer/Publisher's Note: The statements, opinions and data contained in all publications are solely those of the individual author(s) and contributor(s) and not of MDPI and/or the editor(s). MDPI and/or the editor(s) disclaim responsibility for any injury to people or property resulting from any ideas, methods, instructions or products referred to in the content.

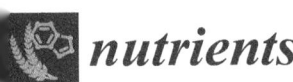

Article

Nutritional Effects of Removing a Serving of Meat or Poultry from Healthy Dietary Patterns—A Dietary Modeling Study

Sanjiv Agarwal [1,*], Kathryn R. McCullough [2] and Victor L. Fulgoni III [3]

1. NutriScience, LLC, East Norriton, PA 19403, USA
2. Foundation for Meat and Poultry Research and Education, Washington, DC 20036, USA; kmccullough@meatinstitute.org
3. Nutrition Impact, LLC, Battle Creek, MI 49014, USA; vic3rd@aol.com
* Correspondence: agarwal47@yahoo.com

Abstract: Meat and poultry are nutrient-dense sources of protein and typically are recommended as part of an overall healthy diet. The objective was to assess the nutritional impact of removing a serving of meat/poultry in Healthy Dietary Patterns (HDPs) using a similar approach to that used by the USDA for Dietary Guidelines for Americans. Composites of minimally processed and further processed meat and poultry were developed and their nutrient profiles were used to accomplish modeling by removing nutrients of each meat and poultry composite from the HDPs. The removal of a 3 oz (85 g) serving of meat or poultry resulted in decreases (10% or more from baseline) in protein and several key micronutrients including iron, phosphorus, potassium, zinc, selenium, thiamine, riboflavin, niacin, vitamin B_6, vitamin B_{12}, and choline as well as cholesterol and sodium in the HDPs, and the decreases were consistent for most nutrients with the removal of either minimally processed (fresh) or further processed meat or poultry and even after adjusting for changes in calories. In conclusion, the results of this dietary modeling study show that the removal of a meat and poultry serving from HDPs resulted in decreases in protein and several key nutrients.

Keywords: Healthy U.S.-Style Dietary Pattern; Healthy Mediterranean-Style Dietary Pattern; beef; pork; chicken; turkey; cold cut; frankfurter; sausages; bacon; protein; micronutrients

Citation: Agarwal, S.; McCullough, K.R.; Fulgoni, V.L., III. Nutritional Effects of Removing a Serving of Meat or Poultry from Healthy Dietary Patterns—A Dietary Modeling Study. *Nutrients* 2023, 15, 1717. https://doi.org/10.3390/nu15071717

Academic Editor: Alaa El-Din A. Bekhit

Received: 7 March 2023
Revised: 27 March 2023
Accepted: 28 March 2023
Published: 31 March 2023

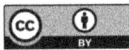

Copyright: © 2023 by the authors. Licensee MDPI, Basel, Switzerland. This article is an open access article distributed under the terms and conditions of the Creative Commons Attribution (CC BY) license (https:// creativecommons.org/licenses/by/ 4.0/).

1. Introduction

Meat, including poultry, is a major component of the US diet and is a predominant source of dietary protein [1]. Dietary Guidelines for Americans (DGA) 2020–2025 [2] and MyPlate [3] recommend the consumption of lean meat and poultry as part of an overall healthy diet. In the U.S., meat comprises a significant portion of the normal diet, contributing more than 15% to daily energy intake, 40% to daily protein intake, and 20% to daily fat intake [4], and over 70% of adults consume red meat or poultry with a mean intake of 14–15 lean oz equivalents (eq)/week [5].

Meat is a dense source of nutrients such as protein, iron, zinc, and B vitamins [6,7]. Animal-sourced protein foods, because of their higher protein quality, are more efficient sources of dietary protein than plant protein foods. Consumption of meat has been criticized from ethical, environmental, and health perspectives in scientific and popular media. However, the meat foods evaluated in these studies as well as the terminology used to describe meat foods in nutrition research has been inconsistent and varies in different studies [8,9]. Meat is generally defined as beef, veal, pork, lamb, and game meat; and poultry is defined as chicken, turkey, Cornish hens, duck, goose, quail, and pheasant (game birds) by USDA [10]. Cured meat (frankfurters, sausages, corned beef, cured ham, and luncheon meat that are made from beef, pork, or poultry) is usually considered a separate food category [10]. While red meat and processed meat have been associated with a variety of chronic diseases in observational studies [11–13], minimally processed meat and poultry were not associated with chronic disease risk or related mortality [14,15].

To help guide individuals in healthy eating, the USDA developed Healthy Food Patterns and released them as part of DGA 2015–2020 [16] and updated them as Healthy Dietary Patterns for release as part of DGA 2020–2025 [2]. These patterns include the characteristics of healthy eating with details on how to follow the DGA guidance within caloric needs, and these can be used by all individuals for meal planning. Three Healthy Dietary Patterns are developed: (1) The Healthy U.S.-Style Dietary Pattern (USP), which is the primary dietary pattern of the USDA based on food types and the proportions Americans typically consume; (2) The Healthy Mediterranean-Style Dietary Pattern (MSP) which more closely reflects Mediterranean-style diets that are associated with positive health outcomes in studies; and (3) the Healthy Vegetarian Dietary Pattern (VDP) to more closely reflect the eating patterns of vegetarians. These Healthy Dietary Patterns are based on the types and proportions of foods Americans of all ages, genders, races, and ethnicities typically consume, but in nutrient-dense forms, and appropriate amounts and servings of lean meat, poultry, and eggs are included as part of protein foods in USP and MSP. DGA 2020–2025 [2] also suggest that a healthy dietary pattern is associated with beneficial outcomes for all-cause mortality, cardiovascular disease, overweight and obesity, type 2 diabetes, bone health, and certain types of cancer (i.e., breast and colorectal).

However, there is a strong push among scientific advocacy groups and policy makers to limit animal-sourced food products in the diet primarily due to environmental concerns [17–22]. Therefore, the aim of this analysis was to examine the potential unintended consequences of limiting meat and poultry by modeling the effect of removing a serving of meat and poultry on nutrient profiles of the healthy dietary patterns identified in the Dietary Guidelines for Americans, 2020–2025, and to assess whether the modeled changes lead to meaningful changes in intake.

2. Materials and Methods

To achieve the objective of this study, four different minimally and further processed meat and poultry composites were developed using a total of 397 food codes in 10 food categories [10] using a similar modeling approach as that used by the USDA. The foods were grouped into minimally processed and further processed foods, and further into meat (beef and pork) and poultry (chicken and turkey). These groups are consistent with the meat science classification of meat products [23]. Minimally processed meat and poultry items include raw, uncooked products that have not been significantly altered compositionally and contain no added ingredients, but may have been reduced in size by fabrication, mincing, grinding, and/or a meat recovery system. Further processed meat and poultry items include those that undergo a transformation beyond minimal processing, contain approved ingredients, and may be subject to a preservation or processing step(s) including salting, curing, fermentation, thermal processing (smoking and cooking), batter/breading, or other processes to enhance sensory, quality, and safety attributes. One or two representative food codes were selected in each category, similar to the approach used by the USDA, and proportions of different foods in a category were based on their population-weighted consumptions for NHANES 2017–2018 participants ($n = 7036$; age 2+ years) [24]. The meat composite used in USDA's Healthy Dietary Patterns [25] was also used as an additional meat option. The following composites were developed and further details are provided in Table 1:

- Meat composite used in USDA's Healthy Dietary Patterns: USDA meat
- Minimally processed meat: 69.30% Beef; and 30.70% Pork
- Minimally processed poultry: 87.73% Chicken; and 12.27% Turkey.
- Further processed meat: 13.27% Beef; 5.09% Pork; and 81.64% Cold cuts/bacon/frankfurters/sausages
- Further processed poultry: 82.49% Chicken; and 17.51% Cold cuts/bacon/frankfurters/sausages.

Table 1. Composition of meat and poultry composites.

Composites	Proportion (%)
USDA Meat Meat composite used in USDA's Healthy Dietary Patterns	100.00
• 23.71% Beef	
• 27.12% Beef, ground	
• 12.76% Pork, fresh	
• 6.35% Pork, cured	
• 6.62% Sausage	
• 8.75% Luncheon meats and bacon, beef	
• 12.34% Luncheon meats and bacon, pork	
• 2.35% Others (game meat, lamb and liver)	
Minimally processed meat Minimally processed beef (total 38 WWEIA food codes in WWEIA categories 2002 and 2004)	69.30
• 83.85% Beef steak, broiled or baked, lean only eaten (WWEIA food code 21101130)	
• 16.15% Beef steak, fried, lean only eaten (WWEIA food code 21102130)	
Minimally processed pork (total 41 WWEIA food codes in WWEIA category 2006)	30.70
• 100% Pork chop, broiled or baked, lean only eaten (WWEIA food code 22101120)	
Minimally processed poultry Minimally processed chicken (total 73 WWEIA food codes in WWEIA categories 2202 and 2204)	87.73
• 53.25% Chicken breast, grilled without sauce, skin not eaten (WWEIA food code 24123301)	
• 39.06% Chicken breast, baked, broiled, or roasted, skin not eaten, from raw (WWEIA food code 24122131)	
• 7.69% Chicken drumstick, sauteed, skin not eaten (WWEIA food code 24144301)	
Minimally processed turkey (total 26 WWEIA food codes in WWEIA category 2206)	12.27
• 100% Turkey, light meat, roasted, skin not eaten (WWEIA food code 24201120)	
Further processed meat Further processed Beef (total 10 WWEIA food codes in WWEIA categories 2002 and 2004)	13.27
• 20.90% Beef steak, battered, fried, NS as to fat eaten (WWEIA food code 21104110)	
• 79.10% Ground beef patty, cooked (FDC ID 173113)	
Further processed pork (total 17 WWEIA food codes in WWEIA category 2006)	5.09
• 75.05% Pork chop, breaded or floured, broiled or baked, lean only eaten (WWEIA food code 22101150)	
• 24.95% Pork, spareribs, barbecued, with sauce, lean only eaten (WWEIA food code 22701050)	
Cold cuts, bacon, frankfurters & sausages (total 84 WWEIA food codes in WWEIA categories 2602, 2604, 2606 and 2608)	81.64
• 46.29% Ham, prepackaged or deli, luncheon meat, reduced sodium (WWEIA food code 25230220)	
• 18.05% Pork bacon, NS as to fresh, smoked or cured, reduced sodium, cooked (WWEIA food code 22600210)	
• 27.27% Frankfurter or hot dog, beef, reduced fat or light (WWEIA food code 25210620)	
• 8.39% Pork sausage, reduced sodium (WWEIA food code 25221408)	
Further processed poultry Further processed Chicken/Turkey (total 91 WWEIA food codes in WWEIA categories 2202, 2204 and 2206)	82.49
• 34.54% Chicken breast, grilled with sauce, skin not eaten (WWEIA food code 24123311)	
• 15.27% Chicken breast, rotisserie, skin not eaten (WWEIA food code 24122171)	
• 50.18% Chicken nuggets, from fast food (WWEIA food code 24198731)	
Cold cuts, bacon frankfurters & sausages (total 15 WWEIA food codes in WWEIA categories 2602, 2604, 2606 and 2608)	17.51
• 80.11% Turkey, prepackaged or deli, luncheon meat, reduced sodium (WWEIA food code 25230785)	
• 8.30% Turkey bacon, reduced sodium, cooked (WWEIA food code 24208510)	
• 4.94% Frankfurter or hot dog, chicken (WWEIA food code 25210310)	
• 6.65% Turkey or chicken sausage, reduced sodium (WWEIA food code 25221855)	

USDA meat composite details were obtained from the Food Pattern Modeling Report [25]. Proportions of different foods in minimally processed and further processed meat and poultry composites were based on the population-weighted consumptions for NHANES 2017–2018 participants (n = 7036; age 2+ years). WWEIA: What We Eat in America; NS: not specified; FDC: Food data central.

The nutrient profile for the meat composite used by the USDA was obtained from the Food Pattern Modeling Report [25]. Nutrient profiles for all representative meat and poultry foods (except for ground beef) were obtained from USDA's Food and Nutrient Database for dietary Studies (FNDDS) 2017–2018 specific for NHANES 2017–2018 [26]. Nutrient profile for ground beef (FDC ID 173113, Beef, ground, 97% lean meat /3% fat, patty, cooked, pan-broiled) was obtained using USDA Food Data Central [27]. Nutrient profiles for meat and poultry composites were computed by adding the nutrients of component foods in the proportions as described above and are presented in Table 2.

Table 2. Nutrient profiles per 3 oz (85 g) of meat and poultry composites.

	USDA Meat	Minimally Processed Meat	Minimally Processed Poultry	Further Processed Meat	Further Processed Poultry
Macronutrients					
Energy (kcal)	131	151.27	140.99	166.62	186.43
Protein (g)	20.8	24.83	24.93	18.21	16.73
Total fat (g)	4.38	5.17	3.84	8.51	9.68
Carbohydrate (g)	0.84	0.02	0.00	3.37	7.52
Dietary fiber (g)	0.03	0.00	0.00	0.05	0.37
Cholesterol (mg)	60.2	68.89	81.86	51.56	55.55
Saturated fatty acids (g)	1.44	1.96	0.78	2.79	1.81
Monounsaturated fatty acids (g)	1.74	2.23	1.20	3.67	3.60
Polyunsaturated fatty acids (g)	0.42	0.32	0.88	1.09	2.89
Minerals					
Calcium (mg)	7.41	11.00	6.60	7.86	10.87
Iron (mg)	1.65	1.54	0.44	0.98	0.54
Magnesium (mg)	18.4	21.91	23.72	19.78	20.19
Phosphorus (mg)	191	215.73	191.60	231.02	202.85
Potassium (mg)	279	345.56	284.54	372.02	257.44
Sodium (mg)	299	364.91	318.69	625.03	461.27
Zinc (mg)	3.45	3.92	0.94	2.21	0.65
Copper (mg)	0.15	0.07	0.04	0.09	0.04
Selenium (µg)	24.1	33.18	25.52	28.52	16.71
Vitamins					
Vitamin A, RAE (µg)	41.5	0.59	6.86	2.53	4.58
Vitamin E, ATE (mg)	0.21	0.23	0.63	0.29	0.73
Vitamin D (µg)	0.28	0.16	0.03	0.39	0.11
Vitamin C (mg)	0.09	0.00	0.00	0.06	0.53
Thiamin (mg)	0.18	0.20	0.07	0.26	0.07
Riboflavin (mg)	0.18	0.21	0.18	0.21	0.15
Niacin (mg)	4.89	6.91	8.55	5.49	6.24
Vitamin B_6 (mg)	0.33	0.55	0.70	0.31	0.32
Vitamin B_{12} (µg)	1.74	1.32	0.23	0.67	0.24
Total choline (mg)	78.0	75.05	64.65	66.28	41.12
Vitamin K (µg)	0.90	0.88	1.28	2.21	3.57
Folate, DFE (µg)	NA	4.72	6.09	6.75	8.86

The nutritional profile of USDA meat was obtained from the Food Pattern Modeling Report [25]. Nutrients profiles for all representative meat and poultry foods (except for ground beef) were obtained from USDA's Food and Nutrient Database for dietary Studies (FNDDS) 2017–2018 specific for NHANES 2017–2018 [26]. Nutrient profile for ground beef (FDC ID 173113) was obtained using USDA Food Data Central [27]. Nutrient profiles for meat and poultry composites per 3 oz (85 g) were computed by adding the nutrients of component foods in the proportions as presented in Table 1 (for example: nutrient profile for minimally processed meat was computed as 69.30% minimally processed beef (83.85% Beef steak, broiled or baked, lean only eaten + 16.15% Beef steak, fried, lean only eaten) + 30.70% minimally processed pork (Pork chop, broiled or baked, lean only eaten)). ATE: alpha tocopherol equivalents; DFE, dietary folate equivalents; RAE: retinol activity equivalents.

Base nutritional profiles of Heathy Dietary Patterns: USP and MSP for 2000 kcal were obtained from the Food Pattern Modeling Report [25]. Dietary modeling was accomplished by removing nutrients of a 3 oz (85 g) serving of each meat and poultry composite from the Healthy Dietary Patterns (USP and MSP), and modified nutrient profiles were created using Microsoft Excel (Version 2019, Microsoft, Inc., Redmond, WA, USA). Additional modeling approaches were conducted where calories and nutrients were increased from the rest of the diet to match the baseline calories, thus providing an isocaloric removal of meat and poultry servings (i.e., showing the impact of removing meat and poultry and allowing the remaining diet to increase to meet the planned calorie level). To accomplish this, each nutrient value after removal of the meat and poultry composite was multiplied by the baseline calories and divided by the modified calories (Isocaloric nutrient value = {(baseline nutrient value − composite nutrient value) ÷ (baseline calorie value − composite calorie value)} × baseline calorie value). Basically, all the foods in the existing dietary pattern are increased proportionally to the number of calories of meat removed. A change of 10% or more in nutrients due to dietary modeling analyses of Healthy Dietary Patterns was used as an indicator of meaningful differences.

3. Results

Removal of a 3 oz (85 g) serving of USDA meat composite from USP resulted in a decrease in protein (−23%), iron (−11%), phosphorus (−12%), zinc (−27%), copper (−11%), selenium (−21%), thiamine (10%), niacin (−21%), vitamin B_6 (−15%), vitamin B_{12} (−28%), and choline (−22%) (Table 3). Additionally, cholesterol and sodium also decreased (−28% and −18%, respectively) by removing a 3 oz (85 g) serving of meat. However, the decreases for iron, phosphorus, copper, thiamin, and B_6 were attenuated and became less than 10% from the baseline in the isocaloric scenario (Table 3). Identical results were obtained when a 3 oz (85 g) serving of meat was removed from MSP except that the decrease in thiamin was always less than 10% from the baseline (Table 3).

Table 3. Energy and nutrients in 2000 kcal Healthy Dietary Patterns before and after removal of a 3 oz (85 g) serving of USDA meat.

	2000 kcal Healthy US-Style Pattern			2000 kcal Healthy Mediterranean Style Pattern		
	Baseline	After Removal of 3 oz (85 g) Serving of USDA Meat	After Isocaloric Removal of 3 oz (85 g) Serving of USDA Meat	Baseline	After Removal of 3 oz (85 g) Serving of USDA Meat	After Isocaloric Removal of 3 oz (85 g) Serving of USDA Meat
Macronutrients						
Energy (kcal)	2001	1870	2001	2085	1954	2085
Protein (g)	92	71.2 *	76.2 *	99	78.2 *	83.4 *
Total fat (g)	71	66.6	71.3	72	67.6	72.2
Carbohydrate (g)	259	258	276	271	270	288
Dietary fiber (g)	30	30.0	32.1	31	31.0	33.0
Cholesterol (mg)	214	154 *	165 *	237	177 *	189 *
Saturated fatty acids (g)	18	16.6	17.7	18	16.6	17.7
Monounsaturated fatty acids (g)	25	23.3	24.9	26	24.3	25.9
Polyunsaturated fatty acids (g)	22	21.6	23.1	23	22.6	24.1
Minerals						
Calcium (mg)	1278	1271	1360	1297	1290	1376
Iron (mg)	14	12.4 *	13.2	15	13.4 *	14.2
Magnesium (mg)	358	340	363	377	359	383
Phosphorus (mg)	1654	1463 *	1566	1740	1549 *	1653
Potassium (mg)	3390	3111	3329	3628	3349	3574
Sodium (mg)	1658	1359 *	1454 *	1740	1441 *	1538 *
Zinc (mg)	13	9.55 *	10.2 *	13	9.6 *	10.2 *
Copper (mg)	1.4	1.25 *	1.34	1.5	1.35 *	1.44
Selenium (µg)	113	88.9 *	95.1 *	127	103 *	110 *

Table 3. Cont.

	2000 kcal Healthy US-Style Pattern			2000 kcal Healthy Mediterranean Style Pattern		
	Baseline	After Removal of 3 oz (85 g) Serving of USDA Meat	After Isocaloric Removal of 3 oz (85 g) Serving of USDA Meat	Baseline	After Removal of 3 oz (85 g) Serving of USDA Meat	After Isocaloric Removal of 3 oz (85 g) Serving of USDA Meat
Vitamins						
Vitamin A, RAE (µg)	898	857	917	914	873	931
Vitamin E, ATE (mg)	10	9.79	10.5	11	10.8	11.5
Vitamin D (µg)	7.5	7.22	7.72	9	8.72	9.30
Vitamin C (mg)	129	129	138	145	145	155
Thiamin (mg)	1.8	1.62 *	1.73	1.9	1.72	1.84
Riboflavin (mg)	2	1.82	1.95	2	1.82	1.94
Niacin (mg)	23	18.1 *	19.4 *	25	20.1 *	21.5 *
Vitamin B_6 (mg)	2.2	1.87 *	2.00	2.3	1.97 *	2.10
Vitamin B_{12} (µg)	6.2	4.46 *	4.77 *	7.3	5.56 *	5.93 *
Total choline (mg)	355	277 *	296 *	378	300 *	320 *
Vitamin K (µg)	140	139	149	142	141	151
Folate, DFE (µg)	513	NA	NA	527	NA	NA

Baseline nutritional profiles of 2000 kcal Heathy Dietary Patterns were obtained from Food Pattern Modeling Report [25]. Nutrient profiles after removal of USDA meat were computed by removing the nutrients of USDA meat (Table 2) from the nutrients of the Healthy Dietary Patterns. Calories were adjusted from the rest of the diet to match the baseline calories in the isocaloric removal of USDA meat. ATE: alpha tocopherol equivalents; DFE: dietary folate equivalents; RAE: retinol activity equivalents. * Indicates ≥10% change from baseline.

Removal of a 3 oz (85 g) serving of minimally processed meat from USP resulted in decreases in protein (−27%), iron (−11%), phosphorus (−13%), potassium (−10%), zinc (−30%), selenium (−29%), thiamine (11%), riboflavin (−11%), niacin (−30%), vitamin B_6 (−25%), vitamin B_{12} (−21%), and choline (−21%) (Table 4). Additionally, cholesterol, saturated fat, and sodium also decreased (−32%, −11%, and −22%, respectively) by removing a 3 oz (85 g) serving of minimally processed meat. However, the decreases for iron, phosphorus, potassium, thiamin, riboflavin, and saturated fat were attenuated and became less than 10% from baseline in the isocaloric scenario (Table 4). Identical results were obtained when a 3 oz (85 g) serving of minimally processed meat was removed from MSP (Table 4).

Table 4. Energy and nutrients in 2000 kcal Healthy Dietary Patterns before and after removal of a 3 oz (85 g) serving of minimally processed meat.

	2000 kcal Healthy US-Style Pattern			2000 kcal Healthy Mediterranean Style Pattern		
	Baseline	After Removal of 3 oz (85 g) Serving of Minimally Processed Meat	After Isocaloric Removal of 3 oz (85 g) Serving of Minimally Processed Meat	Baseline	After Removal of 3 oz (85 g) Serving of Minimally Processed Meat	After Isocaloric Removal of 3 oz (85 g) Serving of Minimally Processed Meat
Macronutrients						
Energy (kcal)	2001	1850	2001	2085	1934	2085
Protein (g)	92	67.2 *	72.7 *	99	74.2 *	80 *
Total fat (g)	71	65.8	71.2	72	66.8	72.1
Carbohydrate (g)	259	259	280	271	271	292
Dietary fiber (g)	30	30.0	32.5	31	31.0	33.4
Cholesterol (mg)	214	145 *	157 *	237	168 *	181 *
Saturated fatty acids (g)	18	16.0 *	17.4	18	16.0 *	17.3
Monounsaturated fatty acids (g)	25	22.8	24.6	26	23.8	25.6
Polyunsaturated fatty acids (g)	22	21.7	23.4	23	22.7	24.4

Table 4. *Cont.*

	2000 kcal Healthy US-Style Pattern			2000 kcal Healthy Mediterranean Style Pattern		
	Baseline	After Removal of 3 oz (85 g) Serving of Minimally Processed Meat	After Isocaloric Removal of 3 oz (85 g) Serving of Minimally Processed Meat	Baseline	After Removal of 3 oz (85 g) Serving of Minimally Processed Meat	After Isocaloric Removal of 3 oz (85 g) Serving of Minimally Processed Meat
Minerals						
Calcium (mg)	1278	1267	1371	1297	1286	1387
Iron (mg)	14	12.5 *	13.5	15	13.5 *	14.5
Magnesium (mg)	358	336	364	377	355	383
Phosphorus (mg)	1654	1438 *	1556	1740	1524 *	1644
Potassium (mg)	3390	3044 *	3293	3628	3282 *	3539
Sodium (mg)	1658	1293 *	1399 *	1740	1375 *	1483 *
Zinc (mg)	13	9.08 *	9.83 *	13	9.08 *	9.79 *
Copper (mg)	1.4	1.33	1.44	1.5	1.43	1.55
Selenium (µg)	113	79.8 *	86.3 *	127	93.8 *	101 *
Vitamins						
Vitamin A, RAE (µg)	898	897	971	914	913	985
Vitamin E (ATE) (mg)	10	9.77	10.57	11	10.8	11.6
Vitamin D (µg)	7.5	7.34	7.94	9	8.84	9.53
Vitamin C (mg)	129	129	140	145	145	156
Thiamin (mg)	1.8	1.60 *	1.73	1.9	1.70 *	1.83
Riboflavin (mg)	2	1.79 *	1.94	2	1.79 *	1.93
Niacin (mg)	23	16.1 *	17.4 *	25	18.1 *	19.5 *
Vitamin B_6 (mg)	2.2	1.65 *	1.78 *	2.3	1.75 *	1.89 *
Vitamin B_{12} (µg)	6.2	4.88 *	5.28 *	7.3	5.98 *	6.45 *
Total choline (mg)	355	280 *	303 *	378	303 *	327 *
Vitamin K (µg)	140	139	150	142	141	152
Folate, DFE (µg)	513	508	550	527	522	563

Baseline nutritional profiles of 2000 kcal Heathy Dietary Patterns were obtained from Food Pattern Modeling Report [25]. Nutrient profiles after the removal of minimally processed meat were computed by subtracting the nutrients of minimally processed meat (Table 2) from the nutrients of the Healthy Dietary Patterns. Calories were adjusted from the rest of the diet to match the baseline calories in the isocaloric removal of minimally processed meat. ATE: alpha tocopherol equivalents; DFE, dietary folate equivalents; RAE: retinol activity equivalents. * Indicates ≥10% change from baseline.

Removal of a 3 oz (85 g) serving of minimally processed poultry from USP resulted in decreases in protein (−27%), phosphorus (−12%), selenium (−23%), niacin (−37%), vitamin B_6 (−32%), and choline (−18%) (Table 5). Additionally, cholesterol and sodium also decreased (−38% and −19%, respectively) by removing a 3 oz (85 g) serving of minimally processed poultry. However, the decrease in phosphorus was attenuated and became less than 10% from the baseline in the isocaloric scenario (Table 5). Identical results were obtained when a 3 oz (85 g) serving of minimally processed poultry was removed from MSP (Table 5).

Removal of a 3 oz (85 g) serving of further processed meat from USP resulted in decreases in protein (−20%), MUFA (−15%), phosphorus (−14%), potassium (−11%), zinc (−17%), selenium (−26%), thiamine (−14%), riboflavin (−11%), niacin (−24%), vitamin B_6 (−13%), B_{12} (−11%), and choline (−19%) (Table 6). Additionally, fat, cholesterol, saturated fat, and sodium also decreased (−12%, −24%, −16%, and −38%, respectively) by removing a 3 oz (85 g) serving of further processed meat. However, the decreases for phosphorus, potassium, zinc (only in USP), thiamin, riboflavin, and vitamins B_6, B_{12}, fat, and saturated fat were attenuated and became less than 10% from baseline in the isocaloric scenario (Table 6). Identical results were obtained when a 3 oz (85 g) serving of further processed meat was removed from MSP except that the decrease in vitamin B_{12} was always less than 10% from baseline (Table 6).

Table 5. Energy and nutrients in 2000 kcal Healthy Dietary Patterns before and after removal of a 3 oz (85 g) serving of minimally processed poultry.

	2000 kcal Healthy US-Style Pattern			2000 kcal Healthy Mediterranean Style Pattern		
	Baseline	After Removal of 3 oz (85 g) Serving of Minimally Processed Poultry	After Isocaloric Removal of 3 oz (85 g) Serving of Minimally Processed Poultry	Baseline	After Removal of 3 oz (85 g) Serving of Minimally Processed Poultry	After Isocaloric Removal of 3 oz (85 g) Serving of Minimally Processed Poultry
Macronutrients						
Energy (kcal)	2001	1860	2001	2085	1944	2085
Protein (g)	92	67.1 *	72.1 *	99	74.1 *	79.4 *
Total fat (g)	71	67.2	72.3	72	68.2	73.1
Carbohydrate (g)	259	259	279	271	271	291
Dietary fiber (g)	30	30.0	32.3	31	31.0	33.2
Cholesterol (mg)	214	132 *	142 *	237	155 *	166 *
Saturated fatty acids (g)	18	17.2	18.5	18	17.2	18.5
Monounsaturated fatty acids (g)	25	23.8	25.6	26	24.8	26.6
Polyunsaturated fatty acids (g)	22	21.1	22.7	23	22.1	23.7
Minerals						
Calcium (mg)	1278	1271	1368	1297	1290	1384
Iron (mg)	14	13.6	14.6	15	14.6	15.6
Magnesium (mg)	358	334	360	377	353	379
Phosphorus (mg)	1654	1462 *	1573	1740	1548 *	1661
Potassium (mg)	3390	3105	3341	3628	3343	3586
Sodium (mg)	1658	1339 *	1441 *	1740	1421 *	1524 *
Zinc (mg)	13	12.1	13	13	12.1	12.9
Copper (mg)	1.4	1.36	1.46	1.5	1.46	1.56
Selenium (μg)	113	87.5 *	94.1 *	127	101 *	109 *
Vitamins						
Vitamin A, RAE (μg)	898	891	959	914	907	973
Vitamin E (ATE) (mg)	10	9.37	10.1	11	10.4	11.1
Vitamin D (μg)	7.5	7.47	8.03	9	8.97	9.62
Vitamin C (mg)	129	129	139	145	145	156
Thiamin (mg)	1.8	1.73	1.86	1.9	1.83	1.96
Riboflavin (mg)	2	1.82	1.96	2	1.82	1.95
Niacin (mg)	23	14.4 *	15.5 *	25	16.4 *	17.6 *
Vitamin B_6 (mg)	2.2	1.50 *	1.62 *	2.3	1.60 *	1.72 *
Vitamin B_{12} (μg)	6.2	5.97	6.42	7.3	7.07	7.58
Total choline (mg)	355	290 *	312 *	378	313 *	336 *
Vitamin K (μg)	140	139	149	142	141	151
Folate, DFE (μg)	513	507	545	527	521	559

Baseline nutritional profiles of 2000 kcal Heathy Dietary Patterns were obtained from Food Pattern Modeling Report [25]. Nutrient profiles after removal of minimally processed poultry were computed by subtracting the nutrients of minimally processed poultry (Table 2) from the nutrients of the Healthy Dietary Patterns. Calories were adjusted from the rest of the diet to match the baseline calories in the isocaloric removal of minimally processed poultry. ATE: alpha tocopherol equivalents; DFE, dietary folate equivalents; RAE: retinol activity equivalents. * Indicates ≥10% change from baseline.

Removal of a 3 oz (85 g) serving of further processed poultry from USP resulted in decreases in protein (−18%), monounsaturated fatty acids (−14%), polyunsaturated fatty acids (−13%), phosphorus (−12%), selenium (−15%), niacin (−27%), vitamin B_6 (−15%), and choline (−12%) (Table 7). Additionally, fat, cholesterol, saturated fat, and sodium also decreased (−14%, −26%, −10%, and −28%, respectively) by removing a 3 oz (85 g) serving of further processed poultry. However, the decreases for fat, saturated fat, monounsaturated fatty acids, polyunsaturated fatty acids, phosphorus, selenium, B_6, and choline were attenuated and became less than 10% from baseline in the isocaloric scenario (Table 7). Generally identical results were obtained when a 3 oz (85 g) serving of further processed poultry was removed from MSP, however, with isocaloric removal of further processed poultry vitamin A and C in USP and vitamin C in MSP also increased by ≥10% from baseline (Table 7).

Table 6. Energy and nutrients in 2000 kcal Healthy Dietary Pattern before and after removal of a 3 oz (85 g) serving of further processed meat.

	2000 kcal Healthy US-Style Pattern			2000 kcal Healthy Mediterranean Style Pattern		
	Baseline	After Removal of 3 oz (85 g) Serving of Further Processed Meat	After Isocaloric Removal of 3 oz (85 g) Serving of Further Processed Meat	Baseline	After Removal of 3 oz (85 g) Serving of Further Processed Meat	After Isocaloric Removal of 3 oz (85 g) Serving of Further Processed Meat
Macronutrients						
Energy (kcal)	2001	1834	2001	2085	1918	2085
Protein (g)	92	73.8 *	80.5 *	99	80.8 *	87.8
Total fat (g)	71	62.5 *	68.2	72	63.5 *	69.0
Carbohydrate (g)	259	256	279	271	268	291
Dietary fiber (g)	30	30.0	32.7	31	31.0	33.6
Cholesterol (mg)	214	162 *	177 *	237	185 *	202 *
Saturated fatty acids (g)	18	15.2 *	16.6	18	15.2 *	16.5
Monounsaturated fatty acids (g)	25	21.3 *	23.3	26	22.3 *	24.3
Polyunsaturated fatty acids (g)	22	20.9	22.8	23	21.9	23.8
Minerals						
Calcium (mg)	1278	1270	1386	1297	1289	1401
Iron (mg)	14	13.0	14.2	15	14.0	15.2
Magnesium (mg)	358	338	369	377	357	388
Phosphorus (mg)	1654	1423 *	1552	1740	1509 *	1640
Potassium (mg)	3390	3018 *	3292	3628	3256 *	3539
Sodium (mg)	1658	1033 *	1127 *	1740	1115 *	1212 *
Zinc (mg)	13	10.8 *	11.8	13	10.8 *	11.7 *
Copper (mg)	1.4	1.31	1.43	1.5	1.41	1.54
Selenium (µg)	113	84 *	92 *	127	98 *	107 *
Vitamins						
Vitamin A, RAE (µg)	898	895	977	914	911	991
Vitamin E (ATE) (mg)	10	9.71	10.59	11	10.7	11.6
Vitamin D (µg)	7.5	7.11	7.75	9	8.61	9.35
Vitamin C (mg)	129	129	141	145	145	158
Thiamin (mg)	1.8	1.54 *	1.68	1.9	1.64 *	1.78
Riboflavin (mg)	2	1.79 *	1.95	2	1.79 *	1.95
Niacin (mg)	23	17.5 *	19.1 *	25	19.5 *	21.2 *
Vitamin B_6 (mg)	2.2	1.89 *	2.07	2.3	1.99 *	2.17
Vitamin B_{12} (µg)	6.2	5.53 *	6.03	7.3	6.63	7.20
Total choline (mg)	355	289 *	315 *	378	312 *	339 *
Vitamin K (µg)	140	138	150	142	140	152
Folate, DFE (µg)	513	506	552	527	520	565

Baseline nutritional profiles of 2000 kcal Heathy Dietary Patterns were obtained from Food Pattern Modeling Report [25]. Nutrient profiles after removal of further processed meat were computed by subtracting the nutrients of further processed meat (Table 2) from the nutrients of the Healthy Dietary Patterns. Calories were adjusted from the rest of the diet to match the baseline calories in the isocaloric removal of further processed meat. ATE: alpha tocopherol equivalents; DFE, dietary folate equivalents; RAE: retinol activity equivalents. * Indicates ≥10% change from baseline.

Table 7. Energy and nutrients in 2000 kcal Healthy Dietary Pattern before and after removal of a 3 oz (85 g) serving of further processed poultry.

	2000 kcal Healthy US-Style Pattern			2000 kcal Healthy Mediterranean Style Pattern		
	Baseline	After Removal of 3 oz (85 g) Serving of Further Processed Poultry	After Isocaloric Removal of 3 oz (85 g) Serving of Further Processed Poultry	Baseline	After Removal of 3 oz (85 g) Serving of Further Processed Poultry	After Isocaloric Removal of 3 oz (85 g) Serving of Further Processed Poultry
Macronutrients						
Energy (kcal)	2001	1815	2001	2085	1899	2085
Protein (g)	92	75.3 *	83 *	99	82.3 *	90.3
Total fat (g)	71	61.3 *	67.6	72	62.3 *	68.4
Carbohydrate (g)	259	251	277	271	263	289
Dietary fiber (g)	30	29.6	32.7	31	30.6	33.6
Cholesterol (mg)	214	158 *	175 *	237	181 *	199 *
Saturated fatty acids (g)	18	16.2 *	17.9	18	16.2 *	17.8
Monounsaturated fatty acids (g)	25	21.4 *	23.6	26	22.4 *	24.6
Polyunsaturated fatty acids (g)	22	19.1 *	21.1	23	20.1 *	22.1
Minerals						
Calcium (mg)	1278	1267	1397	1297	1286	1412
Iron (mg)	14	13.5	14.8	15	14.5	15.9
Magnesium (mg)	358	338	373	377	357	392
Phosphorus (mg)	1654	1451 *	1600	1740	1537 *	1688
Potassium (mg)	3390	3133 *	3454	3628	3371	3702
Sodium (mg)	1658	1197 *	1320 *	1740	1279 *	1404 *
Zinc (mg)	13	12.3	13.6	13	12.3	13.6
Copper (mg)	1.4	1.36	1.50	1.5	1.46	1.60
Selenium (μg)	113	96 *	106	127	110 *	121
Vitamins						
Vitamin A, RAE (μg)	898	893	985 *	914	909	999
Vitamin E (ATE) (mg)	10	9.27	10.2	11	10.3	11.3
Vitamin D (μg)	7.5	7.39	8.15	9	8.89	9.77
Vitamin C (mg)	129	128	142 *	145	144	159 *
Thiamin (mg)	1.8	1.73	1.91	1.9	1.83	2.01
Riboflavin (mg)	2	1.85	2.03	2	1.85	2.03
Niacin (mg)	23	16.8 *	18.5 *	25	18.8 *	20.6 *
Vitamin B_6 (mg)	2.2	1.88 *	2.08	2.3	1.98 *	2.18
Vitamin B_{12} (μg)	6.2	5.96	6.57	7.3	7.06	7.75
Total choline (mg)	355	314 *	346	378	337 *	370
Vitamin K (μg)	140	136	150	142	138	152
Folate, DFE (μg)	513	504	556	527	518	569

Baseline nutritional profiles of 2000 kcal Heathy Dietary Patterns were obtained from Food Pattern Modeling Report [25]. Nutrient profiles after removal of further processed poultry were computed by subtracting the nutrients of further processed poultry (Table 2) from the nutrients of the Healthy Dietary Patterns. Calories were adjusted from the rest of the diet to match the baseline calories in the isocaloric removal of further processed poultry. ATE: alpha tocopherol equivalents; DFE, dietary folate equivalents; RAE: retinol activity equivalents. * Indicates ≥10% change from baseline.

4. Discussion

The results of this dietary modeling analysis show that the removal of a serving of meat or poultry resulted in decreases (10% or more from baseline) in protein and several key micronutrients including iron, phosphorus, potassium, zinc, selenium, thiamine, riboflavin, niacin, vitamin B_6, vitamin B_{12}, and choline as well as cholesterol and sodium in the Healthy Dietary Patterns. It is interesting to note that the decreases were consistent for most nutrients with the removal of either minimally processed or further processed meat or poultry and even after adjusting for the decreases in calories associated with removing meat/poultry servings.

Minimally processed meat used in our study included lean beef steaks and lean pork chops; minimally processed poultry included chicken breasts, drumsticks, and turkey; further processed meat included battered/fried beef steaks, breaded pork chops, spareribs, deli ham, pork bacon, beef hot dogs, and pork sausages; and further processed poultry included grilled and rotisserie chicken breasts, chicken nuggets, deli turkey, turkey bacon, chicken hot dogs, and turkey sausages (see Table 1). Beef is a staple food in the Western diet and is an important source of high-quality protein and several key micronutrients including highly bioavailable iron, zinc, and B vitamins in the American diet [6,7,28,29]. We recently reported that beef also contributes significant amounts of several key micronutrients such as zinc, iron, vitamin B_{12}, vitamin B_6, and choline in the diets of American adults [30]. Pork is one of the most widely consumed meats in the world and accounts for over 30% of global meat production and intake. Pork is a nutrient-rich source of high-quality protein and select nutrients such as potassium, phosphorus, zinc, selenium, thiamin, riboflavin, niacin, and vitamins B_6 and B_{12} [31,32]. Poultry meat is also high in protein and B-group vitamins (mainly thiamin, vitamin B_6, and pantothenic acid), and minerals (like iron, zinc, and copper) [33,34].

In the present analysis, removal of a 3 oz (85 g) serving of minimally processed meat from the Healthy Dietary Patterns resulted in $\geq$10% decreases from baseline in protein, iron, phosphorus, potassium, zinc, selenium, thiamine, riboflavin, niacin, vitamin B_6, vitamin B_{12}, and choline. Similarly, removal of a 3 oz (85 g) serving of minimally processed poultry also resulted in $\geq$10% decreases in protein, phosphorus, selenium, niacin, vitamin B_6 and choline. Although there was a consequent small decrease in energy with the removal of meat or poultry from healthy dietary patterns, the decrease was less than 10% from baseline. Interestingly, the decreases in protein, zinc, selenium, niacin, vitamin B_6, vitamin B_{12}, and choline from the removal of meat; and protein, selenium, niacin, vitamin B_6, and choline from the removal of poultry remained $\geq$10% from baseline when the decrease in energy was adjusted (isocaloric scenario) by adding back energy/nutrients from the rest of the healthy dietary pattern. This suggests that the meat and poultry are more nutrient-dense foods than other foods in the Healthy Dietary Patterns. Indeed, minimally processed meat or poultry provides about three times more protein, four times more zinc (for meat only), three to four times more selenium, three to four times more niacin, three to four times more vitamin B_6, and two to three times more choline than Healthy Dietary Patterns on a per 100 kcal basis. However, meat and poultry also provide over four times more cholesterol, ~70% more saturated fat (for meat only), and about three times more sodium.

While lean and fresh/unprocessed meat and poultry are recommended as part of healthy diets [2,3] and are not associated with adverse health outcomes [14,15], intake of processed meat has been reported to be associated with risk for several chronic disease outcomes in scientific research [11–13]. On a per 3 oz (85 g) serving basis, further processed meat or poultry provide more calories, less protein and other key micronutrients, and more saturated fat and sodium than their minimally processed counterparts. DGA 2020–2025 has identified saturated fat and sodium as nutrients to limit, as their current intake is more than recommended based on their suspected role in chronic disease outcomes [2]. Additionally, heme iron, N-nitroso compounds in processed meat, as well as heterocyclic aromatic amines and polycyclic aromatic hydrocarbons formed during high-temperature processing are also considered, by some, as potential carcinogens in processed meat [35]. However, the removal of further processed meat and poultry such as ground beef, fried steaks, pork chops, spareribs, chicken nuggets, cold cuts, bacon, frankfurters, and sausages, also resulted in $\geq$10% decreases in protein, selenium, and choline. In a recently published analysis of NHANES 2001–2018, we reported that beef including processed and ground beef contributed to the intake of protein and several key micronutrients [30]. In an earlier analysis of NHANES, intake of lunch meat (deli, cold cuts, or cured meat) did not adversely affect diet quality or physiological parameters in children and adults [36]. Although there is some evidence that high meat consumption (especially red and processed meat) may increase the risk for some types of chronic disease [37], meat (fresh and lean meat) can be an important source of nutrients, especially for people with limited availability of foods.

There has been a consistent ongoing discussion and increasing concerns about the environmental impact of animal-sourced foods and policymakers are increasingly concerned with the environmental consequences of meat consumption in addition to the effect on human health. Some studies show that meat production results in anthropogenic greenhouse gas emissions including CO_2, methane, and nitrous oxide and is the single most important source of methane [17,18]. Consequently, there has been a strong push to limit or eliminate animal-based foods to minimize environmental impacts [19–22]. However, such recommendations do not account for their potential effect on food availability and nutrient intake. While removing or limiting animal foods from the diet may help lower greenhouse gas emissions, nutritional inadequacies may occur as potential trade-offs. Thus, recommending limiting animal-sourced foods could have potential unintended consequences [38–40]. Our results clearly show that the removal of a serving of meat or poultry could cause decreases in protein and several key nutrients in the Healthy Dietary Patterns.

While we used USDA's dietary modeling approach for menu modeling of Healthy Dietary Patterns, there are some key aspects to consider when interpreting our results. Firstly, the representative foods for different meat or poultry composites were selected in each category using USDA's approach, and proportions of different food in a category were based on their population-weighted consumptions using the most recent nationally representative database (NHANES 2017–2018). However, our results are dependent on foods selected in our meat and poultry composites and changes in the items selected for each composite may impact modeling results. Additionally, the results presented here are based on dietary modeling to evaluate the maximum effect of removing meat and/or poultry and may not reflect actual individual dietary behavior; however, such dietary modeling offers a technique to test the potential nutritional impact of dietary guidance. Finally, our results may not apply to non-US cultures as dietary recommendations and current dietary patterns may be different.

5. Conclusions

In conclusion, the results of this dietary modeling study show that the removal of a meat and poultry serving from Healthy Dietary Patterns resulted in decreases in protein and several key nutrients associated with meat intake like iron, zinc, and vitamin B_{12} but also phosphorus, potassium, selenium, thiamine, riboflavin, niacin, vitamin B_6, and choline with considerable consistency in results whether removing minimally processed or further processed meat and poultry. The results also provide insight into the nutritional consequences of removing meat and poultry from Healthy Dietary Patterns and identifies nutrient amounts that may need to be replaced by other foods.

Author Contributions: S.A.: participated in project conception, research design, overall research plan, analysis and interpretation of the data, manuscript preparation; K.R.M.: reviewed and classified meat and poultry items; V.L.F.III: participated in project conception, research design, overall research plan, analysis and interpretation of the data, manuscript preparation; All authors have read and agreed to the published version of the manuscript.

Funding: The study and the writing of the manuscript were supported by Beef Checkoff and the Foundation for Meat and Poultry Research and Education.

Institutional Review Board Statement: Not applicable.

Informed Consent Statement: Not applicable.

Data Availability Statement: All data obtained for this study are publicly available at: https://www.dietaryguidelines.gov/sites/default/files/2020-07/FoodPatternModeling_Report_2YearsandOlder.pdf; http://www.cdc.gov/nchs/nhanes/; https://fdc.nal.usda.gov/ (accessed on 7 May 2022).

Conflicts of Interest: S.A. as Principal of NutriScience LLC performs nutrition science consulting for various food and beverage companies and related entities; K.R.M. is an employee of Foundation for Meat and Poultry Research and Education; V.L.F.III as Senior Vice President of Nutrition Impact, LLC performs consulting and database analyses for various food and beverage companies and related entities.

References

1. Pasiakos, S.M.; Agarwal, S.; Lieberman, H.R.; Fulgoni, V.L., 3rd. Sources and Amounts of Animal, Dairy, and Plant Protein Intake of US Adults in 2007–2010. *Nutrients* **2015**, *7*, 7058–7069. [CrossRef] [PubMed]
2. U.S. Department of Agriculture; U.S. Department of Health and Human Services. *Dietary Guidelines for Americans, 2020–2025*, 9th ed.; December 2020. Available online: https://DietaryGuidelines.gov (accessed on 2 November 2022).
3. U.S. Department of Agriculture. Choose My Plate. Available online: https://www.choosemyplate.gov (accessed on 2 November 2022).
4. Daniel, C.R.; Cross, A.J.; Koebnick, C.; Sinha, R. Trends in meat consumption in the USA. *Public Health Nutr.* **2011**, *14*, 575–583. [CrossRef] [PubMed]
5. O'Connor, L.E.; Herrick, K.A.; Parsons, R.; Reedy, J. Heterogeneity in Meat Food Groups Can Meaningfully Alter Population-Level Intake Estimates of Red Meat and Poultry. *Front. Nutr.* **2021**, *8*, 778369. [CrossRef]
6. Klurfeld, D.M. Research gaps in evaluating the relationship of meat and health. *Meat Sci.* **2015**, *109*, 86–95. [CrossRef]
7. Pereira, P.M.; Vicente, A.F. Meat nutritional composition and nutritive role in the human diet. *Meat Sci.* **2013**, *93*, 586–592. [CrossRef] [PubMed]
8. Dietary Guidelines Advisory Committee. *Scientific Report of the 2020 Dietary Guidelines Advisory Committee: Advisory Report to the Secretary of Agriculture and the Secretary of Health and Human Services*; U.S. Department of Agriculture, Agricultural Research Service: Washington, DC, USA, 2020. Available online: https://doi.org/10.52570/DGAC2020 (accessed on 2 November 2022).
9. O'Connor, L.E.; Gifford, C.L.; Woerner, D.R.; Sharp, J.L.; Belk, K.E.; Campbell, W.W. Dietary meat categories and descriptions in chronic disease research are substantively different within and between experimental and observational studies: A systematic review and landscape analysis. *Adv. Nutr.* **2020**, *11*, 41–51. [CrossRef] [PubMed]
10. U.S. Department of Agriculture. *What We Eat in America*. Available online: https://www.ars.usda.gov/northeast-area/beltsville-md-bhnrc/beltsville-human-nutrition-research-center/food-surveys-research-group/docs/wweianhanes-overview/ (accessed on 14 June 2022).
11. Boada, L.D.; Henríquez-Hernández, L.A.; Luzardo, O.P. The impact of red and processed meat consumption on cancer and other health outcomes: Epidemiological evidences. *Food Chem. Toxicol.* **2016**, *92*, 236–244. [CrossRef]
12. Wang, X.; Lin, X.; Ouyang, Y.Y.; Liu, J.; Zhao, G.; Pan, A.; Hu, F.B. Red and processed meat consumption and mortality: Dose-response meta-analysis of prospective cohort studies. *Public Health Nutr.* **2016**, *19*, 893–905. [CrossRef]
13. Wolk, A. Potential health hazards of eating red meat. *J. Intern. Med.* **2017**, *281*, 106–122. [CrossRef]
14. van den Brandt, P.A. Red meat, processed meat, and other dietary protein sources and risk of overall and cause-specific mortality in The Netherlands Cohort Study. *Eur. J. Epidemiol.* **2019**, *34*, 351–369. [CrossRef]
15. Micha, R.; Michas, G.; Mozaffarian, D. Unprocessed red and processed meats and risk of coronary artery disease and type 2 diabetes–an updated review of the evidence. *Curr. Atheroscler. Rep.* **2012**, *14*, 515–524. [CrossRef] [PubMed]
16. U.S. Department of Health and Human Services; U.S. Department of Agriculture. *2015–2020 Dietary Guidelines for Americans*, 8th ed.; December 2015. Available online: http://health.gov/dietaryguidelines/2015/guidelines/ (accessed on 2 November 2022).
17. Gerber, P.J.; Steinfeld, H.; Henderson, B.; Mottet, A.; Opio, C.; Dijkman, J.; Falcucci, A.; Tempio, G. *Tackling Climate Change through Livestock: A Global Assessment of Emissions and Mitigation Opportunities*; Food and Agriculture Organization of the United Nations (FAO): Rome, Italy, 2013.
18. Herrero, M.; Gerber, P.; Vellinga, T.; Garnett, T.; Leip, A.; Opio, C.; Westhoek, H.J.; Thornton, P.K.; Olesen, J.; Hutchings, N.; et al. Livestock and greenhouse gas emissions: The importance of getting the numbers right. *Anim. Feed Sci. Technol.* **2011**, *166–167*, 779–782. [CrossRef]
19. IOM. *Sustainable Diets: Food for Healthy People and a Healthy Planet*; Workshop Summary; The National Academies Press: Washington, DC, USA, 2014.
20. Willett, W.; Rockström, J.; Loken, B.; Springmann, M.; Lang, T.; Vermeulen, S.; Garnett, T.; Tilman, D.; DeClerck, F.; Wood, A.; et al. Food in the Anthropocene: The EAT-Lancet Commission on healthy diets from sustainable food systems. *Lancet* **2019**, *393*, 447–492. [CrossRef] [PubMed]
21. Westhoek, H.; Lesschen, J.P.; Rood, T.; Wagner, S.; De Marco, A.; Murphy-Bokern, D.; Leip, A.; van Grinsven, H.; Sutton, M.A.; Oenema, O. Food choices, health and environment: Effects of cutting Europe's meat and dairy intake. *Glob Environ. Chang.* **2014**, *26*, 196–205. [CrossRef]
22. Hedenus, F.; Wirsenius, S.; Johansson, D.J.A. The importance of reduced meat and dairy consumption for meeting stringent climate change targets. *Clim. Chang.* **2014**, *124*, 79–91. [CrossRef]
23. Seman, D.L.; Boler, D.D.; Carr, C.; Dikeman, M.E.; Owens, C.M.; Keeton, J.T.; Pringle, T.; Sindelar, J.J.; Woerner, D.R.; de Mello, A.S.; et al. Meat Science Lexicon. *Meat Muscle Biol.* **2018**, *2*. [CrossRef]
24. Centers for Disease Control and Prevention; National Center for Health Statistics. *National Health and Nutrition Examination Survey*; National Center for Health Statistics: Hyattsville, MD, USA, 2021. Available online: https://www.cdc.gov/nchs/nhanes/index.htm (accessed on 14 June 2022).
25. 2020 Dietary Guidelines Advisory Committee and Food Pattern Modeling Team. *Food Pattern Modeling: Ages 2 Years and Older. 2020 Dietary Guidelines Advisory Committee Project*; U.S. Department of Agriculture: Washington, DC, USA, 2020. Available online: https://www.dietaryguidelines.gov/sites/default/files/2020-07/FoodPatternModeling_Report_2YearsandOlder.pdf (accessed on 14 June 2022).

26. U.S. Department of Agriculture. Food and Nutrient Database for Dietary Studies. 2021. Available online: https://www.ars.usda.gov/northeast-area/beltsville-md-bhnrc/beltsville-humannutrition-research-center/food-surveys-research-group/docs/fndds/ (accessed on 14 June 2022).
27. USDA; ARS. FoodData Central. 2019. Available online: https://fdc.nal.usda.gov/ (accessed on 14 June 2022).
28. Biesalski, H.K. Meat as a component of a healthy diet—Are there any risks or benefits if meat is avoided in the diet? *Meat Sci.* **2005**, *70*, 509–524. [CrossRef]
29. Wyness, L.; Weichselbaum, E.; O'Connor, A.; Williams, E.B.; Benelam, B.; Riley, H.; Stanner, S. Red meat in the diet: An update. *Nutr. Bull.* **2011**, *36*, 34–77. [CrossRef]
30. Agarwal, S.; Fuilgoni, V.L., 3rd. Contribution of beef to key nutrient intakes in American adults: An updated analysis with NHANES 2011–2018. *Nutr. Res.* **2022**, *105*, 105–112. [CrossRef]
31. Murphy, M.M.; Spungen, J.H.; Bi, X.; Barraj, L.M. Fresh and fresh lean pork are substantial sources of key nutrients when these products are consumed by adults in the United States. *Nutr. Res.* **2011**, *31*, 776–783. [CrossRef]
32. An, R.; Nickols-Richardson, S.M.; Alston, R.; Clarke, C. Fresh and lean pork consumption in relation to nutrient intakes and diet quality among US adults, NHANES 2005–2016. *Health Behav. Policy Rev.* **2019**, *6*, 570–581. [CrossRef]
33. Marangoni, F.; Corsello, G.; Cricelli, C.; Ferrara, N.; Ghiselli, A.; Lucchin, L.; Poli, A. Role of poultry meat in a balanced diet aimed at maintaining health and wellbeing: An Italian consensus document. *Food Nutr. Res.* **2015**, *59*, 27606. [CrossRef]
34. Donma, M.M.; Donma, O. Beneficial Effects of Poultry Meat Consumption on Cardiovascular Health and the Prevention of Childhood Obesity. *MED ONE* **2017**, *2*, e170018. [CrossRef]
35. Bouvard, V.; Loomis, D.; Guyton, K.Z.; Grosse, Y.; Ghissassi, F.E.; Benbrahim-Tallaa, L.; Guha, N.; Mattock, H.; Straif, K.; International Agency for Research on Cancer Monograph Working Group. Carcinogenicity of consumption of red and processed meat. *Lancet Oncol.* **2015**, *16*, 1599–1600. [CrossRef]
36. Agarwal, S.; Fulgoni, V.L., 3rd; Berg, E.P. Association of lunch meat consumption with nutrient intake, diet quality and health risk factors in U.S. children and adults: NHANES 2007–2010. *Nutr. J.* **2015**, *14*, 128. [CrossRef]
37. GBD 2013 Risk Factors Collaborators. Global, regional, and national comparative risk assessment of 79 behavioural, environmental and occupational, and metabolic risks or clusters of risks in 188 countries, 1990–2013: A systematic analysis for the Global Burden of Disease Study 2013. *Lancet* **2015**, *386*, 2287–2323. [CrossRef]
38. Springmann, M.; Wiebe, K.; Mason-D'Croz, D.; Sulser, T.B.; Rayner, M.; Scarborough, P. Health and nutritional aspects of sustainable diet strategies and their association with environmental impacts: A global modelling analysis with country-level detail. Lancet Planet. *Health* **2018**, *2*, e451–e461. [CrossRef]
39. Tso, R.; Forde, C.G. Unintended Consequences: Nutritional Impact and Potential Pitfalls of Switching from Animal- to Plant-Based Foods. *Nutrients* **2021**, *13*, 2527. [CrossRef] [PubMed]
40. Salomé, M.; Huneau, J.F.; Le Baron, C.; Kesse-Guyot, E.; Fouillet, H.; Mariotti, F. Substituting Meat or Dairy Products with Plant-Based Substitutes Has Small and Heterogeneous Effects on Diet Quality and Nutrient Security: A Simulation Study in French Adults (INCA3). *J. Nutr.* **2021**, *151*, 2435–2445. [CrossRef] [PubMed]

Disclaimer/Publisher's Note: The statements, opinions and data contained in all publications are solely those of the individual author(s) and contributor(s) and not of MDPI and/or the editor(s). MDPI and/or the editor(s) disclaim responsibility for any injury to people or property resulting from any ideas, methods, instructions or products referred to in the content.

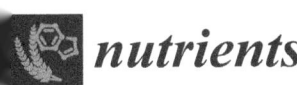

Article

The Consumption of Animal and Plant Foods in Areas of High Prevalence of Stroke and Colorectal Cancer

Kellie E. Mayfield [1,*], Julie Plasencia [2], Morgan Ellithorpe [3], Raeda K. Anderson [4] and Nicole C. Wright [5]

1. Department of Nutrition, Georgia State University, Atlanta, GA 30302, USA
2. Department of Dietetics and Human Nutrition, University of Kentucky, Lexington, KY 40506, USA
3. Department of Communication, University of Delaware, Newark, DE 19716, USA
4. Virginia C. Crawford Research Institute, Shepherd Center and Department of Sociology, Georgia State University, Atlanta, GA 30302, USA
5. Department of Epidemiology, School of Public Health, University of Alabama at Birmingham, Birmingham, AL 35294, USA
* Correspondence: kmayfield@gsu.edu; Tel.:+1-404-413-1080

Abstract: Diets of red and processed meat have been reported as important risk factors for developing colorectal cancer. Given the racial and ethnic differences in the incidence of colorectal cancer, patterns of food consumption, and areas of residence, particularly in the South, more data is needed on the relationship between residing in a high stroke area, colorectal cancer incidence levels, and red meat and processed meat consumption. We created online surveys to ascertain meat, red meat, and healthy food consumption levels. We used OLS regression to evaluate the association between residence in Stroke Belt states and colorectal cancer incidence quartiles with food consumption. We further used path analysis using structural equation modeling to evaluate if age, sex, race/ethnicity, income, and comorbidity index mediated the association between residence in the eight-state Stroke Belt, colorectal cancer incidence groups, and meat consumption. Our sample included 923 participants, with 167 (18.1%) residing in the Stroke Belt and 13.9% being in the highest colorectal cancer incidence group. The findings show that residing in a Stroke Belt state is predictive of the consumption of overall meat 0.93 more days per week or red meat 0.55 more days per week compared to those not residing in a Stroke Belt state. These data can be used to develop future diet interventions in these high-risk areas to reduce rates of colorectal cancer and other negative health outcomes.

Keywords: stroke; colorectal cancer; meat consumption; health outcomes; mediation; racial and ethnic disparities

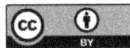

1. Introduction

Chronic diseases associated with meat consumption are costly and unequally distributed. Overconsumption of red and processed meat is a well-established risk factor for multiple types of cancers, particularly colorectal cancer [1–15], obesity [16], type 2 diabetes, [17] and cardiovascular disease [14]. In the US, colorectal cancer is the second costliest cancer, accounting for 12.6% of all cancer treatment costs [18]. Red and processed meat (e.g., beef, pork, sausages, and hot dogs) are strongly associated with risk of multiple cancers and mortality [8,9,11,12,14]. Studies show that more than 100–120 g of red meat per day increases the risk of colorectal cancer by up to 24%, and more than 25–30 g of processed meat daily increases colorectal cancer risk by up to 49% [1,19,20].

On average, Americans consumed 186 g of processed meat per week and 284 g of unprocessed red meat per week in 2016 [21]. Consumption volumes differ due to numerous factors, particularly race and ethnicity. Studies show that Black and Hispanic Americans consume more meat, especially red and processed meat, than other groups [22,23]. Non-Hispanic Black Americans consumed the lowest level of unprocessed red meat, whereas

Hispanics consumed the highest level of unprocessed red meat [21]. Similarly, cancer incidence and mortality rates differ by type of cancer, ethnicity, and race. Hispanic Americans have a greater risk for liver and stomach cancers compared to White Americans [24], and they have equal or lower risk for colorectal [25], breast [26], and ovarian cancers [27]. Hispanic Americans have a higher risk than non-Hispanic White Americans for obesity [28–31] and diabetes [28,32,33]. However, Black Americans and Hispanic Americans have greater risk than non-Hispanic White Americans for obesity [28–30,34,35], diabetes [33,35–37], cardiovascular disease [28,35,38–40], and both cancer incidence and mortality [41,42].

Certain U.S. regions have higher rates of diet-related diseases. Evidence regarding the concomitant incidence of colorectal cancer and heart disease by region is limited. Stroke is a leading cause of mortality and is of particular concern in what is now labeled the Stroke Belt, which is composed of southern U.S. states. Treatments for stroke is expensive, costing over 50 billion between 2017 and 2018, and it is a contributing factor to long-term disability [43]. The highest concentrations of stroke deaths are mostly in the southeast region, with some of the heaviest concentration in the Deep South, a region of eight states that includes Alabama, Arkansas, Georgia, Louisiana, Mississippi, North Carolina, South Carolina, and Tennessee [44]. Geographic location matters because the south and southeast regions of the U.S. are also where the majority of its Black and Hispanic populations reside [45,46]. Evidence also shows that red meat consumption is a leading risk factor for type 2 diabetes in the U.S. and other parts of the world, such as Australasia [47].

The consumption of healthy foods, such as leafy greens and starches, is associated with reduced stroke risk [48], and evidence regarding the contribution of meat consumption, especially red and processed meat, to risk of stroke is weak [49]. Furthermore, adoption of alternative and plant-based diets such as pescatarian (no meats, except seafood), vegetarian (no meat, but eggs and dairy are included), and vegan (no animal or foods that are sourced from animals) are associated with lower morbidity and mortality from cancer, diabetes, and cardiovascular disease, as well as with reduced diet-related risk factors such as body mass index (BMI), cholesterol, and blood pressure [50–52].

Studies show that healthier diet patterns consisting of plant foods can reduce the risk and prevalence of chronic diseases such as cardiovascular disease, hypertension, and some cancers. However, the relationship between living in the Stroke Belt, CRC rates, and diet-related diseases to race/ethnicity is less clear. Therefore, using a nationally representative sample of Hispanics, Blacks, and non-Hispanic Whites, this cross-sectional study examined the association between Stroke Belt residence and colorectal cancer incidence and diet, and it evaluated if age, race/ethnicity, income, and number of health conditions mediates the association between Stroke Belt residence and colorectal cancer incidence with food consumption.

2. Materials and Methods

The study was conducted in accordance with the Declaration of Helsinki, and it was determined exempt (category 2) by the Institutional Review Board of Michigan State University. A priori, our intention was to recruit a stratified sample of approximately equal numbers of Black, Hispanic, and non-Hispanic White participants. We first used Amazon's Mechanical Turk (MTurk) [53], but data has found that the MTurk participant pool tends to overrepresent Whites compared to the general U.S. population [54]; thus, we also employed a second survey tool from Qualtrics Research Suite (Qualtrics, 2009, Provo, UT, USA. Version 12.018). Qualtrics maintains a non-probability, nationally representative panel based on airline lists, online shopping centers, and targeted customer profiles. Participants of this sample are compensated based on their preferred method of compensation (e.g., points redeemable for flyer miles, shopping points, and cash rewards). An e-mail was sent to their panelists who identified themselves as non-Hispanic White, non-Hispanic Black, and Hispanics living in the U.S. For both MTurk and Qualtrics, eligible and interested participants were provided with the link to the informed consent form for participation followed by the web-based survey that included sociodemographic questions. The combined datasets yielded a total of n = 1069. After combining samples, we excluded participants with missing demographic, state, or diet data. The final sample size was 923 total participants; 661 (71.6%) identified as female, the median age was 38.3 years (SD = 15.0, range 18 to 86), 261 (28.3%) were non-Hispanic Black or African American, 278 (30.1%) were Hispanic, and 384 (41.6%) were non-Hispanic White. For additional participant statistics, please see Table 1.

Table 1. Participant demographics and characteristics. Note: colorectal cancer is abbreviated in this and all other tables as "CRC".

	Total n = 923
Sample Source, n (%)	
MTurk	262 (28.4)
Qualtrics	661 (71.6)
Age, mean years (range)	38.3 (18–86)
Female, n (%)	661 (71.61)
Race and ethnicity, n (%)	
Non-Hispanic White	384 (41.6)
Black Americans	261 (28.3)
Hispanic	278 (30.1)
Income, n (%)	
<$25,000	243 (26.3)
$25,000–$50,000	307 (33.3)
$50,001–$75,000	191 (20.7)
$75,001–$100,000	84 (9.1)
>$100,000	98 (10.6)
Residence in Stroke Belt, n (%)	167 (18.1)
Health conditions, mean (SD)	0.49 (0.82)
CRC incidence quartile, n (%)	
1	233 (25.2)
2	359 (38.9)
3	203 (22.0)
4	128 (13.9)

Colorectal cancer Incidence. Colorectal cancer incidence data was based on colorectal cancer rates per 100,000 people from 2015 data. We grouped states into quartiles based on colorectal cancer incidence, which included the following: Q4, the highest colorectal cancer incidence ($\geq$42.3), included Alaska, Alabama, Mississippi, Louisiana, Arkansas, West Virginia, Ohio, Kentucky, Illinois, Iowa, North Dakota, and Nebraska; Q3, the second-highest colorectal cancer incidence (41.9–38.7), included Montana, South Dakota, Oklahoma, Missouri, Indiana, Tennessee, Georgia, South Carolina, Pennsylvania, Delaware, New Jersey, and New York; Q2, the second-lowest colorectal cancer incidence (38.4–35.0), included California, Idaho, Texas, Kansas, Minnesota, Wisconsin, Michigan, North Carolina, Maryland, Connecticut, Massachusetts, New Hampshire, and Maine; Q1, the lowest colorectal cancer incidence (<34.9), included Florida, New Mexico, Arizona, Nevada, Oregon, Washington, Wyoming, Utah, Colorado, Virginia, Vermont, and Rhode Island.

Stroke belt states. Participants provided their state of residence, and this information was used to delineate whether a participant was living in a Stroke Belt state, which was defined as residing in one of the following eight states: Alabama, Arkansas, Georgia,

Louisiana, Mississippi, North Carolina, South Carolina, or Tennessee; n = 167 (18.1%) of the sample resided in a Stroke Belt state.

Food consumption. Participants were provided with a list of food categories and were asked to indicate in how many days in the past week they had consumed each food. We grouped foods into the following categories: (1) meat (beef, pork, poultry, fish, and venison), (2) red meat (beef, pork, and venison only), and (3) healthy foods (fruits, leafy green vegetables, starchy vegetables, grains, nuts and seeds, tofu, seitan, and tempeh). We calculated the sum of the days each food group was consumed in the past week. This means that the more foods in each category a person reported consuming over more days in the past week, the higher their score was on the measure. Eggs and dairy were also measured but were not included in these measures due to their controversiality in being included in measures of healthy foods, and they do not belong in either meat category.

Health condition diagnoses. Participants were asked to indicate whether they had ever been diagnosed with any of the following health conditions: heart disease, diabetes, high blood pressure, high cholesterol, liver disease, or kidney disease. These conditions were selected as being some that are well-known to be associated with meat consumption. The number of "yes" responses was summed to create an overall measure of health conditions. Those who responded yes to more than three were coded together with those who had three, as only one or two people had scores of four, five, or six; therefore, the final measure was scaled from zero to three as a count of the number of health conditions previously demonstrated to be associated with meat consumption (M = 0.59, SD = 0.87).

Covariates. Other variables of interest included age, gender, race/ethnicity, annual household income, and history of any of the following health conditions: heart disease, diabetes, high blood pressure, high cholesterol, liver disease, or kidney disease, which were self-reported by the participants. We counted the number of conditions reported and summed them together to create an overall measure of health conditions ranging from 0 to 3. Sample source (Qualtrics, n = 661, 71.6%, and MTurk, n = 262, 28.4%) was also included as a covariate in the analyses.

Statistical Analysis. The characteristics of the sample were compared, and the means and standard deviations (SD) for continuous variables and the frequency and proportion for categorical variables are reported. The sum of the days in which the participants ate each food group in the past week (meat, red meat, and healthy foods) overall, by Stroke Belt residence, and by CRC incidence quartile were estimated, and a t-test or ANOVA was used to compare the means within each variable. OLS regressions were used to evaluate the association between Stroke Belt residence and CRC incidence with food consumption. Models for each food group were ran separately. Models were adjusted for age, sex, race/ethnicity, income, and comorbidity score. Subsequently, a path analysis was conducted using structural equation modeling to test mediation effects. Models for overall meat and red meat were ran separately due to the nested nature of the measures. Indirect effects were assessed using 5000 bias-corrected bootstrap samples. We used Stata v.17 (College Station, TX, USA) for all analyses, with the level of significance set to 0.05. The full statistical results can be found in Table 2.

Table 2. Dietary habits of participants.

	Overall Meat Mean Days (Range)	p-Value	Red Meat Mean Days (Range)	p-Value	Healthy Food Mean Days (Range)	p-Value
Overall	6.95 (0–35)		3.42 (0–21)		15.4 (0–42)	
Stroke Belt Residence, mean (SD)		0.047		0.050		0.643
Yes	7.60 (5.55)		3.83 (3.61)		15.23 (8.09)	
No	6.84 (4.43)		3.35 (2.85)		15.53 (7.84)	

Table 2. Cont.

	Overall Meat Mean Days (Range)	p-Value	Red Meat Mean Days (Range)	p-Value	Healthy Food Mean Days (Range)	p-Value
CRC Incidence Quartile, mean (SD)		0.961		0.708		0.015
1	7.01 (4.24)		3.44 (2.79)		14.93 (8.42)	
2	7.00 (4.67)		3.48 (2.99)		16.36 (7.66)	
3	6.91 (4.99)		3.23 (3.17)		15.01 (7.34)	
4	6.77 (5.12)		3.58 (5.18)		14.09 (8.19)	

3. Results

After excluding 397 participants with missing data, our final sample included 923 participants, of which the mean age was 38.3 years (SD = 15.0, range 18 to 86), 661 (71.6%) were female, 262 (28.4%) were male, 261 (28.3%) were Black, 278 (30.1%) were Hispanic, 384 (41.6%) were non-Hispanic White, 167 (18.1%) resided in the Stroke Belt, 25.2% were in the lowest colorectal cancer incidence group, and 13.9% were in the highest colorectal cancer incidence group (Table 1).

3.1. Dietary Habits

Overall, participants consumed 6.95 servings of meat on average in the previous week, with red meat accounting for 3.42 of those servings. About 15.4 servings of healthy foods were consumed in the previous week. As shown in Table 2, Stroke Belt state residence was significantly associated with increased overall meat consumption and red meat consumption but not with healthy food consumption. Colorectal cancer state residence was not significantly associated with meat or red meat consumption, but residence in the second quartile colorectal cancer states was associated with the highest healthy food consumption.

3.2. Relationship between Stroke Belt Residence, Colorectal Cancer Incidence, and Food Consumption

Residing in a Stroke Belt state was significantly associated with consuming more meat overall, as well as more red meat, in the past week. There was no significant relationship between Stroke Belt states and healthy food consumption. Colorectal state quartile was not significantly associated with any food consumption outcome, except for living in a second quartile state was associated with higher healthy food consumption, but once covariates were accounted for this relationship was no longer significant. Overall meat consumption and red meat consumption were both significantly associated with increased health conditions reported. The indirect effect of residing in a Stroke Belt state on health conditions was significant when mediated by overall meat consumption ($b = 0.02$, 95% CI (0.002, 0.04)) and by red meat consumption ($b = 0.01$, 95% CI (0.0002, 0.04)) but not by healthy food consumption ($b = -0.003$, 95% CI (-0.02, 0.002)). This suggests that the relationship between residing in a Stroke Belt state and health outcomes may be at least partially mediated by meat consumption. There was not, however, a relationship between CRC quartile and health outcomes.

In the crude analyses, Stroke Belt state residence was associated with more overall meat and red meat consumption. Residing in a Stroke Belt state was significantly associated with consuming more meat overall ($b = 0.76$ (0.38)) and more red meat ($b = 0.48$ (0.25)) in the past week (Table 3). After adjusting for age, sex, income, health conditions, and sample source, we found similar results.

Table 3. Relationship between Stroke Belt residence, colorectal cancer incidence group, and food consumption.

	Overall Meat		Red Meat		Healthy Food	
	Crude b (95% CI)	Adjusted b (95% CI)	Crude b (95% CI)	Adjusted b (95% CI)	Crude b (95% CI)	Adjusted b (95% CI)
Stroke Belt Residence	0.76 (0.01, 1.52)	1.00 (0.14, 1.86)	0.48 (0.00, 0.97)	0.65 (0.09, 1.21)	−0.30 (−1.59, 0.98)	0.87 (−0.58, 2.31)
CRC Quartile						
1	Ref.	Ref.	Ref.	Ref.	Ref.	Ref.
2	−0.01 (−0.77, 0.75)	0.09 (−0.66, 0.85)	0.04 (−0.045, 0.52)	0.07 (−0.42, 0.56)	1.42 (0.15, 2.69)	1.14 (−0.13, 2.41)
3	−0.10 (−0.97, 0.77)	−0.48 (−1.40, 0.45)	−0.22 (−0.78, 0.34)	−0.41 (−1.00, 0.19)	0.07 (−1.38, 1.52)	−0.12 (−1.67, 1.43)
4	−0.24 (−1.25, 0.76)	−0.24 (−1.28, 0.80)	0.14 (−0.51, 0.78)	0.15 (−0.53, 0.82)	−0.84 (−2.53, 0.84)	−0.74 (−2.49, 1.00)

B: unstandardized coefficient; CI: confidence interval; CRC: colorectal cancer. Adjusted for age, sex, income, health conditions, and sample source.

Sample source was included as a covariate after independent-samples t-tests found a significant difference between sample sources in the frequency of healthy food consumption (Qualtrics M = 14.44, SD = 7.95; MTurk M = 17.70, SD = 7.03; t (921) = −5.80, $p < 0.001$). There was not a significant difference between sample sources for amounts of meat consumed (Qualtrics M = 6.88, SD = 4.82; MTurk M = 7.11, SD = 4.34, t (921) = −0.65, $p = 0.51$,) or for amount of red meat consumed (Qualtrics M = 3.36, SD = 3.07; MTurk M = 3.56, SD = 2.92, t (921) = −0.91, $p = 0.36$). Of the other covariates, age, gender, race/ethnicity, and income were all significant covariates predicting meat consumption and red meat consumption, but only income was a significant covariate for healthy food consumption. The measures of these covariates are as follows: age on meat, b = −0.04, 95% confidence interval (CI) (−0.06, −0.01); age on red meat, b = −0.03, 95% CI (−0.05, −0.02); age on healthy food, b = 0.01, 95% CI (−0.02, 0.05); gender on meat, b = −1.57, 95% CI (−2.25, −0.88); gender on red meat, b = −1.14, 95% CI (−1.58 −0.70); gender on healthy food, b = −0.01, 95% CI (−1.15, 1.13); Black compared to White on meat, b = 1.54, 95% CI (0.78, 2.30); Black compared to White on red meat, b = 0.55, 95% CI (0.06, 1.04); Black compared to White on healthy food, b = −0.34, 95% CI (−1.62, 0.94); Hispanic compared to White on meat, b = 1.09, 95% CI (0.31, 1.87); Hispanic compared to White on red meat, b = 0.46, 95% CI (−0.05, 0.96); Hispanic compared to White on healthy food, b = 0.45, 95% CI (−0.85, 1.76); income on meat, b = 0.34, 95% CI (0.16, 0.53); income on red meat, b = 0.15, 95% CI (0.03, 0.27); income on healthy food, b = 0.75, 95% CI (0.44, 1.06).

4. Discussion

In this cross-sectional study of a representative U.S. sample of non-Hispanic Black Americans, non-Hispanic White Americans, and Hispanic Americans, we found that living in the eight-state Stroke Belt region was associated with eating more meat, especially red meat. The same associations were not seen for colorectal cancer quartiles and meat consumption, nor were there associations between the Stroke Belt region and healthy food consumption. The key findings in this study were that Stroke Belt residency was associated with meat and red meat consumption but not with healthy food consumption, and colorectal cancer state residency was not associated with the diet patterns assessed in this study.

In addition to the findings regarding residence in a Stroke Belt or colorectal cancer state and meat consumption, our results also showed that the health conditions of heart disease, diabetes, high blood pressure, high cholesterol, liver disease, and kidney disease were associated with Stroke Belt residence as mediated by overall meat consumption.

These findings are consistent with findings from other, larger studies where a review of epidemiological studies found an association between cardiovascular disease and type 2 diabetes as well as long-term consumption of red and processed meat [55]. Although studies show associations, there is a lack of evidence for the specific components of meat products that increase risks for cardiovascular disease and type 2 diabetes. There is an opening for future research to investigate this finding in more detail in order to better pinpoint the mechanisms and boundary conditions at play in this context.

Compared to White participants, Black participants did report significantly more overall meat and red meat consumption. The results were greater for Black participants compared to the Hispanic participants for both types of meat consumption, though the difference in overall meat consumption was not significant for Hispanics (see Table 2). Other studies showed that when compared to White women, Black women were significantly more likely to eat more total meat [56]. Additionally, compared to White Americans, Black Americans consumed more pork, and Mexican Americans consumed more beef compared to White Americans [23]. These findings were among a youth sample of over 14,000, ages 2 to 18 years, which is much younger than our sample, which had a median age of 38 years [23]. In this study, Hispanic youth did not report significantly more red meat consumption compared to White participants [23]. This is counter to literature reporting that Hispanics eat slightly more red meat than Whites or Blacks [57]. There are many complex factors at play in disparities in meat consumption by racial and ethnic identity. This includes the multifaceted relationships between identity and socioeconomic status, health care access, likelihood of residing in a food- and nutrition-insecure area, lifetime experience of allostatic stress and discrimination, and cultural differences in beliefs and practices surrounding food and nutrition.

A study examining household purchasing patterns, including the effect of spending on red meat on greenhouse gas emissions and diet quality [58] found that greenhouse gas emissions were lower and diet quality was higher in households that spent the least on red meat [58]. Although this study found no differences across race and ethnicity, lower education and study participants enrolled in SNAP were spending a larger percentage of their food income on red meat [58]. Similar to our findings, as income increases, healthier foods are preferred, and thus, a higher diet quality is attained.

When examining cultural factors, traditional or heritage foods may be influential in dietary practices. Within Hispanic ethnic groups, differences in meat consumption exist, and the risk of diet-related diseases differs. For example, in a study conducted in Costa Rica, there was a positive association between unprocessed and processed red meat and abdominal obesity, but this relationship only existed for overall meat consumption and metabolic syndrome [59]. Although this was not a U.S.-based study, immigrants and other ethnic groups build dietary practices around their heritage or traditional foods and are largely dependent on access and affordability. The percent of income spent on food in 2021 in the U.S. was 6.7% versus 31.6% in Costa Rica [60]. These differences may also be seen based on the type of retailers where Americans shop for food. Structural inequities may be more impactful risk factors on diet quality and health due to their impact on the food environment.

Some limitations should be considered. First, the retrospective, self-reported measure of meat consumption has limitations. Research participants often underreport diet information due to reliance on memory of prior intake [61]. The format of the measure was also not ideal, as averaging the number of days that each type of meat was consumed could be interpreted as the variety of meat consumption in addition to the amount or frequency. Although the measure is not ideal as a measure of absolute meat consumption, prior work examining the diet compositions of U.S. ethnic groups supports the self-reported food intake in the current study [23]. Second, we did not specifically ask about processed meat such as hot dogs, sausages, or bacon, nor did we collect information on preparation methods. According to the International Agency for Research on Cancer, red meat consumption and processed meat consumption are probably carcinogenic and carcinogenic to humans, respectively [62]. Although processed meat could not be analyzed in concert with red meat, evidence exists showing that the consumption of red meat is associated with cardiovascular disease mortality [63]. Additionally, a recent study showed that a higher intake of red and processed meat was associated with higher risk of cardiovascular events, but not poultry [63]. Third, dairy foods were not included as part of the analysis of the Stroke Belt and colorectal cancer. Dairy consumption is inversely associated with colorectal cancer and stroke [64,65], and data was not accessed nor was dairy included in our list of healthy foods. Fourth, we did not ask about disability status. A stroke-associated disability may have yielded higher gender differences in the southern Stroke Belt region, which is telling because the percentage of people with disabilities is highest in the southern U.S. [66]. Future studies are needed to address these important issues.

Colorectal cancer and Stroke Belt states are also some of the states with poor access to healthcare, making prevention through not only diet but also regular medical screenings more challenging [67]. Future studies should examine how access to preventative medical care and healthcare professionals confounds poor dietary choices associated with chronic diseases.

5. Conclusions

Health outcomes such as cancer and heart disease have a multitude of public health factors that predict their occurrence. It is known from previous research that meat consumption, especially red and processed meat, is one such factor [55,62]. Geographic location, such as state of residence in the U.S., can also be implicated as a risk factor in many related health outcomes, such as stroke and colorectal cancer incidence [44]. The present study suggests that overall and red meat consumption is associated with geographic location. Public health interventions aimed at reducing diet-related health disparities should consider the confluence of location and meat consumption in the development of lifestyle behavior change strategies and targeting practices. Dietary habits are inextricably linked to systemic and structural influences, which highlights the importance of not only continuing to examine the association of diet choices linked to diet-related health issues, but also to identify protective factors that can be incorporated in public health interventions.

Author Contributions: Conceptualization, K.E.M., M.E. and J.P.; data curation, M.E. and J.P.; Formal analysis, R.K.A. and N.C.W.; funding acquisition, M.E.; investigation, M.E. and J.P.; methodology, M.E. and R.K.A.; project administration, M.E. and J.P.; resources, M.E., J.P. and R.K.A.; supervision, K.E.M., M.E. and J.P.; validation, M.E. and R.K.A.; visualization, M.E., J.P. and K.E.M.; writing—original draft, K.E.M., J.P., M.E., R.K.A. and N.C.W.; writing—review & editing, K.E.M., J.P., M.E. and N.C.W. All authors have read and agreed to the published version of the manuscript.

Funding: This manuscript was funded in part by the Health and Risk Communication Center at Michigan State University.

Institutional Review Board Statement: The study was conducted in accordance with the Declaration of Helsinki and was determined exempt (category 2) by the Institutional Review Board of Michigan State University.

Informed Consent Statement: Informed consent was obtained from all subjects involved in the study.

Data Availability Statement: Data described in the manuscript will be made available upon request from the corresponding author.

Conflicts of Interest: The authors declare no conflict of interest.

References

1. Norat, T.; Lukanova, A.; Ferrari, P.; Riboli, E. Meat consumption and colorectal cancer risk: Dose-response meta-analysis of epidemiological studies. *Int. J. Cancer* **2002**, *98*, 241–256. [CrossRef]
2. Norat, T.; Bingham, S.; Ferrari, P.; Slimani, N.; Jenab, M.; Mazuir, M.; Overvad, K.; Olsen, A.; Tjønneland, A.; Clavel, F.; et al. Meat, fish, and colorectal cancer risk: The European Prospective Investigation into cancer and nutrition. *J. Natl. Cancer Inst.* **2005**, *97*, 906–916. [CrossRef] [PubMed]

3. Larsson, S.C.; Wolk, A. Meat consumption and risk of colorectal cancer: A meta-analysis of prospective studies. *Int. J. Cancer* **2006**, *119*, 2657–2664. [CrossRef] [PubMed]
4. Zhao, Z.; Feng, Q.; Yin, Z.; Shuang, J.; Bai, B.; Yu, P.; Guo, M.; Zhao, Q. Red and processed meat consumption and colorectal cancer risk: A systematic review and meta-analysis. *Oncotarget* **2017**, *8*, 83306. [CrossRef] [PubMed]
5. World Cancer Research Fund/American Institute for Cancer Research. Diet, Nutrition, Physical Activity and Colorectal Cancer. 2018. In *Continuous Update Project Expert Report 2018*; World Cancer Research Fund/American Institute for Cancer: Washington, DC, USA, 2018.
6. González, C.A.; Jakszyn, P.; Pera, G.; Agudo, A.; Bingham, S.; Palli, D.; Ferrari, P.; Boeing, H.; Del Giudice, G.; Plebani, M.; et al. Meat intake and risk of stomach and esophageal adenocarcinoma within the European Prospective Investigation Into Cancer and Nutrition (EPIC). *J. Natl. Cancer Inst.* **2006**, *98*, 345–354. [CrossRef] [PubMed]
7. Salehi, M.; Moradi-Lakeh, M.; Salehi, M.H.; Nojomi, M.; Kolahdooz, F. Meat, fish, and esophageal cancer risk: A systematic review and dose-response meta-analysis. *Nutr. Rev.* **2013**, *71*, 257–267. [CrossRef]
8. Choi, Y.; Song, S.; Song, Y.; Lee, J.E. Consumption of red and processed meat and esophageal cancer risk: Meta-analysis. *World J. Gastroenterol.* **2013**, *19*, 1020. [CrossRef] [PubMed]
9. Lam, T.K.; Cross, A.J.; Consonni, D.; Randi, G.; Bagnardi, V.; Bertazzi, P.A.; Caporaso, N.E.; Sinha, R.; Subar, A.F.; Landi, M.T. Intakes of red meat, processed meat, and meat mutagens increase lung cancer risk. *Cancer Res.* **2009**, *69*, 932–939. [CrossRef]
10. Tasevska, N.; Sinha, R.; Kipnis, V.; Subar, A.F.; Leitzmann, M.F.; Hollenbeck, A.R.; Caporaso, N.E.; Schatzkin, A.; Cross, A.J. A prospective study of meat, cooking methods, meat mutagens, heme iron, and lung cancer risks. *Am. J. Clin. Nutrit.* **2009**, *89*, 1884–1894. [CrossRef]
11. Larsson, S.; Wolk, A. Red and processed meat consumption and risk of pancreatic cancer: Meta-analysis of prospective studies. *Br. J. Cancer* **2012**, *106*, 603. [CrossRef]
12. Larsson, S.C.; Orsini, N.; Wolk, A. Processed meat consumption and stomach cancer risk: A meta-analysis. *J. Natl. Cancer Inst.* **2006**, *98*, 1078–1087. [CrossRef] [PubMed]
13. Cross, A.J.; Peters, U.; Kirsh, V.A.; Andriole, G.L.; Reding, D.; Hayes, R.B.; Sinha, R. A prospective study of meat and meat mutagens and prostate cancer risk. *Cancer Res.* **2005**, *65*, 11779–11784. [CrossRef] [PubMed]
14. Pan, A.; Sun, Q.; Bernstein, A.M.; Schulze, M.B.; Manson, J.E.; Stampfer, M.J.; Willett, W.C.; Hu, F.B. Red meat consumption and mortality: Results from 2 prospective cohort studies. *Arch. Intern. Med.* **2012**, *172*, 555–563. [PubMed]
15. Marmot, M.; Atinmo, T.; Byers, T. *Food, Nutrition, Physical Activity, and the Prevention of Cancer: A Global Perspective*; World Cancer Research Fund/American Institute for Cancer Research: Washington, DC, USA, 2007.
16. Wang, Y.; Beydoun, M.A. Meat consumption is associated with obesity and central obesity among US adults. *Int. J. Obes.* **2009**, *33*, 621. [CrossRef]
17. Aune, D.; Ursin, G.; Veierød, M. Meat consumption and the risk of type 2 diabetes: A systematic review and meta-analysis of cohort studies. *Diabetologia* **2009**, *52*, 2277. [CrossRef]
18. Health and Economic Benefits of Colorectal Cancer Interventions. 21 December 2022. Available online: https://www.cdc.gov/chronicdisease/programs-impact/pop/colorectal-cancer.htm (accessed on 26 January 2023).
19. Gonzalez, C.A. Nutrition and cancer: The current epidemiological evidence. *Br. J. Nutr.* **2006**, *96*, S42–S45. [CrossRef]
20. Sandhu, M.S.; White, I.R.; McPherson, K. Systematic review of the prospective cohort studies on meat consumption and colorectal cancer risk: A meta-analytical approach. *Cancer Epidemiol. Biomark. Prev.* **2001**, *10*, 439–446.
21. Zeng, L.; Ruan, M.; Liu, J.; Wilde, P.; Naumova, E.N.; Mozaffarian, D.; Zhang, F.F. Trends in processed meat, unprocessed red meat, poultry, and fish consumption in the United States, 1999–2016. *J. Acad. Nutr. Diet.* **2019**, *119*, 1085–1098. [CrossRef]
22. Gossard, M.H.; York, R. Social structural influences on meat consumption. *Hum. Ecol. Rev.* **2003**, *10*, 1–9.
23. Guenther, P.M.; Jensen, H.H.; Batres-Marquez, S.P.; Chen, C.-F. Sociodemographic, knowledge, and attitudinal factors related to meat consumption in the United States. *J. Am. Diet. Assoc.* **2005**, *105*, 1266–1274. [CrossRef]
24. Miller, K.D.; Goding Sauer, A.; Ortiz, A.P.; Fedewa, S.A.; Pinheiro, P.S.; Tortolero-Luna, G.; Martinez-Tyson, D.; Jemal, A.; Siegel, R.L. Cancer statistics for hispanics/latinos, 2018. *CA Cancer J. Clin.* **2018**, *68*, 425–445. [CrossRef] [PubMed]
25. Siegel, R.L.; Miller, K.D.; Goding Sauer, A.; Fedewa, S.A.; Butterly, L.F.; Anderson, J.C.; Cercek, A.; Smith, R.A.; Jemal, A. Colorectal cancer statistics, 2020. *CA Cancer J. Clin.* **2020**, *70*, 145–164. [CrossRef] [PubMed]
26. DeSantis, C.E.; Ma, J.; Gaudet, M.M.; Newman, L.A.; Miller, K.D.; Goding Sauer, A.; Jemal, A.; Siegel, R.L. Breast cancer statistics, 2019. *CA Cancer J. Clin.* **2019**, *69*, 438–451. [CrossRef] [PubMed]
27. Torre, L.A.; Trabert, B.; DeSantis, C.E.; Miller, K.D.; Samimi, G.; Runowicz, C.D.; Gaudet, M.M.; Jemal, A.; Siegel, R.L. Ovarian cancer statistics, 2018. *CA Cancer J. Clin.* **2018**, *68*, 284–296. [CrossRef] [PubMed]
28. Romero, C.X.; Romero, T.E.; Shlay, J.C.; Ogden, L.G.; Dabelea, D. Changing trends in the prevalence and disparities of obesity and other cardiovascular disease risk factors in three racial/ethnic groups of USA adults. *Adv. Prev. Med.* **2012**, *2012*, 172423. [CrossRef]
29. Ogden, C.; Carroll, M.D.; Kit, B.K.; Flegal, K.M. Prevalence of childhood and adult obesity in the United States, 2011–2012. *J. Am. Med. Assoc.* **2014**, *311*, 806–814. [CrossRef]
30. Skinner, A.C.; Skelton, J.A. Prevalence and trends in obesity and severe obesity among children in the United States, 1999–2012. *JAMA Pediatr.* **2014**, *168*, 561–566. [CrossRef]

31. Hales, C.M.; Carroll, M.D.; Fryar, C.D.; Ogden, C.L. Prevalence of obesity among adults and youth: United States, 2015–2016. *NCHS Data Brief.* **2017**, *288*, 1–8.
32. Diabetes Report Card 2019. 2020. Available online: https://stacks.cdc.gov/view/cdc/103877 (accessed on 24 January 2023).
33. Golden, S.H.; Brown, A.; Cauley, J.A.; Chin, M.H.; Gary-Webb, T.L.; Kim, C.; Sosa, J.A.; Sumner, A.E.; Anton, B. Health disparities in endocrine disorders: Biological, clinical, and nonclinical factors—An Endocrine Society scientific statement. *J. Clin. Endocrinol. Metab.* **2012**, *97*, E1579–E1639. [CrossRef]
34. Pan, L.; Galuska, D.A.; Sherry, B.; Hunter, A.S.; Rutledge, G.E.; Dietz, W.H.; Balluz, L.S. Differences in prevalence of obesity among black, white, and Hispanic adults-United States, 2006–2008. *Morb. Mortal. Wkly. Rep.* **2009**, *58*, 740–744.
35. Chang, S.H.; Yu, Y.C.; Carlsson, N.P.; Liu, X.; Colditz, G.A. Racial disparity in life expectancies and life years lost associated with multiple obesity-related chronic conditions. *Obesity* **2017**, *25*, 950–957. [CrossRef] [PubMed]
36. Centers for Disease Control and Prevention. National Diabetes Fact Sheet. 2011. Available online: http://www.cdc.gov/diabetes/pubs/pdf/ndfs_2011.pdf (accessed on 5 April 2018).
37. Kirk, J.K.; D'Agostino, R.B., Jr.; Bell, R.A.; Passmore, L.V.; Bonds, D.E.; Karter, A.J.; Narayan, K.V. Disparities in HbA1c levels between African-American and non-Hispanic white adults with diabetes: A meta-analysis. *Diabetes Care* **2006**, *29*, 2130–2136. [CrossRef]
38. Hollar, D.; Agatston, A.S.; Hennekens, C.H. Hypertension: Trends, risks, drug therapies and clinical challenges in African Americans. *Ethn. Dis.* **2004**, *14*, S2–S23. [PubMed]
39. Davidson, J.A.; Kannel, W.B.; Lopez-Candales, A.; Morales, L.; Moreno, P.R.; Ovalle, F.; Rodriguez, C.J.; Rodbard, H.W.; Rosenson, R.S.; Stern, M. Avoiding the looming Latino/Hispanic cardiovascular health crisis: A call to action. *J. Cardiometab. Syndr.* **2007**, *2*, 238–243. [CrossRef] [PubMed]
40. Brown, A.F.; Liang, L.J.; Vassar, S.D.; Escarce, J.J.; Merkin, S.S.; Cheng, E.; Richards, A.; Seeman, T.; Longstreth, W.T., Jr. Trends in Racial/Ethnic and Nativity Disparities in Cardiovascular Health Among Adults Without Prevalent Cardiovascular Disease in the United States, 1988 to 2014. *Ann. Intern. Med.* **2018**, *168*, 541–549. [CrossRef]
41. Siegel, R.L.; Miller, K.D.; Jemal, A. Cancer statistics, 2017. *CA Cancer J. Clin.* **2017**, *67*, 7–30. [CrossRef]
42. Ward, E.; Jemal, A.; Cokkinides, V.; Singh, G.K.; Cardinez, C.; Ghafoor, A.; Thun, M. Cancer disparities by race/ethnicity and socioeconomic status. *CA Cancer J. Clin.* **2004**, *54*, 78–93. [CrossRef]
43. Tsao, C.W.; Aday, A.W.; Almarzooq, Z.I.; Alonso, A.; Beaton, A.Z.; Bittencourt, M.S.; Boehme, A.K.; Buxton, A.E.; Carson, A.P. Heart Disease and Stroke Statistics-2022 Update: A Report From the American Heart Association. *Circulation* **2022**, *145*, e153–e639.
44. Stroke Death Rates, Total Population 35+, by County. Available online: https://www.cdc.gov/dhdsp/maps/national_maps/stroke_all.htm (accessed on 15 December 2022).
45. Pew Research Center. Hispanics Have Accounted for More Than Half of Total U.S. Population Growth Since 2010. Available online: https://www.pewresearch.org/fact-tank/2020/07/10/hispanics-have-accounted-for-more-than-half-of-total-u-s-population-growth-since-2010/ (accessed on 9 December 2022).
46. Pew Research Center. Facts about the U.S. Black Population. Available online: https://www.pewresearch.org/social-trends/fact-sheet/facts-about-the-us-black-population/ (accessed on 9 December 2022).
47. Nanda, M.; Sharma, R.; Mubarik, S.; Aashima, A.; Zhang, K. Type-2 Diabetes mellitus (T2DM): Spatial-temporal patterns of incidence, mortality and attributable risk factors from 1990 to 2019 among 21 world regions. *Endocrine* **2022**, *77*, 444–454. [CrossRef]
48. Larsson, S.C. Dietary approaches for stroke prevention. *Stroke* **2017**, *48*, 2905–2911. [CrossRef]
49. Lescinsky, H.; Afshin, A.; Ashbaugh, C.; Bisignano, C.; Brauer, M.; Ferrara, G.; Hay, S.I.; He, J.; Iannucci, V.; Marczak, L.B.; et al. Health effects associated with consumption of unprocessed red meat: A Burden of Proof study. *Nat. Med.* **2022**, *28*, 2075–2082. [CrossRef] [PubMed]
50. Craig, W.J. Health effects of vegan diets. *Am. J. Clin. Nutr.* **2009**, *89*, 1627S–1633S. [CrossRef] [PubMed]
51. Key, T.J.; Appleby, P.N.; Rosell, M.S. Health effects of vegetarian and vegan diets. *Proc. Nutr. Soc.* **2006**, *65*, 35–41. [CrossRef] [PubMed]
52. Tilman, D.; Clark, M. Global diets link environmental sustainability and human health. *Nature* **2014**, *515*, 518. [CrossRef]
53. Buhrmester, M.; Kwang, T.; Gosling, S.D. Amazon's Mechanical Turk: A new source of inexpensive, yet high-quality data? *Perspect. Psychol. Sci.* **2011**, *6*, 3–5. [CrossRef]
54. Burnham, M.J.; Le, Y.K.; Piedmont, R.L. Who is Mturk? Personal characteristics and sample consistency of these online workers. *Ment. Health Relig. Cult.* **2018**, *21*, 934–944. [CrossRef]
55. Richi, E.B.; Baumer, B.; Conrad, B.; Darioli, R.; Schmid, A.; Keller, U. Health risks associated with meat consumption: A review of epidemiological studies. *Int. J. Vitam. Nutr. Res.* **2015**, *85*, 70–78. [CrossRef]
56. Choi, S.E.; Lee, K.J. Ethnic differences in attitudes, beliefs, and patterns of meat consumption among American young women meat eaters. *Nutr. Res. Pract.* **2022**, *16*, e48. [CrossRef]
57. Daniel, C.R.; Cross, A.J.; Koebnick, C.; Sinha, R. Trends in meat consumption in the USA. *Public Health Nutr.* **2011**, *14*, 575–583. [CrossRef]
58. Boehm, R.; Ver Ploeg, M.; Wilde, P.E.; Cash, S.B. Greenhouse gas emissions, total food spending and diet quality by share of household food spending on red meat: Results from a nationally representative sample of US households. *Public Health Nutr.* **2019**, *22*, 1794–1806. [CrossRef]

49. Luan, D.; Wang, D.; Campos, H.; Baylin, A. Red meat consumption and metabolic syndrome in the Costa Rica Heart Study. *Eur. J. Nutr.* **2020**, *59*, 185–193. [CrossRef] [PubMed]
50. Share of Consumer Expenditure Spent on Food vs. Total Consumer Expenditure. 2021. Available online: https://ourworldindata.org/grapher/food-expenditure-share-gdp?country=~CRI (accessed on 2 February 2023).
51. Subar, A.F.; Freedman, L.S.; Tooze, J.A.; Kirkpatrick, S.I.; Boushey, C.; Neuhouser, M.L.; Thompson, F.E.; Potischman, N.; Guenther, P.M.; Tarasuk, V.; et al. Addressing Current Criticism Regarding the Value of Self-Report Dietary Data. *J. Nutr.* **2015**, *145*, 2639–2645. [CrossRef] [PubMed]
52. IARC Working Group on the Evaluation of Carcinogenic Risks to Humans. *Red Meat and Processed Meat*; International Agency for Research on Cancer: Lyon, France, 2018.
53. Zhong, V.W.; Van Horn, L.; Greenland, P.; Carnethon, M.R.; Ning, H.; Wilkins, J.T.; Lloyd-Jones, D.M.; Allen, N.B. Associations of processed meat, unprocessed red meat, poultry, or fish intake with incident cardiovascular disease and all-cause mortality. *JAMA Intern. Med.* **2020**, *180*, 503–512. [CrossRef] [PubMed]
54. Barrubés, L.; Babio, N.; Becerra-Tomás, N.; Rosique-Esteban, N.; Salas-Salvadó, J. Association Between Dairy Product Consumption and Colorectal Cancer Risk in Adults: A Systematic Review and Meta-Analysis of Epidemiologic Studies. *Adv. Nutr.* **2019**, *10* (Suppl. 2), S190–S211. [CrossRef] [PubMed]
55. De Goede, J.; Soedamah-Muthu, S.S.; Pan, A.; Gijsbers, L.; Geleijnse, J.M. Dairy Consumption and Risk of Stroke: A Systematic Review and Updated Dose-Response Meta-Analysis of Prospective Cohort Studies. *J. Am. Heart Assoc.* **2016**, *5*, e002787. [CrossRef] [PubMed]
56. Disability Impacts Us All. 2022. Available online: https://www.cdc.gov/ncbddd/disabilityandhealth/infographic-disability-impacts-all.html (accessed on 13 October 2022).
57. United Health Foundation (UHF) & American Public Health Association (APHA). A Call to Action for Individuals and Their Communities. *Am. Health Rankings* **2017**. Available online: https://assets.americashealthrankings.org/app/uploads/ahrannual17_complete-121817.pdf (accessed on 23 January 2023).

Disclaimer/Publisher's Note: The statements, opinions and data contained in all publications are solely those of the individual author(s) and contributor(s) and not of MDPI and/or the editor(s). MDPI and/or the editor(s) disclaim responsibility for any injury to people or property resulting from any ideas, methods, instructions or products referred to in the content.

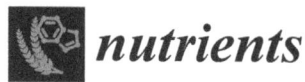 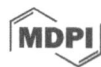

Article

Nutrients and Dementia: Prospective Study

Hikaru Takeuchi [1,*] and Ryuta Kawashima [1,2,3]

[1] Division of Developmental Cognitive Neuroscience, Institute of Development, Aging and Cancer, Tohoku University, Sendai 980-8575, Japan
[2] Smart Aging Research Center, Tohoku University, Sendai 980-8575, Japan
[3] Department of Advanced Brain Science, Institute of Development, Aging and Cancer, Tohoku University, Sendai 980-8575, Japan
* Correspondence: takehi@idac.tohoku.ac.jp

Abstract: The association of diet and nutrients with dementia risk is an interesting research topic. Middle-aged and older Europeans not diagnosed with dementia within two years of baseline were followed up and their data were analysed until 2021. The association between the nutrient quintiles measured by the web-based 24 h dietary and the risk of developing dementia was examined using a Cox proportional hazard model after adjusting for potential confounding factors. Approximately 160,000 subjects and 1200 cases were included in the analysis of each nutrient. A greater risk of dementia was associated with (a) no alcohol intake (compared with moderate to higher intake), (b) higher intake of total sugars and carbohydrates (compared with lower intake), (c) highest or lowest fat intake (compared with moderate intake), (d) quintiles of highest or lowest magnesium intake (compared with the quintile of the second highest intake), and (e) highest protein intake (compared with moderate intake). Overall, the present results are congruent with the importance of a moderate intake of certain nutrients.

Keywords: nutrients; dementia; magnesium; protein; sugar

Citation: Takeuchi, H.; Kawashima, R. Nutrients and Dementia: Prospective Study. *Nutrients* 2023, 15, 842. https://doi.org/10.3390/nu15040842

Academic Editor: Joanna Stadnik

Received: 13 November 2022
Revised: 2 February 2023
Accepted: 2 February 2023
Published: 7 February 2023

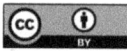

Copyright: © 2023 by the authors. Licensee MDPI, Basel, Switzerland. This article is an open access article distributed under the terms and conditions of the Creative Commons Attribution (CC BY) license (https://creativecommons.org/licenses/by/4.0/).

1. Introduction

The increasing incidence of dementia is an important social issue in this current ageing society. No effective treatment has been developed for dementia; thus, the preventive effects of various lifestyle factors, including nutrition and diet, are currently being investigated as they hold great importance. Numerous cohort studies have been conducted on the association between the intake of different nutrients and the risk of dementia. In addition, meta-analyses revealed that a higher risk of dementia is associated with a lower intake of unsaturated fatty acids [1], folate [2], vitamin D [1], vitamin E [3], and minimal or no alcohol intake [4]. However, some reports are inconsistent (e.g., findings on vitamin E) [5]. In addition, the association between the lower risk of dementia and the intake of magnesium, proteins, other nutrients, and some forms of sugars was observed only in individual observational studies using a relatively smaller sample size than those using UK Biobank data [6–9].

These observational studies have various problems. First, they were generally small in size (compared with those of UK Biobank studies). Although meta-analyses can compensate for this limitation, they are not free from publication bias. Second, the abundant potential confounding factors have a potential impact. For instance, our previous study showed that body mass index (BMI) and the risk of dementia are significantly affected by adjusting for educational history [10]. Although previous meta-analyses linked obesity in middle age to a higher risk of dementia [11], recent large studies found the opposite effect [12,13]. The underlying reason is uncertain and may be partly due to the increase in effective coping strategies for stroke. Thus, investigating relevant associations using modern data is important.

To address these issues, we used data from the UK Biobank to reveal the association between dietary nutrients and the risk of dementia in a large cohort after adjusting for a wide range of confounding factors. Our hypothesis was that a lower risk of dementia is associated with a higher intake of polyunsaturated fatty acids, protein, vitamins B, D, and E, and magnesium; a moderate alcohol intake; and a low sugar intake. We also conducted an exploratory investigation of nutrients and dementia risk. The increasing incidence of dementia is an important issue for the modern ageing society, and the identification of dietary habits associated with its prevention and risk is an important scientific topic. Further, the strengths of this study are summarized as follows: First, the large sample and careful adjustment for confounding factors attempt to provide robust answers to an important research topic (nutrition and dementia risk) on which previous findings have been mixed. Second, this study aims to confirm the findings in a modern sample. Finally, we are investigating nutrients not well investigated previously.

2. Methods

2.1. Participants

The UK Biobank provided a dataset obtained from a prospective cohort study of a middle-aged population in the United Kingdom [http://www.ukBiobank.ac.uk/wp-content/uploads/2011/11/UK-Biobank-Protocol.pdf, (accessed on 5 July 2021)]. The North–West Multi-Centre Research Ethics Committee approved these experiments, and each participant provided written informed consent.

The online dietary survey was administered five times between 2009 and 2012. The data of subjects who participated in the survey at least once were used in the analysis. For subjects who participated in the survey more than once, the average of each data type was used. A total of 211,013 subjects participated in the online dietary survey at least once.

In addition, each participant attended to one of the 22 assessment sites in the United Kingdom for data collection; baseline data were received from 502,505 participants in this cohort. Our analysis also included data from the first assessment visit (2006–2010) for the covariates of the analysis. We conducted each analysis using data from all participants for whom valid data for all independent and dependent variables were available.

The descriptions in this subsection are largely reproduced from our previous study using data from the UK Biobank [14].

2.2. Assessment of Nutrients

Nutrient item data were derived from the web-based 24 h dietary assessment "Oxford WebQ" [15]. The questionnaire was administered from 2009 to 2012. Oxford WebQ contains questions on the consumption of 206 foods and 32 beverages over the past 24 h. Subjects enlisted in the last year of the UK Biobank's subject recruitment list were not enrolled through the web but rather through their email information when they were invited to participate in the study and took the survey 1–4 times between 2009 and 2012. The nutrients were calculated from the intake frequency, standard portion size, and nutrient composition of each food and beverage type. For subjects who took the survey more than once, the average value was used.

2.3. Sociodemographic and Lifestyle Measurements as Covariates

Self-reported gender data were used. From the UK Biobank database, the neighbourhood-level socioeconomic status at recruitment (cov1), education level at recruitment (cov2), household income at baseline (cov3), employment status at baseline (cov4), metabolic equivalent of task hours (MET) (cov5), number of people in the household (cov6), height (cov7), BMI category (cov8), self-reported health status (cov9), category of duration of sleep (cov10), category of diastolic blood pressure (cov11), current tobacco smoking level (cov12), ethnicity (cov13), diagnosis of diabetes, heart attack, angina, stroke, cancer, and other serious medical conditions (cov14–cov19), visuospatial memory task performance (number of errors: performance worse than 2SD were excluded) (cov20), depression score (cov21), antihypertensive medication (cov22), and statin use (cov23) were extracted or calculated and included as covariates together with age and sex. Additional information can be found in the Supplemental Methods.

The reason for including covariates for disease and health status in the analysis is to prevent, as far as possible, health status from being a confounding factor in the association between dementia and nutrients. That is, poor health leads to certain eating habits, such as eating small meals, and poor health is a risk for dementia, and the association between nutritional intake and dementia as a result of these two factors is prevented as much as possible by this model. Height was also included as a covariate to avoid the possibility of height being a confounding factor in the association between dementia and nutrients, as height is related to nutrient intake but also to dementia risk [16].

When all explanatory variables were treated as continuous variables and the correlation coefficients between explanatory variables calculated, the single correlation coefficient r was >|0.5| for the association between sex and standing height, and the association between age and current employment status and these associations did not include nutritional variables. Thus, multicollinearity did not appear to affect the association between nutritional variables and dementia. To confirm this, we excluded standing height and current employment status from the covariates and found that the adjusted hazard ratios of each group of nutrient intake level were barely affected and the significance (FDR-corrected) of the overall group differences was not affected.

2.4. Statistical Data Analysis

Predictive Analysis Software version 22.0.0 (SPSS Inc., Chicago, IL, USA; 2010) was used for statistical analyses. Cox proportional hazard models were used to investigate the relationship between diet type and the risk of all-cause dementia over time [17]. All-cause dementia was determined using hospital inpatient records and connections to death registry data. Additional information can be found in the Supplemental Methods. This method of determining dementia was adopted from a representative study that assessed lifestyle and risk of incident dementia over time using UK Biobank data [17] and from our previous work [14]. The descriptions in this subsection are largely reproduced from our previous study using the same methods [14].

Exclusion criteria were as follows: (a) self-reported dementia, Alzheimer's disease, or cognitive impairment without a diagnosis of all-cause dementia in either hospital inpatient records or death register data; (b) a diagnosis of dementia at baseline or within two years after providing the answer to the first diet type question; (c) death within two years after baseline; and (d) visuospatial memory performance <2SD. The observation period started when each participant had first completed the diet type questionnaire and continued until death, dementia diagnosis, or until 30 September 2021. For each analysis, sex, age at completion of the first diet type questionnaire, and cov1–cov24 values were all used as covariates. People who developed dementia within two years were excluded from the analysis to eliminate the possibility that certain behaviour patterns are already being observed as a result of dementia. This approach has been previously applied in other studies on dementia [18].

Results with a $p < 0.05$ corrected for false-discovery rates using the two-stage sharpened method [19] in the analyses of group differences in each nutrition type were considered statistically significant. This correction was applied to the p values of the 23 main analyses of group differences for each type of nutrition.

In this study, we included subjects with complete data of covariates and nutritional data among those not excluded according to the four exclusion criteria of dementia. The UK Biobank, like any cohort study, involves participants with specific characteristics; therefore, it is likely that the subjects who took part in the online dietary survey also have specific characteristics. Moreover, participants in the online dietary survey, for whom complete covariates' data are available, may also have specific characteristics. However, this study is an analysis within those specific cohorts, and all samples have the same conditions; in that respect, the removal of participants with a lack of data is unlikely to be a confounding factor (however, the generalizability of the results or their sensitivity may be altered). Among the participants in the UK Biobank not excluded according to the four exclusion criteria of dementia that completed the online survey and had nutritional data, the subjects who lacked ≥1 covariate (those excluded in the analysis) tended to be systematically different from those with complete covariate data. The former is particularly characterized (effect size: Cohen's d > 0.3 or odds ratio >1.3 or <0.7) by low education level, low household income, non-current employment, female sex, non-white ethnicity, doctor diagnosis of diabetes, and doctor diagnosis of angina. These data are provided in Supplemental Table S1.

3. Results

3.1. Basic Baseline Data

Table 1 shows the baseline psychological variables of the participants. A total of 161,376 subjects participated in the online dietary survey, provided all data used in the analysis, and failed to meet the exclusion criteria. Among them, 160,170 (mean age of 58.5 [SD: 8.0] years) did not develop dementia, and 1206 (mean age of 66.3 [SD: 5.2] years) developed dementia.

Table 1. Baseline characteristics of participants with and without incident dementia.

	No Incident Dementia (n = 160,170)	Incident Dementia (n = 1206)
	Mean	
Age	58.51 (8.01)	66.27 (5.19)
Townsend deprivation index	−1.62 (2.84)	−1.48 (2.94)
Education length	15.49 (4.79)	14.3 (5.07)
MET *	30.27 (32.04)	32.1 (36.08)
Height	169.66 (9.17)	169.48 (9.13)
Depression score	5.42 (1.87)	5.47 (1.94)
Visuospatial memory (errors)	3.5 (2.36)	3.93 (2.5)
	Number	
Male number	74,596 (46.6%)	699 (58%)
Household income (a) Less than £18,000 (b) £18,000 to £30,999 (c) £31,000 to £5,1999 (d) £52,000 to £100,000 (e) Greater than £100,000	22,864 (14.3%) 37,766 (23.6%) 46,066 (28.8%) 41,033 (25.6%) 12,441 (7.8%)	359 (29.8%) 404 (33.5%) 266 (22.1%) 140 (11.6%) 37 (3.1%)
Currently employed	102,800 (64.2%)	337 (27.9%)
BMI Underweight (x ≤ 18.5) Normal (18.5 < x ≤ 25) Overweight (25 < x ≤ 30) Obesity (x < 30)	819 (0.5%) 59,474 (37.1%) 66,943 (41.8%) 32,934 (20.6%)	10 (0.8%) 409 (33.9%) 476 (39.5%) 311 (25.8%)
Household number (a) 1 (b) 2 (c) 3 (d) 4≤	28,380 (17.7%) 73,416 (45.8%) 25,180 (15.7%) 33,194 (20.7%)	281 (23.3%) 754 (62.5%) 101 (8.4%) 70 (5.8%)

Table 1. *Cont.*

	No Incident Dementia (*n* = 160,170)	Incident Dementia (*n* = 1206)
Overall health (4 levels)		
(a) Poor	4326 (2.7%)	88 (7.3%)
(b) Fair	26,009 (16.2%)	287 (23.8%)
(c) Good	95,771 (59.8%)	673 (55.8%)
(d) Excellent	34,064 (21.3%)	158 (13.1%)
Sleep duration		
(a) ≤ 4 h,	911 (0.6%)	11 (0.9%)
(b) 5 h or 6 h,	34,352 (21.4%)	266 (22.1%)
(c) 7 h or 8 h,	114,998 (71.8%)	816 (67.7%)
(d) 9 h$\leq$	9909 (6.2%)	113 (9.4%)
Current smoking level (3 levels)		
(a) No	147,642 (92.2%)	1111 (92.1%)
(b) Only occasionally	4021 (2.5%)	29 (2.4%)
(c) On most or all days	8507 (5.3%)	66 (5.5%)
Diastolic BP		
$x < 65$	5626 (3.5%)	47 (3.9%)
$65 \leq x < 90$	121,089 (75.6%)	918 (76.1%)
$90 \leq 30$	33,455 (20.9%)	241 (20%)
Ethnicity (non-white)	5631 (3.5%)	19 (1.6%)
Antihypertensive drug intake	27,627 (17.2%)	431 (35.7%)
Statin intake	15,590 (9.7%)	239 (19.8%)
Diabetes	6159 (3.8%)	120 (10%)
Heart attack	2535 (1.6%)	59 (4.9%)
Angina	3270 (2%)	95 (7.9%)
Stroke	1589 (1%)	52 (4.3%)
Cancer	12,781 (8%)	128 (10.6%)
Other serious medical conditions	31,084 (19.4%)	408 (33.8%)

* MET: metabolic equivalent of task hours (MET). Physical activity level.

3.2. Prospective Dementia Analysis

A total of 211,013 subjects participated at least once in the online diet survey. Among them, 28 who had a record of only self-reported dementia or cognitive impairment, 53 who had dementia diagnosis before baseline, and 69 who were diagnosed with dementia within two years after their last participation in the online dietary survey were excluded. A total of 1431 participants who died without a dementia diagnosis within two years after baseline were also excluded. Analyses were conducted using only the data of subjects who had all covariates, including those with visuospatial memory performance >2SD.

A Cox proportional hazard model split the subjects into five categories according to the nutrient intake level (mostly quintiles) to correct for a wide range of potential confounding factors. A correction for multiple comparisons was conducted as well. One analysis per nutrient was performed for a total of 23. The results showed significant group differences for alcohol, fat, carbohydrate, protein, total sugars, and magnesium. However, no group differences existed for calcium, carotene, energy, energy dietary fibre, folate, food weight, potassium, polyunsaturated fat, iron retinol, starch, saturated fat, and vitamins B6, B12 C, D, and E. Statistical values and adjusted rates, as well as the number of cases and samples in each group in each analysis, are provided in Table 2.

Table 2. Nutrient intake level (amount, adjusted HR, and case ratio) for each group and uncorrected and corrected p values of overall group differences.

Nutrients		Amount (Upper), Adjusted HR (Middle), Case Number/Entire Sample (%)					p (FDR)
(Unit)	Level 1	Level 2	Level 3	Level 4	Level 5		
alcohol	$x \leq 0$	$0 < x \leq 3.2533$	$3.2533 < x \leq 14.74$	$14.74 < x \leq 30.45$	$30.45 < x$		
(g)	reference	0.79 (0.62,1.02)	0.85 (0.72,1)	0.77 (0.65,0.9)	0.79 (0.67,0.93)		0.026
	462/52,407 (0.9%)	71/9352 (0.8%)	226/32,299 (0.7%)	215/33,446 (0.6%)	232/33,872 (0.7%)		
calcium	$x \leq 688.02$	$688.02 < x \leq 853.05$	$853.05 < x \leq 1011.97$	$1011.97 < x \leq 1226.67$	$1226.67 < x$		
(mg)	reference	1.11 (0.92,1.34)	1.07 (0.89,1.29)	1.01 (0.84,1.23)	1.21 (1.01,1.45)		0.324
	200/31,483 (0.6%)	237/32,560 (0.7%)	241/32,671 (0.7%)	239/32,663 (0.7%)	289/31,999 (0.9%)		
carbohydrate	$x \leq 187.33$	$187.33 < x \leq 227.05$	$227.05 < x \leq 263.84$	$263.84 < x \leq 312.90$	$312.90 < x$		
(g)	reference	0.86 (0.71,1.04)	0.91 (0.76,1.1)	1.07 (0.89,1.28)	1.18 (0.98,1.4)		0.026
	225/31,682 (0.7%)	200/32,274 (0.6%)	218/32,544 (0.7%)	265/32,813 (0.8%)	298/32,063 (0.9%)		
carotene	$x \leq 991.92$	$991.92 < x \leq 1996.76$	$1996.76 < x \leq 3107.49$	$3107.49 < x \leq 4748.76$	$4748.76 < x$		
(μg)	reference	0.93 (0.78,1.12)	0.9 (0.75,1.08)	0.91 (0.76,1.1)	1.07 (0.9,1.27)		0.328
	240/31,192 (0.8%)	225/32,817 (0.7%)	225/32,932 (0.7%)	231/32,641 (0.7%)	285/31,794 (0.9%)		
energy	$x \leq 6757.23$	$6757.23 < x \leq 7976.07$	$7976.07 < x \leq 9124.26$	$9124.26 < x \leq 10,674.42$	$10,674.42 < x$		
(KJ)	reference	1.01 (0.84,1.21)	0.96 (0.8,1.16)	0.89 (0.73,1.07)	1.15 (0.96,1.38)		0.126
	224/30,924 (0.7%)	235/32,216 (0.7%)	236/32,667 (0.7%)	221/33,035 (0.7%)	290/32,534 (0.9%)		
Englyst dietary fibre	$x \leq 11.10$	$11.10 < x \leq 14.22$	$14.22 < x \leq 17.19$	$17.19 < x \leq 21.14$	$21.14 < x$		
(g)	reference	0.94 (0.78,1.13)	0.83 (0.69,1)	0.98 (0.82,1.18)	0.99 (0.83,1.18)		0.336
	224/31,504 (0.7%)	227/32,513 (0.7%)	209/32,632 (0.6%)	263/32,718 (0.8%)	283/32,009 (0.9%)		
fat	$x \leq 52.97$	$52.97 < x \leq 67.44$	$67.44 < x \leq 81.38$	$81.38 < x \leq 100.03$	$100.03 < x$		
(g)	reference	0.8 (0.67,0.95)	0.83 (0.69,0.99)	0.76 (0.64,0.91)	1 (0.84,1.18)		0.025
	266/31,328 (0.8%)	219/32,136 (0.7%)	232/32,681 (0.7%)	213/32,695 (0.7%)	276/32,536 (0.8%)		
folate	$x \leq 213.92$	$213.92 < x \leq 265.13$	$265.13 < x \leq 314.08$	$314.08 < x \leq 381.53$	$381.53 < x$		
(μg)	reference	0.84 (0.69,1.01)	0.8 (0.66,0.96)	0.88 (0.74,1.06)	0.98 (0.82,1.17)		0.126
	231/31,317 (0.7%)	216/32,488 (0.7%)	213/32,643 (0.7%)	250/32,654 (0.8%)	296/32,274 (0.9%)		

Table 2. Cont.

Nutrients	Amount (Upper), Adjusted HR (Middle), Case Number/Entire Sample (%)					p (FDR)
(Unit)	Level 1	Level 2	Level 3	Level 4	Level 5	
food weight	x ≤ 2552.33	2552.33 < x ≤ 2940.00	2940.00 < x ≤ 3302.85	3302.85 < x ≤ 3782.00	3782.00 < x	0.35
(g)	reference	0.95 (0.79,1.14)	0.89 (0.74,1.07)	0.93 (0.78,1.12)	1.07 (0.9,1.28)	
	247/31,082 (0.8%)	237/32,243 (0.7%)	225/32,558 (0.7%)	233/32,805 (0.7%)	264/32,688 (0.8%)	
iron	x ≤ 10.08	10.08 < x ≤ 12.30	12.30 < x ≤ 14.34	14.34 < x ≤ 16.96	16.96 < x	0.132
(mg)	reference	0.92 (0.77,1.11)	0.85 (0.7,1.02)	0.83 (0.69,1)	1.02 (0.86,1.22)	
	231/30,826 (0.7%)	228/32,230 (0.7%)	219/32,464 (0.7%)	229/33,002 (0.7%)	299/32,854 (0.9%)	
magnesium	x ≤ 263.40	263.40 < x ≤ 313.92	313.92 < x ≤ 360.46	360.46 < x ≤ 422.92	422.92 < x	0.025
(mg)	reference	0.98 (0.81,1.18)	0.91 (0.76,1.1)	0.81 (0.67,0.98)	1.14 (0.95,1.36)	
	225/30,903 (0.7%)	237/32,185 (0.7%)	228/32,590 (0.7%)	213/32,937 (0.6%)	303/32,761 (0.9%)	
polyunsaturated fat	x ≤ 8.32	8.32 < x ≤ 11.55	11.55 < x ≤ 14.91	14.91 < x ≤ 19.51	19.51 < x	0.078
(g)	reference	0.87 (0.73,1.04)	0.89 (0.75,1.06)	0.74 (0.61,0.89)	0.89 (0.75,1.06)	
	275/31,462 (0.9%)	242/32,390 (0.7%)	244/32,726 (0.7%)	202/32,515 (0.6%)	243/32,283 (0.8%)	
potassium	x ≤ 2821.42	2821.42 < x ≤ 3377.58	3377.58 < x ≤ 3893.73	3893.73 < x ≤ 4571.70	4571.70 < x	0.18
(mg)	reference	0.86 (0.71,1.04)	0.92 (0.76,1.1)	0.87 (0.73,1.05)	1.05 (0.88,1.26)	
	222/31,075 (0.7%)	210/32,439 (0.6%)	233/32,666 (0.7%)	238/32,866 (0.7%)	303/32,330 (0.9%)	
protein	x ≤ 62.51	62.51 < x ≤ 74.76	74.76 < x ≤ 85.60	85.60 < x ≤ 99.95	99.95 < x	0.044
(g)	reference	0.98 (0.82,1.18)	0.94 (0.78,1.13)	0.87 (0.72,1.05)	1.17 (0.98,1.4)	
	226/31,191 (0.7%)	238/32,504 (0.7%)	230/32,577 (0.7%)	219/32,710 (0.7%)	293/32,394 (0.9%)	
retinol	x ≤ 176.18	176.18 < x ≤ 259.66	259.66 < x ≤ 345.04	345.04 < x ≤ 459.58	459.58 < x	0.814
(μg)	reference	0.96 (0.8,1.16)	0.94 (0.78,1.14)	1 (0.83,1.2)	0.97 (0.81,1.17)	
	221/31,216 (0.7%)	224/31,751 (0.7%)	228/31,963 (0.7%)	251/32,225 (0.8%)	259/32,048 (0.8%)	
saturated fat	x ≤ 19.28	19.28 < x ≤ 25.25	25.25 < x ≤ 31.14	31.14 < x ≤ 39.24	39.24 < x	0.393
(g)	reference	0.9 (0.75,1.08)	0.95 (0.79,1.14)	1.04 (0.87,1.24)	1.06 (0.89,1.27)	
	232/31,383 (0.7%)	218/32,302 (0.7%)	230/32,601 (0.7%)	257/32,611 (0.8%)	269/32,479 (0.8%)	

Table 2. Cont.

Nutrients	Amount (Upper), Adjusted HR (Middle), Case Number/Entire Sample (%)					p (FDR)
(Unit)	Level 1	Level 2	Level 3	Level 4	Level 5	
starch	x ≤ 84.78	84.78 < x ≤ 108.32	108.32 < x ≤ 129.57	129.57 < x ≤ 156.59	156.59 < x	0.328
(g)	reference	0.93 (0.78,1.11)	0.97 (0.81,1.16)	0.82 (0.68,0.99)	0.97 (0.81,1.16)	
	244/31,383 (0.8%)	240/32,122 (0.7%)	249/32,585 (0.8%)	216/32,807 (0.7%)	257/32,479 (0.8%)	
total sugars	x ≤ 80.88	80.88 < x ≤ 103.52	103.52 < x ≤ 125.50	125.50 < x ≤ 155.11	155.11 < x	0.001
(g)	reference	0.82 (0.68,1)	0.92 (0.76,1.11)	1.07 (0.89,1.28)	1.27 (1.07,1.51)	
	220/31,923 (0.7%)	186/32,566 (0.6%)	214/32,579 (0.7%)	261/32,558 (0.8%)	325/31,750 (1%)	
vitamin B6	x ≤ 1.59	1.59 < x ≤ 1.95	1.95 < x ≤ 2.29	2.29 < x ≤ 2.72	2.72 < x	0.369
(mg)	reference	0.94 (0.77,1.13)	0.97 (0.8,1.16)	0.94 (0.78,1.13)	1.1 (0.92,1.31)	
	213/31,540 (0.7%)	217/32,686 (0.7%)	235/32,843 (0.7%)	242/32,350 (0.7%)	299/31,957 (0.9%)	
vitamin B12	x ≤ 3.18	3.18 < x ≤ 4.65	4.65 < x ≤ 6.31	6.31 < x ≤ 9.07	9.07 < x	0.814
(μg)	reference	1.05 (0.87,1.26)	1 (0.83,1.2)	0.99 (0.83,1.19)	0.98 (0.82,1.18)	
	216/31,639 (0.7%)	247/32,359 (0.8%)	242/32,335 (0.7%)	244/32,617 (0.7%)	257/32,426 (0.8%)	
vitamin C	x ≤ 69.00	69.00 < x ≤ 109.51	109.51 < x ≤ 154.23	154.23 < x ≤ 217.06	217.06 < x	0.549
(mg)	reference	0.97 (0.81,1.17)	1 (0.83,1.21)	1.01 (0.84,1.22)	1.12 (0.93,1.34)	
	221/31,367 (0.7%)	235/32,293 (0.7%)	245/32,419 (0.8%)	246/32,809 (0.7%)	259/32,488 (0.8%)	
vitamin D	x ≤ 0.97	0.97 < x ≤ 1.65	1.65 < x ≤ 2.52	2.52 < x ≤ 4.23	4.23 < x	0.344
(μg)	reference	0.91 (0.76,1.1)	0.87 (0.73,1.04)	0.83 (0.7,1)	0.96 (0.81,1.14)	
	238/31,738 (0.7%)	234/32,610 (0.7%)	232/32,269 (0.7%)	226/32,382 (0.7%)	276/32,377 (0.9%)	
vitamin E	x ≤ 5.73	5.73 < x ≤ 7.64	7.64 < x ≤ 9.54	9.54 < x ≤ 12.19	12.19 < x	0.814
(mg)	reference	0.98 (0.82,1.17)	1 (0.84,1.2)	1.02 (0.85,1.22)	1.02 (0.85,1.22)	
	241/31,182 (0.8%)	235/32,358 (0.7%)	242/32,719 (0.7%)	244/32,728 (0.7%)	244/32,389 (0.8%)	

For alcohol, post hoc analyses revealed that groups with intake levels 3–5 (highest intake levels) showed a significantly lower risk of dementia than that with intake level 1 (lowest intake level and no alcohol intake; Figure 1).

Nutrient	adjusted HR	95% CI upper	95% CI lower	P values (post hoc, unc)	P (post hoc, unc, other comparisons)	P (group, FDR)	N	Cases
Alcohol(g)								
x≤0	reference					0.026	52,407	462
0<x≤3.2533	0.795	0.618	1.022	0.074(Lv1v.s.Lv2)			9352	71
3.2533<x≤14.74	0.847	0.720	0.996	**0.045(Lv1v.s.Lv3)**			32,299	226
14.74<x≤30.45	0.766	0.649	0.904	**0.002(Lv1v.s.Lv4)**			33,446	215
30.45<x	0.788	0.669	0.930	**0.005(Lv1v.s.Lv5)**			33,872	232
Carbohydrate(g)								
x≤187.33	reference					0.026	31,682	225
187.33<x≤227.05	0.863	0.713	1.045	0.131(Lv1v.s.Lv2)	**0.022(Lv2v.s.Lv4)**		32,274	200
227.05<x≤263.84	0.912	0.756	1.100	0.336(Lv1v.s.Lv3)	**0.001(Lv2v.s.Lv5)**		32,544	218
263.84<x≤312.90	1.071	0.894	1.283	0.456(Lv1v.s.Lv4)			32,813	265
312.90<x	1.175	0.984	1.404	0.075(Lv1v.s.Lv5)			32,063	298
Fat(g)								
x≤52.97	reference					0.025	31,328	266
52.97<x≤67.44	0.797	0.666	0.953	**0.013(Lv1v.s.Lv2)**	**0.014(Lv2v.s.Lv5)**		32,136	219
67.44<x≤81.38	0.830	0.695	0.991	**0.039(Lv1v.s.Lv3)**	**0.040(Lv3v.s.Lv5)**		32,681	232
81.38<x≤100.03	0.762	0.635	0.914	**0.003(Lv1v.s.Lv4)**	**0.003(Lv4v.s.Lv5)**		32,695	213
100.03<x	0.998	0.840	1.185	0.979(Lv1v.s.Lv5)			32,536	276
Magnesium(mg)								
x≤263.40	reference					0.025	30,903	225
263.40<x≤313.92	0.978	0.814	1.175	0.815(Lv1v.s.Lv2)	**1.94×10^{-4}(Lv4v.s.Lv5)**		32,185	237
313.92<x≤360.46	0.910	0.756	1.097	0.322(Lv1v.s.Lv3)			32,590	228
360.46<x≤422.92	0.813	0.672	0.983	**0.033(Lv1v.s.Lv4)**			32,937	213
422.92<x	1.135	0.951	1.355	0.16(Lv1v.s.Lv5)			32,761	303
Protein(g)								
x≤62.51	reference					0.026	31,191	226
62.51<x≤74.76	0.982	0.818	1.179	0.848(Lv1v.s.Lv2)	**0.044(Lv2v.s.Lv5)**		32,504	238
74.76<x≤85.60	0.936	0.778	1.126	0.481(Lv1v.s.Lv3)	**0.011(Lv3v.s.Lv5)**		32,577	230
85.60<x≤99.95	0.872	0.723	1.052	0.152(Lv1v.s.Lv4)	**0.001(Lv4v.s.Lv5)**		32,710	219
99.95<x	1.174	0.984	1.400	0.075(Lv1v.s.Lv5)			32,394	293
Total sugars(g)								
x≤80.88	reference					5.17×10^{-4}	31,923	220
80.88<x≤103.52	0.823	0.677	1.001	0.051(Lv1v.s.Lv2)	**0.007(Lv2v.s.Lv4)**		32,566	186
103.52<x≤125.50	0.918	0.759	1.110	0.379(Lv1v.s.Lv3)	**3.0×10^{-6}(Lv2v.s.Lv5)**		32,579	214
125.50<x≤155.11	1.069	0.891	1.282	0.474(Lv1v.s.Lv4)	**2.53×10^{-4}(Lv3v.s.Lv5)**		32,558	261
155.11<x	1.270	1.066	1.512	**0.007(Lv1v.s.Lv5)**	**0.039(Lv4v.s.Lv5)**		31,750	325

Figure 1. Standardized risks of incident dementia over time according to the intake level of each nutrient (alcohol, carbohydrate, fat, magnesium, protein, and total sugars). Cox proportional hazards models were adjusted for potential confounding variables. The adjusted hazard ratios of each intake level group, compared with the group with the lowest intake level and their 95% confidence intervals, are provided. The p values of overall group difference (p (group)) and post hoc comparisons between each group as well as the size of the entire group and the dementia cases included in each group are shown. Bold = $p < 0.05$.

For carbohydrates, post hoc analyses revealed that groups with intake levels 4 and 5 (highest intake levels) showed a significantly higher risk of dementia than that with intake level 2 (second lowest intake level; Figure 1).

For fat, post hoc analyses revealed that groups with intake levels 2–4 (intermediate intake levels) showed a significantly lower risk of dementia than those with intake levels 1 (lowest intake level) and 5 (highest intake level) (Figure 1).

For magnesium, post hoc analyses revealed that the groups with intake levels 1 (lowest intake level) and 5 (highest intake level) showed a significantly higher risk of dementia than that with intake level 4 (second highest intake level; Figure 1).

For protein, post hoc analyses revealed that the groups with intake levels 2–4 (intermediate intake levels) showed a significantly lower risk of dementia than the group with intake level 5 (highest intake level) (Figure 1).

For total sugars, post hoc analyses revealed that the groups with intake levels 1–4 showed a significantly lower risk of dementia compared with that with intake level 5 (highest intake level; Figure 1). In addition, the group with intake level 4 (second highest intake level) showed a significantly higher risk of dementia than that with intake level 2 (second lowest intake level).

3.3. Sensitivity Analyses Controlling for Energy Intake Quintiles

In addition to all other covariates in the main analyses, the quintile of total energy intake was incorporated as a variable in the sensitivity analysis of each nutrient.

The results of the alcohol analysis showed a similar adjusted hazard ratio for each group and a significant p-value for the presence of overall group differences after corrections for multiple comparisons. The results for carbohydrates and total sugars show a larger adjusted hazard ratio for the higher intake groups, with strong significant differences.

The analysis for protein shows a slightly smaller adjusted hazard ratio for the highest intake group ($1.17 \geq 1.15$) and a slightly larger adjusted hazard ratio for the second ($0.87 \leq 0.89$), resulting in a small difference between the two. However, this change does not alter our discussion, as the difference between the two groups was still significant in the post hoc analysis ($p = 0.008$).

Similarly, the results for magnesium show a slightly smaller adjusted hazard ratio for the highest intake group, whereas that for the second highest intake group remains almost the same, resulting in a smaller difference between the groups. However, this change does not change our discussion, as the difference between the two groups is still significant in the post hoc analysis ($p = 0.003$).

Finally, the analysis for fat shows that the adjusted hazard ratio for the highest intake group substantially decreased ($1.00 \geq 0.81$); the result of the energy intake-adjusted analysis shows almost an L-shaped relationship, with the lowest intake only indicating higher risk. Similarly, the adjusted hazard risk for the highest ($0.89 \geq 0.75$) and second highest intake groups ($0.74 \geq 0.067$) in the polyunsaturated fatty acid results decreased; the p-value for the presence of overall group differences was significant after multiple comparison correction. All statistical results are provided in Table 3.

Table 3. Nutrient intake level (amount and adjusted HR as well as 95% CI) of each group and corrected p values of overall group differences after adjusting for the quintiles of energy intake level (left) and P values in the main analyses (right).

Nutrients		Amount (Upper), Adjusted HR (Lower)					p (Group, FDR)
(Unit)	Level 1	Level 2	Level 3	Level 4	Level 5		
alcohol	x ≤ 0	0 < x ≤ 3.2533	3.2533 < x ≤ 14.74	14.74 < x ≤ 30.45	30.45 < x		0.023
(g)	reference	0.79 (0.61,1.02); 0.79 (0.62,1.02)	0.85 (0.72,1); 0.85 (0.72,1)	0.76 (0.65,0.9); 0.77 (0.65,0.9)	0.77 (0.65,0.91); 0.79 (0.67,0.93)		
calcium	x ≤ 688.02	688.02 < x ≤ 853.05	853.05 < x ≤ 1011.97	1011.97 < x ≤ 1226.67	1226.67 < x		0.516
(mg)	reference	1.13 (0.93,1.37); 1.11 (0.92,1.34)	1.1 (0.9,1.34); 1.07 (0.89,1.29)	1.04 (0.84,1.28); 1.01 (0.84,1.23)	1.19 (0.96,1.49); 1.21 (1.01,1.45)		
carbohydrate	x ≤ 187.33	187.33 < x ≤ 227.05	227.05 < x ≤ 263.84	263.84 < x ≤ 312.90	312.90 < x		0.023
(g)	reference	0.9 (0.73,1.11); 0.86 (0.71,1.04)	1.03 (0.82,1.29); 0.91 (0.76,1.1)	1.31 (1.03,1.68); 1.07 (0.89,1.28)	1.44 (1.09,1.91); 1.18 (0.98,1.4)		
carotene	x ≤ 991.92	991.92 < x ≤ 1996.76	1996.76 < x ≤ 3107.49	3107.49 < x ≤ 4748.76	4748.76 < x		0.440
(ug)	reference	0.93 (0.77,1.12); 0.93 (0.78,1.12)	0.89 (0.74,1.08); 0.9 (0.75,1.08)	0.91 (0.75,1.09); 0.91 (0.76,1.1)	1.05 (0.88,1.25); 1.07 (0.9,1.27)		
Englyst diet fiber	x ≤ 11.10	11.10 < x ≤ 14.22	14.22 < x ≤ 17.19	17.19 < x ≤ 21.14	21.14 < x		0.440
(g)	reference	0.94 (0.78,1.13); 0.94 (0.78,1.13)	0.82 (0.68,1); 0.83 (0.69,1)	0.97 (0.8,1.17); 0.98 (0.82,1.18)	0.94 (0.77,1.15); 0.99 (0.83,1.18)		
fat	x ≤ 52.97	52.97 < x ≤ 67.44	67.44 < x ≤ 81.38	81.38 < x ≤ 100.03	100.03 < x		0.032
(g)	reference	0.75 (0.61,0.91); 0.8 (0.67,0.95)	0.76 (0.61,0.94); 0.83 (0.69,0.99)	0.68 (0.53,0.87); 0.76 (0.64,0.91)	0.81 (0.62,1.07); 1 (0.84,1.18)		
folate	x ≤ 213.92	213.92 < x ≤ 265.13	265.13 < x ≤ 314.08	314.08 < x ≤ 381.53	381.53 < x		0.248
(ug)	reference	0.83 (0.69,1.01); 0.84 (0.69,1.01)	0.79 (0.65,0.96); 0.8 (0.66,0.96)	0.87 (0.71,1.05); 0.88 (0.74,1.06)	0.93 (0.76,1.14); 0.98 (0.82,1.17)		
food weight	x ≤ 2552.33	2552.33 < x ≤ 2940.00	2940.00 < x ≤ 3302.85	3302.85 < x ≤ 3782.00	3782.00 < x		0.614
(g)	reference	0.95 (0.79,1.14); 0.95 (0.79,1.14)	0.89 (0.74,1.08); 0.89 (0.74,1.07)	0.92 (0.76,1.12); 0.93 (0.78,1.12)	1.02 (0.84,1.25); 1.07 (0.9,1.28)		
iron	x ≤ 10.08	10.08 < x ≤ 12.30	12.30 < x ≤ 14.34	14.34 < x ≤ 16.96	16.96 < x		0.328
(mg)	reference	0.9 (0.75,1.1); 0.92 (0.77,1.11)	0.82 (0.67,1.01); 0.85 (0.7,1.02)	0.8 (0.64,1); 0.83 (0.69,1)	0.93 (0.74,1.17); 1.02 (0.86,1.22)		
magnesium	x ≤ 263.40	263.40 < x ≤ 313.92	313.92 < x ≤ 360.46	360.46 < x ≤ 422.92	422.92 < x		0.111
(mg)	reference	0.97 (0.8,1.18); 0.98 (0.81,1.18)	0.9 (0.73,1.12); 0.91 (0.76,1.1)	0.8 (0.64,1.01); 0.81 (0.67,0.98)	1.07 (0.84,1.37); 1.14 (0.95,1.36)		
polyunsaturated fat	x ≤ 8.32	8.32 < x ≤ 11.55	11.55 < x ≤ 14.91	14.91 < x ≤ 19.51	19.51 < x		0.023
(g)	reference	0.84 (0.7,1.01); 0.87 (0.73,1.04)	0.84 (0.7,1.02); 0.89 (0.75,1.06)	0.67 (0.55,0.83); 0.74 (0.61,0.89)	0.75 (0.6,0.93); 0.89 (0.75,1.06)		
potassium	x ≤ 2821.42	2821.42 < x ≤ 3377.58	3377.58 < x ≤ 3893.73	3893.73 < x ≤ 4571.70	4571.70 < x		0.440
(mg)	reference	0.86 (0.71,1.05); 0.86 (0.71,1.04)	0.92 (0.75,1.13); 0.92 (0.76,1.1)	0.87 (0.7,1.09); 0.87 (0.73,1.05)	1.01 (0.8,1.27); 1.05 (0.88,1.26)		

Table 3. Cont.

Nutrients		Amount (Upper), Adjusted HR (Lower)					p (Group, FDR)
(Unit)	Level 1	Level 2	Level 3	Level 4	Level 5		
protein	x ≤ 62.51	62.51 < x ≤ 74.76	74.76 < x ≤ 85.60	85.60 < x ≤ 99.95	99.95 < x		0.248
(g)	reference	0.99 (0.82,1.2): 0.98 (0.82,1.18)	0.95 (0.78,1.17): 0.94 (0.78,1.13)	0.89 (0.71,1.11): 0.87 (0.72,1.05)	1.15 (0.91,1.45): 1.17 (0.98,1.4)		
retinol	X ≤ 176.18	176.18 < x ≤ 259.66	259.66 < x ≤ 345.04	345.04 < x ≤ 459.58	459.58 < x		0.790
(μg)	reference	0.96 (0.8,1.16): 0.96 (0.8,1.16)	0.94 (0.77,1.14): 0.94 (0.78,1.14)	0.99 (0.81,1.2): 1 (0.83,1.2)	0.92 (0.75,1.13): 0.97 (0.81,1.17)		
saturated fat	X ≤ 19.28	19.28 < x ≤ 25.25	25.25 < x ≤ 31.14	31.14 < x ≤ 39.24	39.24 < x		0.629
(g)	reference	0.92 (0.76,1.12): 0.9 (0.75,1.08)	0.99 (0.8,1.21): 0.95 (0.79,1.14)	1.08 (0.87,1.35): 1.04 (0.87,1.24)	1.03 (0.81,1.32): 1.06 (0.89,1.27)		
starch	X ≤ 84.78	84.78 < x ≤ 108.32	108.32 < x ≤ 129.57	129.57 < x ≤ 156.59	156.59 < x		0.328
(g)	reference	0.91 (0.76,1.1): 0.93 (0.78,1.11)	0.94 (0.77,1.14): 0.97 (0.81,1.16)	0.78 (0.63,0.96): 0.82 (0.68,0.99)	0.85 (0.68,1.06): 0.97 (0.81,1.16)		
total sugars	X ≤ 80.88	80.88 < x ≤ 103.52	103.52 < x ≤ 125.50	125.50 < x ≤ 155.11	155.11 < x		0.001
(g)	reference	0.85 (0.7,1.04): 0.82 (0.68,1)	0.98 (0.8,1.19): 0.92 (0.76,1.11)	1.17 (0.96,1.43): 1.07 (0.89,1.28)	1.4 (1.13,1.73): 1.27 (1.07,1.51)		
iron	x ≤ 10.08	10.08 < x ≤ 12.30	12.30 < x ≤ 14.34	14.34 < x ≤ 16.96	16.96 < x		0.328
(mg)	reference	0.9 (0.75,1.1): 0.92 (0.77,1.11)	0.82 (0.67,1.01): 0.85 (0.7,1.02)	0.8 (0.64,1): 0.83 (0.69,1)	0.93 (0.74,1.17): 1.02 (0.86,1.22)		
vitamin B6	X ≤ 3.18	3.18 < x ≤ 4.65	4.65 < x ≤ 6.31	6.31 < x ≤ 9.07	9.07 < x		0.666
(mg)	reference	0.94 (0.78,1.15): 0.94 (0.77,1.13)	0.98 (0.8,1.19): 0.97 (0.8,1.16)	0.95 (0.78,1.16): 0.94 (0.78,1.13)	1.07 (0.87,1.31): 1.1 (0.92,1.31)		
vitamin B12	X ≤ 1.59	1.59 < x ≤ 1.95	1.95 < x ≤ 2.29	2.29 < x ≤ 2.72	2.72 < x		0.790
(μg)	reference	1.04 (0.87,1.26): 1.05 (0.87,1.26)	0.99 (0.82,1.2): 1 (0.83,1.2)	0.98 (0.81,1.18): 0.99 (0.83,1.19)	0.96 (0.8,1.16): 0.98 (0.82,1.18)		
vitamin C	X ≤ 69.00	69.00 < x ≤ 109.51	109.51 < x ≤ 154.23	154.23 < x ≤ 217.06	217.06 < x		0.666
(mg)	reference	0.97 (0.81,1.17): 0.97 (0.81,1.17)	1 (0.83,1.21): 1 (0.83,1.21)	1.01 (0.84,1.22): 1.01 (0.84,1.22)	1.1 (0.91,1.33): 1.12 (0.93,1.34)		
vitamin D	X ≤ 0.97	0.97 < x ≤ 1.65	1.65 < x ≤ 2.52	2.52 < x ≤ 4.23	4.23 < x		0.398
(μg)	reference	0.91 (0.76,1.09): 0.91 (0.76,1.1)	0.86 (0.71,1.03): 0.87 (0.73,1.04)	0.82 (0.68,0.99): 0.83 (0.7,1)	0.94 (0.78,1.12): 0.96 (0.81,1.14)		
Vitamin E	X ≤ 5.73	5.73 < x ≤ 7.64	7.64 < x ≤ 9.54	9.54 < x ≤ 12.19	12.19 < x		0.800
(mg)	reference	0.98 (0.81,1.18): 0.98 (0.82,1.17)	1 (0.82,1.21): 1 (0.84,1.2)	1 (0.82,1.23): 1.02 (0.85,1.22)	0.95 (0.76,1.18): 1.02 (0.85,1.22)		

4. Discussion

We used a large dataset of middle-aged and older people in the UK to examine the relationship between the intake level of various nutrients and the risk of developing dementia >2 years after baseline while adjusting for a wide range of confounding factors. The present results were partly consistent with our hypothesis; that is, a moderately high intake of basic nutrients, such as protein, and fat, is associated with a lower risk of incident dementia, and no alcohol intake is associated with a higher risk of dementia over time. In addition, we confirmed our hypothesis that a higher magnesium intake is associated with a lower risk of dementia. We generally confirmed the association between a higher intake of total sugars or carbohydrates and a greater risk of incident dementia. Meanwhile, polyunsaturated fat, folate, and vitamins D and E were not significantly associated with the risk of dementia over time, although some results showed a statistical tendency. Many studies have shown that people taking a little to a moderate level of alcohol have a lower risk of dementia than those taking no alcohol at all, though the dose–response relationship was L-shaped in some studies [20] and U-shaped in others [4]; this study could well replicate this finding. The replication of these findings seems to indicate the robustness of these and other findings (as discussed below).

The link between a higher magnesium intake and a lower risk of dementia in this study was partly consistent with previous research and may be due to the intrinsic properties of this nutrient. The second-highest magnesium intake group in this study had a lower risk of dementia than the lowest and highest intake groups, respectively. This was partly consistent with previous research on the association between moderate to higher intakes of magnesium or magnesium oxide and a lower risk of dementia [7,8,21]; our findings strengthened the evidence thanks to a large sample size. Another study found that the highest and lowest quintiles of plasma magnesium levels are associated with a subsequent higher risk of vascular dementia [22], a result consistent with the current findings.

One possible mechanism for the association between moderate magnesium intake and the lower risk of dementia is related to magnesium's effect on neuronal excitability. N-methyl-D-aspartate receptors are permeable to calcium but can be blocked by sodium and magnesium ions to prevent the excitotoxicity induced by excessive neuronal activity [23,24]. We speculated that these relationships may be related to magnesium's ability to suppress excessive neural activity; appropriate levels of neural activity are necessary for proper brain activity. Another possible mechanism is magnesium's association with insulin resistance and diabetes. Magnesium supplementation improves the insulin resistance state [25] and a lower dietary intake of magnesium is linked to a greater risk of type 2 diabetes, which is robustly associated with a greater dementia risk [26]. Furthermore, a chronic magnesium deficiency increases the production of free radicals, which in turn increases the risk of a wide range of ageing-related diseases, including stroke and cardiovascular diseases [27]. Magnesium depletion increases the production of oxygen-derived free radicals, hydrogen peroxide, and superoxide anions by inflammatory cells [27]; aggravates oxygen stress; and weakens antioxidant defence [28,29]. Moreover, magnesium is required for the proper function of the γ-glutamine transpeptidase, which plays an important role in the synthesis of glutathione, an antioxidant; hence, magnesium may have a mild antioxidant effect [30,31]. However, whether adequate magnesium levels can prevent dementia must be investigated in future randomized clinical trials (RCTs).

The relationship between a higher intake of total sugars and a higher risk of dementia and the concomitant association of carbohydrates in this work was consistent with previous cohort studies and with the adverse effects of persistently higher blood sugar levels on the brain and nervous system. In the present study, a higher risk of dementia was found in the higher sugar intake groups than in the lower intake groups. This finding is consistent with previous reports stating that a higher risk of dementia is associated with a higher fructose intake [6] and a higher sugar intake from beverages [32]. In addition, animal studies revealed that the long-term consumption of sucrose-sweetened water causes insulin resistance, impairs memory function, and causes amyloid-β deposition [33], and a diet supplemented with liquid sucrose is associated with hippocampal inflammation and memory impairment [34]. In addition, diets high in fat, and sugar can reduce BDNF expression, which is associated with memory impairment [34]. In general, a higher sugar intake is linked to microvascular damage [35] and impaired glucose metabolism [36], which can damage the nervous system. Based on the above, a higher sugar intake may be associated with greater dementia risk. However, as certain dementia patients show sugar-preferring dietary patterns [37], future RCTs must focus on demonstrating a causal relationship, by implementing sugar restriction, for instance.

The link found in this study between the highest or lowest quintiles of fat intake and a higher risk of dementia was consistent with previous findings, which indicated that a higher fat intake is linked to an increased risk of cardiovascular disease and stroke and fat is an important nutrient for nerve cells. In the present work, a moderate fat intake was associated with a lower risk of dementia. This finding may be partly consistent with one study using a relatively smaller sample size than that of the present study (N = 937), which reported that a diet rich in protein and fat is associated with a lower subsequent risk of dementia [9]. A closer look at this relationship revealed that polyunsaturated fats may account for this association: saturated fats did not show a substantial association with dementia risk, whereas polyunsaturated fats showed a similar association with dementia risk. The lack of association found between saturated fats and increased dementia risk over time was not consistent with the findings of a middle-sized meta-analysis (8630 participants and 633 cases from four independent prospective cohort studies) [38]. The results obtained for polyunsaturated fat were not significant after multiple comparison correction, but a trend toward a lower risk of dementia was observed in the group with the second-highest polyunsaturated fat intake compared with that in the group with the lowest intake. This finding is consistent with previous studies showing that moderate fish intake or high unsaturated fat intake is associated with a lower risk of dementia [1,14]. In addition, a previous meta-analysis revealed a dose-dependent decline in the intake level of polyunsaturated fat correlated with mild cognitive impairment risk [39]. Moreover, fish consumption is associated with a lower risk of cardiovascular diseases [40]. Among polyunsaturated fats, docosahexaenoic and eicosapentaenoic acids are considered protective against neurodegeneration [41]. However, fish consumption can lead to an excessive intake of methylmercury [42], which has neurotoxic effects. Accordingly, a moderate fat intake may be associated with the lowest risk of dementia.

The association between moderate protein levels and a lower risk of dementia in this work is consistent with previous research and may be related to the importance of proteins in maintaining brain tissue integrity and the link of excessive meat intake to higher stroke and cardiovascular risk. One study using a sample size relatively smaller than that of the present study (N = 937) reported that a protein-rich diet is associated with a lower subsequent risk of dementia [9]. Similarly, our previous study using UK Biobank data showed that an overall moderate intake of meat and fish is linked to a lower risk of dementia [14]. Given that meat and fish are important protein sources, the present results are consistent with the above previous studies. Possible reasons why adequate protein levels are linked to a lower risk of dementia include the following: first, proteins are essential for the maintenance of neuronal membranes and neuronal integrity and second, certain amino acids are precursors of neurotransmitters [43]. Another possible mechanism is that proteins are important for muscle retention [43]. Further, a higher meat intake has been associated with an increased risk of cardiovascular diseases and stroke [43]. These findings may explain the observed association between moderate protein intake and the lower risk of dementia. However, these findings are only speculative and should be confirmed by future intervention and animal studies.

Although some results were not significant after correcting for multiple comparisons, their tendencies were consistent with previous studies. Additional research and RCT data are warranted for a more comprehensive understanding. For folate, the highest or lowest intake quintile was also linked to an increased risk of dementia. This finding was partly consistent with a meta-analysis linking a higher folate intake to a lower risk of dementia. However, previous results, even among meta-analyses, remain contradictory. For instance, another meta-analysis failed to find an association between higher folate intake and dementia [2]. Similarly, some meta-analyses found an association between higher vitamin E intake and a lower dementia risk [3] and others failed to find a connection [5]. The present results are consistent with the latter. Thus, the lack of cohesion between previous studies and the trends in the present work prevented us from drawing conclusions about the existence of a relationship. Although previous meta-analyses consistently found an association between vitamin D deficiency and greater dementia risk, we failed to find such a connection [1]. However, groups with intermediate vitamin D intake showed an uncorrected tendency to a lower risk of dementia risk over time. Perhaps, the present results may suggest the effect of an insufficient sample size. Further research is warranted to corroborate or disprove the existence of these relationships.

This study has several limitations. First, its prospective observational design. Although we corrected for a wide range of potentially confounding variables, the observed associations may have been influenced by the type of diet chosen by people at risk of developing dementia. In addition, this study excluded subjects who had developed dementia before two years after the online survey of the diet from the analysis. However, the neuropathological process underlying Alzheimer's disease begins 20 years before the onset of the disease [44]. Therefore, specific eating behaviours may also be an expression of some preclinical behaviours. Moreover, there were a few years between the time when the subjects visited the facility for baseline measurements to when they completed the online survey on diet. Therefore, the time when the covariate data were measured and when the data on the variables of interest (i.e., diet) differed. These discrepancies suggested that our correction for covariates may not have been accurate. Finally, although the dietary data from the online diet survey are from 2009 to 2012, this study aimed to predict the onset of dementia up to 2021 but did not consider any changes in dietary habits after the survey. Although true for all subjects, this may have reduced the sensitivity of the statistical analysis.

This study investigated the relationship between the intake of 23 nutrients and the risk of dementia using modern data and a sufficient sample size after adjusting for a wide range of potential confounding factors. The main results were: (a) compared with no alcohol intake, any level of alcohol intake was associated with a lower risk of dementia; (b) compared with a higher protein intake, a moderate intake was associated with a lower risk of dementia; (c) compared with the highest or lowest quintiles of fat intake, a moderate intake was associated with a lower risk of dementia; the same trend was exhibited by polyunsaturated fatty acids (rather consistent with previous studies) but not by saturated fatty acids (not consistent with previous studies); (d) compared with a lower sugar intake, a higher total intake was associated with a higher risk of dementia. The same trend was found for carbohydrates with sugar components; (e) compared with the highest and lowest magnesium intakes, a moderately higher intake was associated with a lower risk of dementia; (f) other than folic acid, which showed a certain association with dementia, the overall association between vitamin intake and dementia described in previous studies could not be replicated; (g) we found no trend of associations between nutrients such as calcium, retinol, etc., and dementia. Points (b), (c), (e–g) are findings that had not been previously established. The association between nutrients and dementia risk was previously reported in studies with relatively smaller sample sizes than that of the present study. However, the unprecedentedly large sample size and the correction for confounding factors are important points of the present study. Overall, the present findings are congruent with the importance of a moderate intake of certain nutrients.

Supplementary Materials: The following supporting information can be downloaded at: https://www.mdpi.com/article/10.3390/{n}u15040842/s1, Table S1: Characteristics of the subjects who lack ≥1 covariates and those who have complete covariate data among the participants in the UK Biobank not excluded according to the four excluding criteria of dementia who completed the online survey and had nutritional data; Method S1: Supplemental Methods Supplemental Table S1. Characteristics of the subjects who lack ≥1 covariates and those who have complete covariate data among the participants in the UK Biobank not excluded according to the four excluding criteria of dementia who completed the online survey and had nutritional data [14,17,45–52].

Author Contributions: H.T. conceptualized the study, preprocessed and analysed the data, and wrote the manuscript. R.K. played a key role in obtaining the relevant funding and supervising the study. All authors have read and agreed to the published version of the manuscript.

Funding: The UK Biobank was supported by the Wellcome Trust, Medical Research Council, Department of Health, Scottish government, and the Northwest Regional Development Agency. It has also received funding from the Welsh Assembly government and the British Heart Foundation. This particular study of the authors was supported by JST/RISTEX, JST/CREST (no particular research number exists). The research was designed, conducted, analysed, and interpreted by the authors entirely independently of the funding sources.

Institutional Review Board Statement: Approval for these experiments was obtained from the Northwest Multi-Centre Research Ethics Committee. Written informed consent was obtained from each participant.

Informed Consent Statement: Patients and the public are not involved in any part of the design of this study. The manuscript's guarantors affirm that the manuscript is an honest, accurate, and transparent account of the study being reported; that no important aspects of the study have been omitted; and that any discrepancies from the study as planned (and, if relevant, registered) have been explained.

Data Availability Statement: Researchers can apply to use the UK Biobank resource (https://www.ukbiobank.ac.uk/ (accessed on 9 September 2022)) and access the data used in this study.

Acknowledgments: We thank all of our colleagues at the Institute of Development, Aging, and Cancer and at Tohoku University for their support. This study was supported by JST/RISTEX, JST/CREST. We are grateful to the UK Biobank participants. This research was conducted using the UK Biobank resource under application number 56726.

Conflicts of Interest: The authors declare no conflict of interest.

References

1. Cao, L.; Tan, L.; Wang, H.-F.; Jiang, T.; Zhu, X.-C.; Lu, H.; Tan, M.-S.; Yu, J.-T. Dietary patterns and risk of dementia: A systematic review and meta-analysis of cohort studies. *Mol. Neurobiol.* **2016**, *53*, 6144–6154. [CrossRef] [PubMed]
2. Zhou, J.; Sun, Y.; Ji, M.; Li, X.; Wang, Z. Association of Vitamin B Status With Risk of Dementia in Cohort Studies: A Systematic Review and Meta-analysis. *J. Am. Med. Dir. Assoc.* **2022**, *23*, 1826.e21–1826.e35. [CrossRef] [PubMed]
3. Zhao, R.; Han, X.; Zhang, H.; Liu, J.; Zhang, M.; Zhao, W.; Jiang, S.; Li, R.; Cai, H.; You, H. Association of vitamin E intake in diet and supplements with risk of dementia: A meta-analysis. *Front. Aging Neurosci.* **2022**, *14*, 955878. [CrossRef] [PubMed]
4. Sabia, S.; Fayosse, A.; Dumurgier, J.; Dugravot, A.; Akbaraly, T.; Britton, A.; Kivimäki, M.; Singh-Manoux, A. Alcohol consumption and risk of dementia: 23 year follow-up of Whitehall II cohort study. *BMJ* **2018**, *362*, k2927. [CrossRef]
5. Wang, W.; Li, J.; Zhang, H.; Wang, X.; Zhang, X. Effects of vitamin E supplementation on the risk and progression of AD: A systematic review and meta-analysis. *Nutr. Neurosci.* **2021**, *24*, 13–22. [CrossRef]
6. Stephan, B.; Wells, J.; Brayne, C.; Albanese, E.; Siervo, M. Increased fructose intake as a risk factor for dementia. *J. Gerontol. Ser. A Biomed. Sci. Med. Sci.* **2010**, *65*, 809–814. [CrossRef]
7. Lo, K.; Liu, Q.; Madsen, T.; Rapp, S.; Chen, J.-C.; Neuhouser, M.; Shadyab, A.; Pal, L.; Lin, X.; Shumaker, S. Relations of magnesium intake to cognitive impairment and dementia among participants in the Women's Health Initiative Memory Study: A prospective cohort study. *BMJ Open* **2019**, *9*, e030052. [CrossRef]
8. Ozawa, M.; Ninomiya, T.; Ohara, T.; Hirakawa, Y.; Doi, Y.; Hata, J.; Uchida, K.; Shirota, T.; Kitazono, T.; Kiyohara, Y. Self-Reported Dietary Intake of Potassium, Calcium, and Magnesium and Risk of Dementia in the J apanese: The H isayama Study. *J. Am. Geriatr. Soc.* **2012**, *60*.
9. Roberts, R.O.; Roberts, L.A.; Geda, Y.E.; Cha, R.H.; Pankratz, V.S.; O'Connor, H.M.; Knopman, D.S.; Petersen, R.C. Relative intake of macronutrients impacts risk of mild cognitive impairment or dementia. *J. Alzheimer's Dis.* **2012**, *32*, 329–339. [CrossRef]
10. Takeuchi, H.; Kawashima, R. Effects of Body Mass Index on Brain Structures in the Elderly: Longitudinal Analyses. *Front. Endocrinol.* **2022**, *13*, 824661. [CrossRef]
11. Albanese, E.; Launer, L.J.; Egger, M.; Prince, M.J.; Giannakopoulos, P.; Wolters, F.J.; Egan, K. Body mass index in midlife and dementia: Systematic review and meta-regression analysis of 589,649 men and women followed in longitudinal studies. *Alzheimer's Dement. Diagn. Assess. Dis. Monit.* **2017**, *8*, 165–178. [CrossRef] [PubMed]

12. Qizilbash, N.; Gregson, J.; Johnson, M.E.; Pearce, N.; Douglas, I.; Wing, K.; Evans, S.J.; Pocock, S.J. BMI and risk of dementia in two million people over two decades: A retrospective cohort study. *Lancet Diabetes Endocrinol.* **2015**, *3*, 431–436. [CrossRef]
13. Kivimäki, M.; Singh-Manoux, A.; Shipley, M.J.; Elbaz, A. Does midlife obesity really lower dementia risk? *Lancet Diabetes Endocrinol.* **2015**, *3*, 498. [CrossRef] [PubMed]
14. Takeuchi, H.; Kawashima, R. Diet and Dementia: A Prospective Study. *Nutrients* **2021**, *13*, 4500. [CrossRef] [PubMed]
15. Liu, B.; Young, H.; Crowe, F.L.; Benson, V.S.; Spencer, E.A.; Key, T.J.; Appleby, P.N.; Beral, V. Development and evaluation of the Oxford WebQ, a low-cost, web-based method for assessment of previous 24 h dietary intakes in large-scale prospective studies. *Public Health Nutr.* **2011**, *14*, 1998–2005. [CrossRef]
16. Russ, T.C.; Kivimäki, M.; Starr, J.M.; Stamatakis, E.; Batty, G.D. Height in relation to dementia death: Individual participant meta-analysis of 18 UK prospective cohort studies. *Br. J. Psychiatry* **2014**, *205*, 348–354. [CrossRef]
17. Lourida, I.; Hannon, E.; Littlejohns, T.J.; Langa, K.M.; Hyppönen, E.; Kuźma, E.; Llewellyn, D.J. Association of lifestyle and genetic risk with incidence of dementia. *JAMA* **2019**, *322*, 430–437. [CrossRef]
18. Luojus, M.K.; Lehto, S.M.; Tolmunen, T.; Brem, A.-K.; Lönnroos, E.; Kauhanen, J. Self-reported sleep disturbance and incidence of dementia in ageing men. *J. Epidemiol. Community Health* **2017**, *71*, 329–335. [CrossRef]
19. Benjamini, Y.; Krieger, A.M.; Yekutieli, D. Adaptive linear step-up procedures that control the false discovery rate. *Biometrika* **2006**, *93*, 491–507. [CrossRef]
20. Wei, C.; Zhao, Z.; Li, B.; Sha, F. Alcohol consumption and risk of dementia: 11-year follow-up of UK Biobank cohort study. *Alzheimer's Dement.* **2021**, *17*, e057753. [CrossRef]
21. Juang, C.-L.; Yang, F.S.; Hsieh, M.S.; Tseng, H.-Y.; Chen, S.-C.; Wen, H.-C. Investigation of anti-oxidative stress in vitro and water apparent diffusion coefficient in MRI on rat after spinal cord injury in vivo with Tithonia diversifolia ethanolic extracts treatment. *BMC Complement. Altern. Med.* **2014**, *14*, 447. [CrossRef] [PubMed]
22. Thomassen, J.Q.; Tolstrup, J.S.; Nordestgaard, B.G.; Tybjærg-Hansen, A.; Frikke-Schmidt, R. Plasma Concentrations of Magnesium and Risk of Dementia: A General Population Study of 102 648 Individuals. *Clin. Chem.* **2021**, *67*, 899–911. [CrossRef] [PubMed]
23. Hynd, M.R.; Scott, H.L.; Dodd, P.R. Glutamate-mediated excitotoxicity and neurodegeneration in Alzheimer's disease. *Neurochem. Int.* **2004**, *45*, 583–595. [CrossRef] [PubMed]
24. Parsons, C.G.; Danysz, W.; Quack, G. Glutamate in CNS disorders as a target for drug development: An update. *Drug News Perspect.* **1998**, *11*, 523–569. [CrossRef]
25. Simental-Mendia, L.E.; Sahebkar, A.; Rodriguez-Moran, M.; Guerrero-Romero, F. A systematic review and meta-analysis of randomized controlled trials on the effects of magnesium supplementation on insulin sensitivity and glucose control. *Pharmacol. Res.* **2016**, *111*, 272–282. [CrossRef]
26. Zheng, F.; Zhang, Y.; Xie, W.; Li, W.; Jin, C.; Mi, W.; Wang, F.; Ma, W.; Ma, C.; Yang, Y. Further evidence for genetic association of CACNA1C and schizophrenia: New risk loci in a Han Chinese population and a meta-analysis. *Schizophr. Res.* **2014**, *152*, 105–110. [CrossRef]
27. Barbagallo, M.; Veronese, N.; Dominguez, L.J. Magnesium in aging, health and diseases. *Nutrients* **2021**, *13*, 463. [CrossRef]
28. Mazur, A.; Maier, J.A.; Rock, E.; Gueux, E.; Nowacki, W.; Rayssiguier, Y. Magnesium and the inflammatory response: Potential physiopathological implications. *Arch. Biochem. Biophys.* **2007**, *458*, 48–56. [CrossRef]
29. Weglicki, W.; Mak, I.; Kramer, J.; Dickens, B.; Cassidy, M.; Stafford, R.; Phillips, T. Role of free radicals and substance P in magnesium deficiency. *Cardiovasc. Res.* **1996**, *31*, 677–682. [CrossRef]
30. Tohidi, M.; Ghasemi, A.; Hadaegh, F.; Arbabi, S.; Hosseini Isfahani, F. Intra-erythrocyte magnesium is associated with gamma-glutamyl transferase in obese children and adolescents. *Biol. Trace Elem. Res.* **2011**, *143*, 835–843. [CrossRef]
31. Weglicki, W.; Bloom, S.; Cassidy, M.; Freedman, A.; Atrakchi, A.; Dickens, B. Antioxidants and the cardiomyopathy of Mg-deficiency. *Am. J. Cardiovasc. Pathol.* **1992**, *4*, 210–215. [PubMed]
32. Miao, H.; Chen, K.; Yan, X.; Chen, F. Sugar in Beverage and the Risk of Incident Dementia, Alzheimer's disease and Stroke: A Prospective Cohort Study. *J. Prev. Alzheimer's Dis.* **2021**, *8*, 188–193. [CrossRef]
33. Orr, M.E.; Salinas, A.; Buffenstein, R.; Oddo, S. Mammalian target of rapamycin hyperactivity mediates the detrimental effects of a high sucrose diet on Alzheimer's disease pathology. *Neurobiol. Aging* **2014**, *35*, 1233–1242. [CrossRef]
34. Beilharz, J.E.; Maniam, J.; Morris, M.J. Diet-induced cognitive deficits: The role of fat and sugar, potential mechanisms and nutritional interventions. *Nutrients* **2015**, *7*, 6719–6738. [CrossRef]
35. Chait, A.; Bornfeldt, K.E. Diabetes and atherosclerosis: Is there a role for hyperglycemia? *J. Lipid Res.* **2009**, *50*, S335–S339. [CrossRef] [PubMed]
36. Leão, L.L.; Tangen, G.; Barca, M.L.; Engedal, K.; Santos, S.H.S.; Machado, F.S.M.; de Paula, A.M.B.; Monteiro-Junior, R.S. Does hyperglycemia downregulate glucose transporters in the brain? *Med. Hypotheses* **2020**, *139*, 109614. [CrossRef] [PubMed]
37. Ahmed, R.M.; Irish, M.; Kam, J.; Van Keizerswaard, J.; Bartley, L.; Samaras, K.; Hodges, J.R.; Piguet, O. Quantifying the eating abnormalities in frontotemporal dementia. *JAMA Neurol.* **2014**, *71*, 1540–1546. [CrossRef]
38. Ruan, Y.; Tang, J.; Guo, X.; Li, K.; Li, D. Dietary fat intake and risk of Alzheimer's disease and dementia: A meta-analysis of cohort studies. *Curr. Alzheimer Res.* **2018**, *15*, 869–876. [CrossRef]
39. Zhang, Y.; Chen, J.; Qiu, J.; Li, Y.; Wang, J.; Jiao, J. Intakes of fish and polyunsaturated fatty acids and mild-to-severe cognitive impairment risks: A dose-response meta-analysis of 21 cohort studies–3. *Am. J. Clin. Nutr.* **2015**, *103*, 330–340. [CrossRef]

40. Mozaffarian, D.; Rimm, E.B. Fish intake, contaminants, and human health: Evaluating the risks and the benefits. *JAMA* **2006**, *296*, 1885–1899. [CrossRef]
41. Wu, S.; Ding, Y.; Wu, F.; Li, R.; Hou, J.; Mao, P. Omega-3 fatty acids intake and risks of dementia and Alzheimer's disease: A meta-analysis. *Neurosci. Biobehav. Rev.* **2015**, *48*, 1–9. [CrossRef] [PubMed]
42. Morris, M.C.; Brockman, J.; Schneider, J.A.; Wang, Y.; Bennett, D.A.; Tangney, C.C.; van de Rest, O. Association of seafood consumption, brain mercury level, and APOE ε4 status with brain neuropathology in older adults. *JAMA* **2016**, *315*, 489–497. [CrossRef] [PubMed]
43. Kouvari, M.; Tyrovolas, S.; Panagiotakos, D.B. Red meat consumption and healthy ageing: A review. *Maturitas* **2016**, *84*, 17–24. [CrossRef] [PubMed]
44. Bateman, R.J.; Xiong, C.; Benzinger, T.L.; Fagan, A.M.; Goate, A.; Fox, N.C.; Marcus, D.S.; Cairns, N.J.; Xie, X.; Blazey, T.M. Clinical and biomarker changes in dominantly inherited Alzheimer's disease. *N. Engl. J. Med.* **2012**, *367*, 795–804. [CrossRef]
45. Batty, G.D.; Mcintosh, A.M.; Russ, T.C.; Deary, I.J.; Gale, C.R. Psychological distress, neuroticism, and cause-specific mortality: Early prospective evidence from UK Biobank. *J. Epidemiol. Community Health* **2016**, *70*, 1136–1139. [CrossRef]
46. Cullen, B.; Newby, D.; Lee, D.; Lyall, D.M.; Nevado-Holgado, A.J.; Evans, J.J.; Pell, J.P.; Lovestone, S.; Cavanagh, J. Cross-sectional and longitudinal analyses of outdoor air pollution exposure and cognitive function in UK Biobank. *Sci. Rep.* **2018**, *8*, 1–14. [CrossRef]
47. Khubchandani, J.; Brey, R.; Kotecki, J.; Kleinfelder, J.; Anderson, J. The psychometric properties of PHQ-4 depression and anxiety screening scale among college students. *Arch. Psychiatr. Nurs.* **2016**, *30*, 457–462. [CrossRef]
48. Okbay, A.; Beauchamp, J.P.; Fontana, M.A.; Lee, J.J.; Pers, T.H.; Rietveld, C.A.; Turley, P.; Chen, G.B.; Emilsson, V.; Meddens, S.F.; et al. Genome-wide association study identifies 74 loci associated with educational attainment. *Nature* **2016**, *533*, 539–542. [CrossRef]
49. Sarkar, S.N.; Huang, R.-Q.; Logan, S.M.; Yi, K.D.; Dillon, G.H.; Simpkins, J.W. Estrogens directly potentiate neuronal L-type Ca^{2+} channels. *Proc. Natl. Acad. Sci. USA* **2008**, *105*, 15148–15153. [CrossRef]
50. Shen, X.; Cox, S.R.; Adams, M.J.; Howard, D.M.; Lawrie, S.M.; Ritchie, S.J.; Bastin, M.E.; Deary, I.J.; Mcintosh, A.M.; Whalley, H.C. Resting-state connectivity and its association with cognitive performance, educational attainment, and household income in the UK Biobank. *Biol. Psychiatry Cogn. Neurosci. Neuroimaging* **2018**, *3*, 878–886. [CrossRef]
51. Townsend, P. Deprivation. *J. Soc. Policy* **1987**, *16*, 125–146. [CrossRef]
52. Veldsman, M.; Kindalova, P.; Husain, M.; Kosmidis, I.; Nichols, T.E. Spatial distribution and cognitive impact of cerebrovascular risk-related white matter hyperintensities. *NeuroImage: Clin.* **2020**, *28*, 102405. [CrossRef] [PubMed]

Disclaimer/Publisher's Note: The statements, opinions and data contained in all publications are solely those of the individual author(s) and contributor(s) and not of MDPI and/or the editor(s). MDPI and/or the editor(s) disclaim responsibility for any injury to people or property resulting from any ideas, methods, instructions or products referred to in the content.

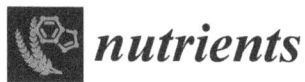 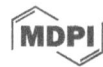

Article

Early Life Beef Consumption Patterns Are Related to Cognitive Outcomes at 1–5 Years of Age: An Exploratory Study

Victoria C. Wilk, Michelle K. McGuire and Annie J. Roe *

Margaret Ritchie School of Family and Consumer Sciences, College of Agricultural and Life Sciences, University of Idaho, Moscow, ID 83844, USA
* Correspondence: aroe@uidaho.edu; Tel.: +1-208-885-1709

Abstract: Protein, iron, zinc, and choline affect early brain development and are found in beef. The aims of this study were to describe (1) early feeding practices related to introduction of beef in the rural US west (Idaho); (2) parental perceptions of beef as a first food, and (3) associations between early beef consumption and child cognition at 1–5 years. A total of 61 children and their parents were enrolled. Parents completed a survey and a food frequency questionnaire to assess perceptions of beef and early feeding practices along with their child's dietary intake at 6–12 months. Children's cognitive function was assessed using the Bayley-4 Scales of Infant and Toddler Development (12–35 months) and the NIH Toolbox for Assessment of Neurological and Behavioral Function (NIHTB) (3–5 years). Parents introduced beef at 7.79 ± 2.65 months of age, primarily so that their children could eat what the family was eating. Higher intake of beef (r = 0.41, p = 0.02), zinc (r = 0.45, p = 0.01), and choline (r = 0.39, p = 0.03) at 6–12 months was associated with better attention and inhibitory control at 3–5 years of age. These findings support the role of beef as an early food for cognitive development, although controlled dietary intervention studies are needed.

Keywords: beef; iron; zinc; choline; protein; infant; cognition; inhibitory control; attention

Citation: Wilk, V.C.; McGuire, M.K.; Roe, A.J. Early Life Beef Consumption Patterns Are Related to Cognitive Outcomes at 1–5 Years of Age: An Exploratory Study. *Nutrients* **2022**, *14*, 4497. https://doi.org/10.3390/nu14214497

Academic Editor: Joanna Stadnik

Received: 30 September 2022
Accepted: 22 October 2022
Published: 26 October 2022

Publisher's Note: MDPI stays neutral with regard to jurisdictional claims in published maps and institutional affiliations.

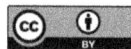

Copyright: © 2022 by the authors. Licensee MDPI, Basel, Switzerland. This article is an open access article distributed under the terms and conditions of the Creative Commons Attribution (CC BY) license (https://creativecommons.org/licenses/by/4.0/).

1. Introduction

Adequate nutrition in utero and the first two years of life is critical for optimal brain development and cognitive function later in life [1]. Suboptimal intake of key nutrients in the first 1000 days may result in cognitive deficits that cannot be reversed through improved intake later in life [2]. The Dietary Guidelines for Americans now include recommendations for children from birth to 2 years of age and highlight the importance of early nutritional needs [3]. A diet composed exclusively of human milk is adequate for most infants during the first 6 months of life [4,5]. Breastfeeding benefits infants by reducing risk of infections [6,7], enhancing neurodevelopment [8,9], and providing a plethora of important nutrients essential for healthy development [10]. Human milk is a nutrient-rich biological system that can sustain an infant for the first 6 months of life, but eventually children require nutrients beyond those provided in breastmilk. To supplement infant feeding, the Dietary Guidelines for Americans and the American Academy of Pediatrics recommend introducing foods (known also as complementary foods) other than human milk and formula at approximately 6 months of age [3,11].

While children obtain diverse nutrition from complementary feeding, nutrients of concern remain. These are nutrients that are not being consumed at recommended levels yet are vital to development. Protein, iron, zinc, and choline are all nutrients that affect early life brain development [12,13]. These nutrients, along with vitamin D and potassium, were noted as nutrients of concern and under-consumption among infants ages 6 to 11 months by the most recent U.S. Dietary Guidelines for Americans Advisory Committee [14]. Iron and zinc deficiency are common in growing children, with mean iron intake among infants in decline [15,16].

Some parents choose to feed their infants fortified infant formulas to prevent nutrient deficiencies, while others incorporate everyday foods in the form of mashing, puree, or liquids into their child's diet. The World Health Organization (WHO) recommends that parents feed their children animal-based products to meet the nutritional needs of children during the first few years of their life [17]. Animal-based products have been shown to reduce iron [18] and zinc [19] deficiencies. Beef, in particular, has been found to provide high levels of both iron and zinc and is a nutrient-dense option for infants as a first food [20,21]. Beef is also high in choline and vitamin B12, both of which play roles in neurodevelopment and cognition [22]. Despite studies showing beef and other meat as a good source of nutrients important for cognitive development, few studies have assessed relationships between early beef intake and child cognition. A systematic review in 2019 reported on only eight studies and concluded inconsistent results, with only one study reporting improved cognitive function with increased intake of beef [23]. This study was not conducted in young children but rather in young women [24].

Research on how parental perceptions of beef as a first food and infant feeding practices influence nutritional status of infants and toddlers is limited. The majority of the research focuses on women with low resources or from developing countries or focuses on weight gain as an outcome [25,26]. A study conducted in August of 2020 by the National Cattlemen's Beef Association investigated the feeding habits of parents with a child who is 6 to 24 months old. The study explored elements considered when choosing food, timing of beef introduction, and knowledge of beef nutritional value. Results suggested that over half of surveyed parents believed that nutritional value was the top benefit of beef, yet only 30% of parents fed their children beef before year one of life [27].

The National Cattlemen's Beef Association's study was very useful for dietitians and nutritionists to understand parents' perceptions of beef throughout the entire nation, but no study has been conducted in the rural west, such as Idaho. According to the U.S. Department of Agriculture (USDA), Idaho had 2.4 million cattle in 2017, outnumbering the human population by over 700,000. The USDA also ranked Idaho 12th among all states in cattle inventory and 11th in cattle sales [28]. Considering that Idaho's beef economy is substantially larger than most states, information needs to be collected to understand the impact of early beef intake on the development and health of Idaho infants and to investigate the perceptions of beef as a first food in infant feeding. This study aimed to describe (1) early feeding practices related to introduction of beef in the rural US west (Idaho); (2) parental perceptions of beef as a first food; and (3) associations between early dietary beef, protein, iron, zinc, and choline intake and child cognition at 1–5 years of age.

2. Materials and Methods

2.1. Study Design

This observational study consisted of a survey assessing perceptions and practices of early beef and feeding practices, a cognitive assessment, and a retrospective food frequency questionnaire. Data were collected from January through June 2022. Idaho parents/caregivers were recruited to participate in this study with their children, all of whom were 1–5 years old. Subjects were recruited using voluntary sampling methods including convenience sampling, which included posting hard-copy and electronic flyers, and snowball sampling, which included asking enrolled subjects to share the recruitment flyer with interested friends or family [29]. Posted flyers gave individuals access to a screening form prior to the study to determine if they met eligibility criteria. Individuals were eligible if they had a child between the ages of 1 and 5 years, were the primary person responsible for feeding the child between ages 6 and 12 months, ≥18 years, and currently resided in Idaho. Once determined eligible, parents were sent an electronic consent form and the parent/child dyad was enrolled.

Once enrolled, parents were sent a 20-min electronic survey administered using Qualtrics software through the University of Idaho (Qualtrics® Software Company Provo, Utah, USA, January 2022). This survey gathered information on perceptions of beef, infant feeding practices, and demographic information. Upon completion of the online survey, parents were contacted to schedule an in-person visit for themselves and their child. At this session, the child completed a cognitive assessment, and height and weight were measured. The parent participated in a researcher-led interview to complete a retrospective food frequency questionnaire. Upon completion of all parts of the study, subject pairs were provided an electronic gift card to compensate for their time and effort in the study. All procedures were approved by the University of Idaho Institutional Review board, and informed consent and assent (as appropriate for age) were obtained.

2.2. Perceptions and Practices Survey

The perceptions and practices survey consisted of five sections: (1) child information; (2) feeding practices and preferences; (3) food purchasing and preparation; (4) sources of information regarding early life feeding; and (5) demographics. The survey took approximately 20 min.

Several questions on the survey were created based on questions asked in the National Cattlemen's Beef Association Early Years Survey conducted in 2020, which assessed beef feeding practices and perceptions in the U.S. [27]. Questions were also created based on conversations with the National Cattlemen's Beef Association, as well as the personal expertise of the research team. The survey was reviewed by two subject-matter experts outside of the research team and revised based on their feedback. A pilot survey was sent to 37 Idaho parents/caregivers before the main study began, which allowed researchers to optimize survey formatting, content, and phrasing. The survey used a variety of questions, both fill-in format and selection format, and Likert-scaling to assess parents' perceptions of beef and their use of beef in infant feeding. To help counteract bias and minimize testing threat with subjects guessing the study was focused on beef feeding practices, the survey also asked questions about other types of meat, such as pork, fish, and chicken.

2.3. Cognitive Assessments

Cognitive assessments were performed between the hours of 8:00 a.m. and 4:00 p.m. Researchers explained the assessments in simple terms to the children and obtained assent. Children were offered a snack before testing to ensure that hunger had minimal effects on scores [30]. Accommodations were made upon participant request, such as having shoes off, changing locations in the room, or having a beverage or snack nearby, in order to minimize discomfort or distractions [30].

The cognitive subtest of the Bayley-4 Scales of Infant and Toddler Development (Bayley-4) was used to assess cognition in children 12 to 35 months of age [31]. This test battery includes items to assess visual performance, attention, memory, sensorimotor, exploration and manipulation, and concept formation. A trained researcher conducted the assessment in a quiet room with a parent present while recording behavioral responses on an iPad. Approximately halfway through the assessment, the researcher gave subjects a break by measuring their height and weight before continuing. The assessment length varied depending on the age and abilities of the child. The Standard score, or overall score, was used to interpret results. This composite score has the highest internal consistency reliability of the scores generated and has a mean of 100 and standard deviation of 15 [32].

The fluid cognition assessment battery of the National Institute of Health Toolbox for Assessment of Neurological and Behavioral Function (NIHTB-CB) was used to assess cognition in children 3–5 years of age [33]. The assessments included in this battery are summarized in Table 1. A trained researcher conducted the assessment in a quiet room using an iPad that was placed within a comfortable reach of the seated participant on a table. After two of the five assessments had been completed, researchers gave subjects a break by measuring their height and weight before continuing with the last three games. The assessment took approximately 50 min, and subjects were able to take a break whenever requested. Parents were allowed to be in the room with the child if needed, although they were asked to not interfere with testing.

Table 1. NIH Toolbox Cognitive Testing Battery.

Construct	Test	Description
Executive Functioning and Attention	Flanker Inhibitory Control and Attention Test	Measures attention and inhibitory control. Participant focuses on a given stimulus while inhibiting attention to stimuli flanking it.
Working Memory	List Sorting Working Memory Test	Measures working memory. Participant recalls and sequences visually and orally presented stimuli.
Executive Function	Dimensional Change Card Sort Test	Measures cognitive flexibility and attention. Pictures are presented varying along two dimensions (e.g., shape and color). The dimension for sorting is indicated by a cue word on the screen.
Processing Speed	Pattern Comparison Processing Speed Test	Measures processing speed. Subjects discern whether two side-by-side pictures are the same or not, with 85 s to respond to as many items as possible. Items are simple to purely measure processing speed.
Episodic Memory	Picture Sequence Memory Test	Measures episodic memory. Subjects are asked to reproduce a sequence of pictures that is shown on the screen. Different practice sequences and test items for subjects of different ages.

The five assessments within the NIHTB-CB were both individually scored by the application and used to generate a fluid cognition composite score. The fully corrected T-score was used to interpret results, which compares the score of the participant to normative national averages, while adjusting for demographic information, including age, gender, race/ethnicity, and parent educational attainment (the score has a mean of 50 and a standard deviation of 10).

2.4. Food Frequency Questionnaire

A retrospective food frequency questionnaire was developed to estimate dietary intake at 6–12 months of age. The food frequency questionnaire was developed based on a previously validated questionnaire designed to estimate dietary intake during the first two years of life [34]. Since the previous questionnaire was developed using foods common in rural Mexico, only the format and organization were used. Many foods were replaced with ones that were more common in Idaho familial households. Foods were chosen based on other U.S. based infant and toddler dietary intake reports [35,36].

The food frequency questionnaire was administered via an interview format. The same researcher conducted all food frequency questionnaire interviews. Six categories of foods were included in the questionnaire: liquids, dairy, cereals and starches, meats, sweets, and other (which included fruits, vegetables, lentils, nuts, and supplements). Parents were asked how often a food/liquid was consumed by the child (per day, week, or month) and how much of it they would eat in one sitting, during months 6–12 of the child's life. If the amount/frequency of the food varied over the span of the 6 months, parents were asked to average the amount/frequency. At the end of each food category, parents were asked if there were any foods not covered in the food frequency questionnaire that they would like to add, and additional foods were added according to each individual participant. Subjects were encouraged to send any future email or text updates about foods they may have forgotten during the interview. Items that represented standard measurement were provided to aid subjects in choosing accurate measurements. The questionnaire lasted approximately 20 min and took place at the Ramsay Research Unit on the University of Idaho campus or via Zoom, if it was more convenient for the participant. Once food frequency questionnaires were conducted, each food item and daily intake amount was entered into the ESHA Research Food Processor, a nutrition analysis software [37]. If food were eaten weekly rather than daily, the amount of food per week was divided by 7 to estimate average daily intake. The ESHA Research Food Processor was then used to estimate the average daily intake of beef, protein, iron, zinc, and choline.

2.5. Data Analysis

Data analysis was conducted using SAS® software, version 9.4 (copyright © 2002–2012, SAS Institute Inc., Cary, NC, USA). Descriptive statistics were used to summarize characteristics of the sample population, including demographic data, cognitive scores, dietary intake data, and data from the perceptions and practices survey. Numerical variables were reported as mean and standard deviation, and categorical variables were reported as frequencies.

Dietary intake data and cognitive scores were evaluated for characteristics of normality by visual evaluation. Outliers for dietary intake (beef, protein, iron, zinc, choline) and cognitive scores were identified if they were 1.5 times the interquartile range greater than the third quartile, or 1.5 times the interquartile range less than the first quartile. Relationships between cognitive scores and dietary intake were assessed via Spearman rank correlation. Missing values were omitted from the final data analysis.

3. Results

3.1. Subject Characteristics

Figure 1 shows the flow of subjects from recruitment to final analysis. A total of 106 individuals completed the screening form and were contacted to enroll in the study. Of these, 5 were ineligible due to state of residency, 1 was a duplicate (2 parents completed separate forms for the same child), and 1 individual did not answer phone calls or respond to attempts to contact. Of the remaining 95 eligible individuals, 29 expressed interest and were sent the link to the consent and perceptions and practices survey but did not complete these documents and so were not scheduled for the in-person assessments, 5 completed the consent and survey but were unable to complete the in-person assessments due to scheduling conflicts or illnesses, 61 individuals completed all aspects of the study. This sample size provided 80% power to detect a correlation of $r = 0.353$, at a significance level of 5% [38].

Subject characteristics are summarized in Table 2. In brief, the sample population was from well-educated, higher-income households. The majority were white and non-Hispanic. Parents introduced beef to their child's diet at an average age of 7.79 ± 2.65 months of age.

3.2. Perceptions and Practices Survey

Parents were asked to rate their agreement with the statement that beef (or chicken, pork, fish, non-meat sources) is a good source of zinc/iron for a baby. Results are summarized in Figure 2. Seventy-eight percent of respondents somewhat agreed or strongly agreed with the statement that beef is a good source of zinc/iron for a baby.

In the sample of 61 Idaho parents/caregivers, 26% of respondents did not introduce meats into their child's diet at 6–12 months of age. Of those who did introduce meat, the most commonly chosen reason for introducing any meat into their child's diet was so that they would eat what the rest of the family eats (see Figure 3). Sixty-three percent of respondents indicated introducing beef so that their child would eat what the rest of the family eats.

Parents were asked to rate the importance of different factors when buying beef. The results are summarized in Figure 4. Over 70% of respondents reported cost, quality, nutrition, and lack of harmful ingredients as somewhat or very important.

Table 2. Subject characteristics. SD indicates standard deviation (*n* = 61).

Variable		n	Mean ± SD
Child age (months)		61	38.06 ± 16.16
Child weight at birth (kg)		60	3.32 ± 0.50
Child length at birth (m)		61	0.50 ± 0.04
Age started solids (months)		59	5.64 ± 1.81
Age stopped breastfeeding (months)		55	16.43 ± 9.76
Age stopped formula (months)		43	8.93 ± 8.87
Age introduced chicken (months)		44	7.67 ± 2.72
Age introduced beef (months)		42	7.79 ± 2.65
Age introduced pork (months)		40	8.28 ± 2.86
Age introduced fish (months)		41	8.73 ± 2.86
Parent 1 Age (years)		61	34.25 ± 4.76
Parent 2 Age (years)		55	36.47 ± 5.8
Number of people in the household		61	4.08 ± 1.02
Number of children in the household		61	2.03 ± 0.84
Variable		**Frequency**	**Percent**
Child sex	Female	32	52%
	Male	29	48%
Parent/caregiver sex	Female	58	95%
	Male	3	5%
Parent/caregiver marital status	Married	56	92%
	Divorced	4	6%
	Single, never married	1	2%
Highest level of education of parent/caregiver	High school/GED	1	2%
	Some college	12	20%
	Associate's degree	5	8%
	Bachelor's degree	16	26%
	Master's degree	21	34%
	Doctorate degree	6	10%
Residence location	Farm/rural	8	13%
	Town less than 5000	2	3%
	Town 5000–10,000	5	8%
	Town/city 10,000–50,000	46	76%
Household income	Less than USD 40,000/year	7	11%
	USD 40,000–50,000/year	10	16%
	USD 60,000–79,000/year	15	25%
	USD 80,000/year or more	29	48%
Race	White	43	71%
	Asian	8	13%
	Two or More Races	2	3%
	Not Reported	8	13%
Ethnicity	Hispanic/Latino	3	5%
	Non-Hispanic/Non-Latino	50	82%
	Not Reported	8	13%

3.3. Retrospective Dietary Intake

Child dietary intake at age 6–12 months was estimated based on the retrospective food frequency questionnaire. Results for dietary intake of beef, protein, iron, zinc, and choline are summarized in Table 3 along with the corresponding Recommended Dietary Allowance or Adequate Intake [39–41].

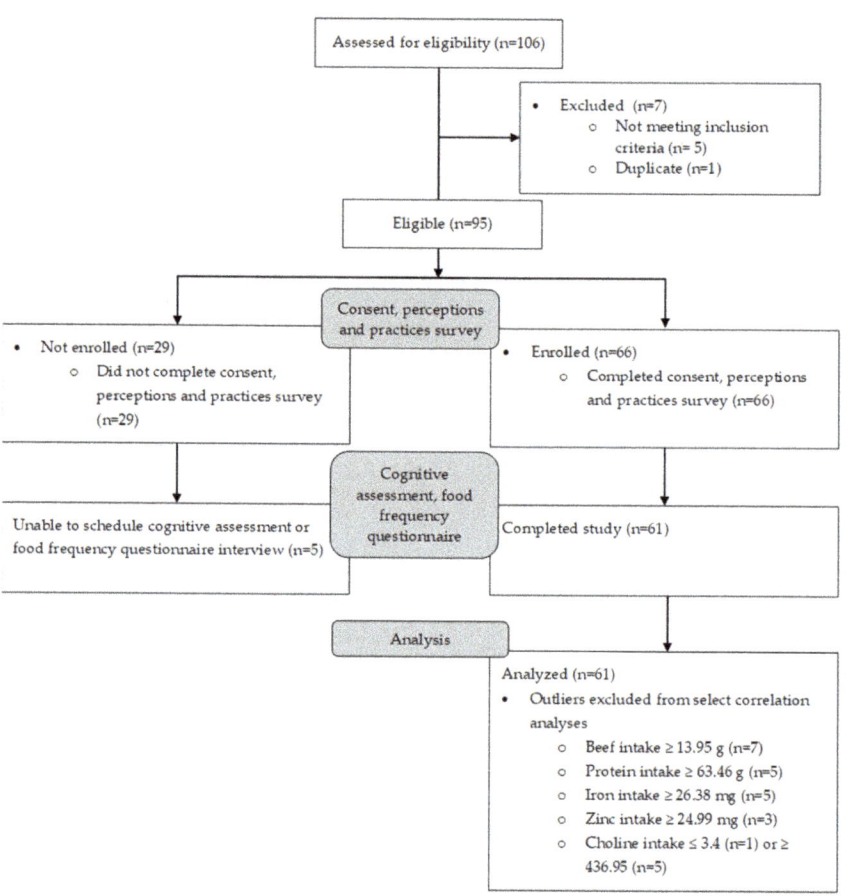

Figure 1. Consort diagram of eligible, enrolled, and analyzed subjects.

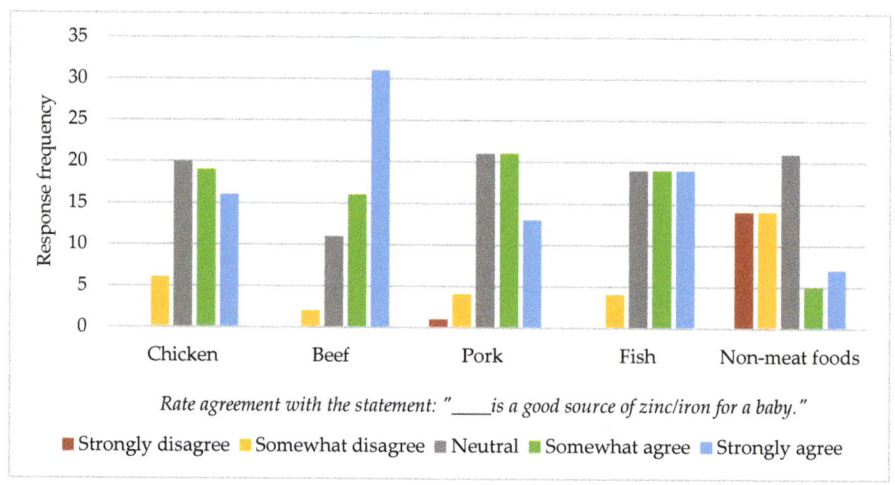

Figure 2. Idaho parent/caregiver's perception of beef and other foods as a good source of zinc/iron for infants. Subjects were asked in the form of an electronic Qualtrics survey ($n = 61$).

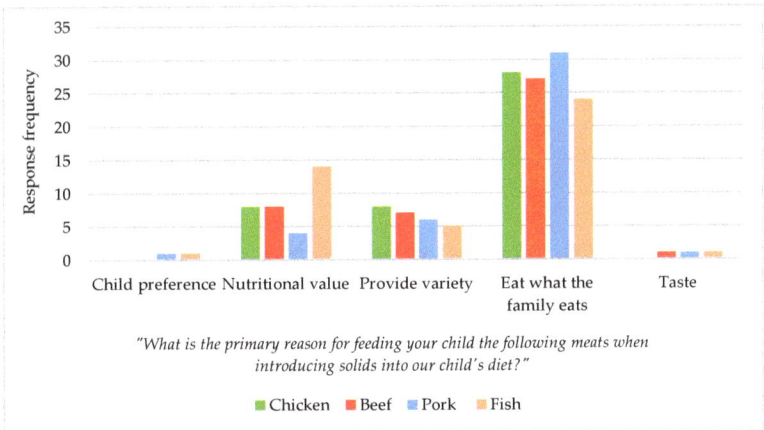

Figure 3. Idaho parent/caregiver primary reason for choosing meat when introducing solids. Subjects were asked in the form of an electronic Qualtrics survey (n = 45).

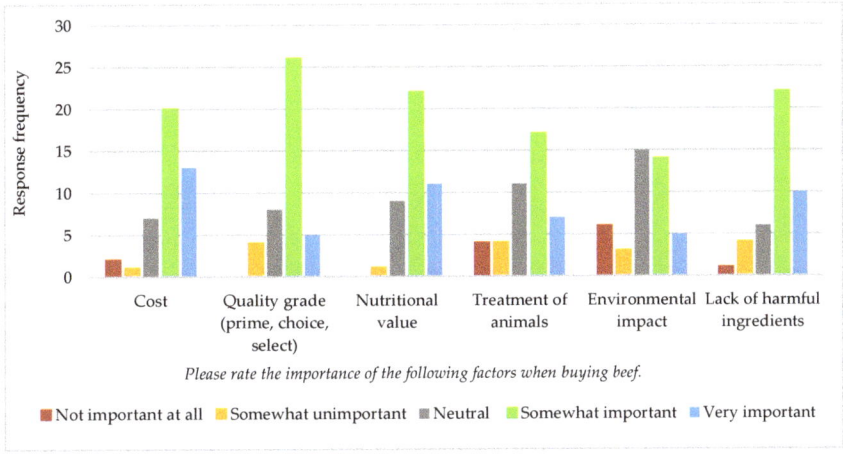

Figure 4. Importance of various factors to Idaho parents when buying beef (n = 43).

Table 3. Estimated dietary intakes of and recommended intakes for beef, protein, iron, zinc, and choline at 6–12 months of age.

Variable	Mean ± SD	Minimum	Maximum	RDA or AI
Beef (g)	4.5 ± 8.5	0.0	48.6	-
Protein (g)	26.5 ± 16.7	0.3	84.6	11
Iron (mg)	9.3 ± 8.7	0.0	39.5	11
Zinc (mg)	6.0 ± 5.3	0.0	25.7	3
Choline (mg)	242.1 ± 166.6	3.4	1212.0	150 *

(n = 61), SD = standard deviation, RDA = Recommended Dietary Allowance, AI = Adequate Intake, * denotes Adequate Intake value.

Relationships between average beef intake and intake of protein, iron, zinc, and choline were assessed by Spearman rank correlation. Higher intake of beef was significantly related to higher intake of protein (r = 0.31, p = 0.01), zinc (r = 0.31, p = 0.02), and choline (r = 0.37, p = 0.004), but not iron (r = 0.15, p = 0.26). The relationships with zinc and choline remained significant when outliers were removed, but the relationship with protein was attenuated.

Using the interquartile range method, outliers were identified as beef intake ≥ 13.93 g (n = 7), protein intake ≥ 63.46 g (n = 5), iron intake ≥ 26.38 mg (n = 5), zinc intake ≥ 24.99 mg (n = 3), and choline intake ≤ 3.4 (n = 1) or ≥ 436.95 (n = 5).

3.4. Cognitive Assessment

Scores on cognitive assessment tests are summarized in Table 4. Children aged 12–35 months of age received a Standard score from the Bayley-4 assessment (the score has a mean of 100 and standard deviation of 15). Children aged 3–5 years of age received individual scores for each of the 5 assessments in the NIHTB-CB, as well as a composite score of overall fluid cognition. The fully corrected T-scores presented in Table 4 are adjusted for age, sex, race/ethnicity, and parental education attainment (the score has a mean of 50 and standard deviation of 10). If subjects were unable to complete the tutorial section of any test, they did not receive a score for that assessment. If a subject did not receive a score on any of the 5 subtests, a Fluid Cognition Composite score was not calculated. This resulted in different sample sizes for each cognitive score. Using the interquartile range method, outliers were identified as a Standard score ≤ 65 (n = 1) and a Picture Sequence Memory score ≥ 78 (n = 1). There were no outliers for any of the other cognitive scores.

Table 4. Child cognitive scores at 1–5 years of age.

Variable	n	Mean ± SD	Minimum	Maximum
Standard	28	102 ± 11	65	115
Fluid	15	41 ± 11	24	61
DCCS	30	50 ± 10	32	70
Flanker	30	48 ± 8	32	67
LSWM	18	42 ± 11	19	57
PCPS	30	32 ± 12	19	65
PSM	26	51 ± 12	33	78

n = sample size, Standard = Bayley-4 Standard score (children age 12–35 months); NIH toolbox assessments were used for children age 3–5 years and included: Fluid = Fluid Cognition Composite score, DCCS = Dimensional Change Card Sort, Flanker = Flanker Inhibitory Control and Attention, LSWM = List Sorting Working Memory, PCPS = Pattern Comparison Processing Speed, PSM = Picture Sequence Memory.

3.5. Relationships between Diet and Cognition

Relationships between dietary intake of beef, protein, iron, zinc, and choline at 6–12 months of age and cognitive scores at age 1–5 years of age are summarized in Table 5. Higher average daily intake of beef, protein, zinc, and choline were significantly correlated with higher scores on the Flanker Inhibitory Control and Attention test. The relationship with beef, zinc, and choline remained significant when removing outliers, while the relationship with protein was attenuated.

Table 5. Relationship between dietary intake at 6–12 months and cognitive scores at 1–5 years of age.

	Beef (g)			Protein (g)			Iron (mg)			Zinc (mg)			Choline (mg)		
	n	r	p	n	r	p	n	r	p	n	r	p	n	r	p
Standard	28	−0.20	0.32	28	0.12	0.54	28	0.05	0.80	28	−0.01	0.96	28	0.12	0.55
Fluid	15	0.13	0.65	15	0.33	0.24	15	0.29	0.29	15	0.36	0.19	15	0.19	0.49
DCCS	30	0.14	0.47	30	0.25	0.18	30	0.09	0.65	30	0.29	0.12	30	0.29	0.12
Flanker	30	0.41	0.02 *	30	0.37	0.05	30	0.28	0.13	30	0.45	0.01 *	30	0.39	0.03 *
LSWM	18	0.19	0.45	18	0.00	0.99	18	0.27	0.28	18	0.25	0.32	18	−0.11	0.67
PCPS	30	0.02	0.90	30	0.14	0.46	30	0.28	0.14	30	0.22	0.24	30	−0.09	0.63
PSM	26	0.34	0.09	26	0.37	0.06	26	0.15	0.47	26	0.32	0.11	26	0.35	0.08

n = sample size, r = Spearman rank correlation coefficient, p = p-value, significance defined as $p \leq 0.05$, * remained significant after removing outliers, Standard = Bayley-4 Standard score, Fluid = Fluid Cognition Composite Score, DCCS = Dimensional Change Card Sort, Flanker = Flanker Inhibitory Control and Attention, LSWM = List Sorting Working Memory, PCPS = Pattern Comparison Processing Speed, PSM = Picture Sequence Memory.

4. Discussion

This observational study captured descriptive data on Idaho parents' perceptions of beef and other types of meat as a first food as well as feeding practices when their children were 6–12 months of age and assessed for relationships between early dietary intake and child cognitive scores at 1–5 years of age. Idaho parents and caregivers reported introducing beef to their children at around 7 months of age, primarily so that their children could eat what the rest of the family was eating. Children whose parents reported higher average daily beef, zinc, and choline intakes at 6–12 months of age scored higher on a test of inhibitory control and attention at 3–5 years of age.

The results of the perceptions and practices survey showed that parents typically followed the Dietary Guidelines for Americans recommendation to introduce complementary foods at the age of six months, with most exclusively breastfeeding their child before the age of six months [14]. Parents also generally followed guidelines with supplementary feedings of breastmilk/formula until at least the age of 1 year. Infant wellbeing was the focus when parents were answering questions about early feeding practices, with nutrition and infant safety being the top values when choosing first foods for their infants, and medical experts being the most common consultants to parents. Idaho parents saw beef favorably as a nutritional food but had worries about their infants chewing and choking on beef as a first food. Parents reported introducing beef when their child was 7.79 ± 2.65 months of age. This was slightly younger than when they introduced pork or fish, but slighter older than when introducing chicken. When buying beef, cost and nutritional value were both highly important for parents of infants. These results were similar to national results, which showed that parents value nutrition when choosing first foods for their infant, and are concerned about choking, chewing, and safety of food [27].

Analysis of the retrospective food frequency questionnaire did not reveal any areas of significant concern for consumption of key nutrients, protein, iron, zinc, and choline in this sample population. However, the variability in the reported intakes makes it difficult to draw clear conclusions. It is also likely that parents overestimated dietary intake, as this is a known limitation of this type of dietary recall data [42].

The Recommended Dietary Allowance (amount needed to meet the nutrition needs for 97–98% of people) of protein for infants ages 6–12 months is 11.0 g/d [41]. The reported average intake for children in our study (26.5 ± 16.7 g/d) was over twice the recommended intake, but only slightly higher than the average daily intake for children aged 6–11.9 months reported in the 2016 Feeding Infants and Toddlers (FITS) database (21 ± 0.2 g/d) [41]. Even when removing outliers, the average reported daily protein intake was high (25.6 ± 10.0 g/d). Similar trends were observed with reported daily intakes of zinc and choline. Parents recalled giving their children, aged 6–12 months, foods containing 6.0 ± 5.3 mg of zinc per day, compared to the RDA of 3 mg/d and the Tolerable Upper Intake Level (UL) of 5 mg/d [40]. When removing outliers, the average zinc intake reported was 5.0 ± 3.0 mg/d. Although above the RDA, the zinc intake reported in this study was similar to the national average of 5.8 ± 0.1 mg/d reported in the 2016 FITS database for infants 6–11.9 months [43]. Similar results were observed with dietary choline intake. Parents reported feeding their children foods containing an average of 242.1 ± 166.6 mg of choline per day. This is above the Adequate Intake of 150 mg/d for children 6–12 months of age [39]. When removing outliers, the mean intake was still high, but the standard deviation was lower (208.9 ± 74.1 mg/d).

Many parents fed their children iron-fortified formulas and iron-fortified baby cereals between the ages of 6–12 months, and the average daily iron intake for infants was estimated to be 9.3 ± 8.7 mg/d. The RDA for daily iron intake in 6–11-month-old infants is 11 mg/day [40]. Average daily iron intake in this study was below the national average reported in the 2016 FITS database of 13 ± 0.2 mg/d in infants 6–11.9 months of age [43]. When removing outliers, the daily iron intake reported in this study was lower (7.5 ± 6.2 mg/d). The large standard deviation in this sample makes it difficult to draw conclusions and warrants further investigation with larger sample sizes. The variability in iron intake may be in part due to the popularity of iron-fortified foods and drinks. The high intake of iron-rich foods other than beef also may be a reason that iron intake was not associated with beef intake, despite beef being a good source of iron [44].

For children aged 12–35 months, the Standard score obtained from the Bayley-4 was categorized as Average and within the 25th–74th percentile of the national validation sample [32]. For children aged 3–5 years who completed the NIHTB-CB, the average scores obtained were all within one standard deviation of the national average with the exception of the Pattern Comparison Processing Speed score which was almost two standard deviations below the average. Estimated daily beef, protein, zinc, and choline intake were all positively correlated with scores on the Flanker Inhibitory Control and Attention test prior to outlier removal, with only the correlation with daily protein intake not remaining significant after outliers were removed. This suggests that beef, or nutrients found in beef, may play a role in attention/inhibitory control. Dietary intakes were not significantly associated with any other cognitive scores.

Finding no significant relationship between dietary intake of iron and cognitive function was unexpected due to the role of iron in early brain development [22]. There was a great deal of iron variability observed in our sample population, so the relationship may not be as clear as if it was more controlled and uniform throughout the cohort. The relationship between beef intake and cognition could be influenced more by zinc, protein, and choline than iron for this reason. Furthermore, other factors are also involved with cognitive development and may be driving these findings. Beef is also a good source of vitamin B12, which has been associated with adverse cognitive outcomes if under-consumed in children [45]. The majority of children in this study were exclusively breastfed early in life, a practice that has been associated with favorable neurodevelopment [46].

Strengths and Limitations

The perceptions and practices survey was designed to be an exploratory tool in nature, looking at the most common selected answers and trends rather than being a determinant of significant relationships. This provided hypothesis-generating data that will help justify further research. However, due to the convenience sample recruiting around the Moscow, Idaho area, our study population was largely white, high income, and well educated. As such, we acknowledge that our data do not represent all of Idaho, nor the entire rural west, which includes even less populated areas with lower income and education levels. In the future, it would be beneficial to repeat this study on a larger scale including additional western states, to include more races, rural areas, and more variability in income and educational obtainment. In addition, while the survey collected data on parent feeding practices, other parenting practices were not assessed. Future studies should collect data on parental involvement or childcare practices in order to assess the role of such variables as mediators or covariates in the relationship between dietary intake and cognition. Better understanding the interplay between other parenting practices and dietary behaviors on cognition may be important to consider when developing interventions to improve child cognitive development.

The retrospective food frequency questionnaire allowed for a longitudinal analysis with relation to cognitive outcomes, without requiring long-term follow-up. However, because we asked parents to recall daily food intake, often years in the past, there are inaccuracies in the dietary intake data, as intakes are likely to be over- or underestimated. While early dietary intake from age 6–12 months was the focus of this study, current dietary intake of subjects may have been a confounding factor that influenced the observed relationships (or lack thereof). Because this is an observational study, cause–effect relationships cannot be made based on these data. Nonetheless, our finding of a positive association between early beef consumption and an indicator of inhibitory control and attention warrants further study.

5. Conclusions

Idaho parents and caregivers reported introducing beef to their children at around 7 months of age, primarily so that their child would eat what the rest of the family was eating. Children whose parents reported higher average daily beef, zinc, and choline intakes at 6–12 months of age scored higher on a test of inhibitory control and attention at 3–5 years of age. It is important to note that these correlational observations do not imply causation. These results need to be confirmed in subjects from lower socioeconomic households and of various racial and ethnic backgrounds in order to make the results generalizable to a larger population. Additionally, prospective cohort and randomized controlled trials also need to be conducted in order to provide insights into causal relationships. Despite the limitations inherent in an observational study with retrospective dietary recall, the findings of this study contribute to the evidence base supporting the role of beef as an early food for cognitive development.

Author Contributions: Conceptualization, V.C.W., M.K.M. and A.J.R.; Data curation, A.J.R.; Formal analysis, A.J.R.; Funding acquisition, M.K.M. and A.J.R.; Investigation, V.C.W. and A.J.R.; Methodology, V.C.W. and A.J.R.; Project administration, A.J.R.; Resources, A.J.R.; Supervision, A.J.R.; Visualization, V.C.W., M.K.M. and A.J.R.; Writing—original draft, V.C.W. and A.J.R.; Writing—review and editing, V.C.W., M.K.M. and A.J.R. All authors have read and agreed to the published version of the manuscript.

Funding: This research was funded by the Idaho Beef Council, grant number AL5329 AL5544. The APC was funded by the University of Idaho.

Institutional Review Board Statement: The study was conducted in accordance with the Declaration of Helsinki and approved by the Institutional Review Board of the University of Idaho (protocol code 21-119 and 5 March 2021).

Informed Consent Statement: Informed consent was obtained from all subjects over the age of 18 involved in the study, and informed assent was obtained from all subjects under the age of 18 involved in the study.

Data Availability Statement: The data presented in this study are available on request from the corresponding author.

Acknowledgments: We thank Janice Fletcher and Hydee Becker for their content review and feedback on our survey. We also thank Miranda Collet, Abril Correa, Megan Follett, Breanna Harmon, Carol Morrison, Maxine Moulton, Jolene Whiteley, and Destiny Whitmire for their assistance with subject recruitment and data collection.

Conflicts of Interest: The authors declare no conflict of interest.

References

1. Prado, E.L.; Dewey, K.G. Nutrition and brain development in early life. *Nutr. Rev.* **2014**, *72*, 267–284. [CrossRef] [PubMed]
2. Schwarzenberg, S.J.; Georgieff, M.K.; Committee on Nutrition; Daniels, S.; Corkins, M.; Golden, N.H.; Kim, J.H.; Lindsey, C.W.; Magge, S.N. Advocacy for Improving Nutrition in the First 1000 Days to Support Childhood Development and Adult Health. *Pediatrics* **2018**, *141*, e20173716. [CrossRef] [PubMed]
3. U.S. Department of Agriculture; U.S. Department of Health and Human Services. *Dietary Guidelines for Americans, 2020–2025*, 9th ed.; December 2020. Available online: https://www.pcrm.org/good-nutrition/nutrition-programs-policies/2020-2025-dietary-guidelines (accessed on 7 January 2021).
4. Kramer, M.S.; Kakuma, R. The optimal duration of exclusive breastfeeding: A systematic review. *Adv. Exp. Med. Biol.* **2004**, *554*, 63–77. [PubMed]
5. Kramer, M.S.; Kakuma, R. Optimal duration of exclusive breastfeeding. *Cochrane Database Syst. Rev.* **2012**, *2012*, Cd003517. [CrossRef]
6. Quigley, M.A.; Carson, C.; Sacker, A.; Kelly, Y. Exclusive breastfeeding duration and infant infection. *Eur. J. Clin. Nutr.* **2016**, *70*, 1420–1427. [CrossRef]
7. Pandolfi, E.; Gesualdo, F.; Rizzo, C.; Carloni, E.; Villani, A.; Concato, C.; Linardos, G.; Russo, L.; Ferretti, B.; Campagna, I.; et al. Breastfeeding and Respiratory Infections in the First 6 Months of Life: A Case Control Study. *Front. Pediatr.* **2019**, *7*, 152. [CrossRef]

8. Belfort, M.B.; Rifas-Shiman, S.L.; Kleinman, K.P.; Guthrie, L.B.; Bellinger, D.C.; Taveras, E.M.; Gillman, M.W.; Oken, E. Infant feeding and childhood cognition at ages 3 and 7 years: Effects of breastfeeding duration and exclusivity. *JAMA Pediatr.* **2013**, *167*, 836–844. [CrossRef]
9. Choi, H.J.; Kang, S.K.; Chung, M.R. The relationship between exclusive breastfeeding and infant development: A 6- and 12-month follow-up study. *Early Hum. Dev.* **2018**, *127*, 42–47. [CrossRef]
10. Dror, D.K.; Allen, L.H. Overview of Nutrients in Human Milk. *Adv. Nutr. Int. Rev. J.* **2018**, *9*, 278S–294S. [CrossRef]
11. American Academy of Pediatrics Committee on Nutrition. *Pediatric Nutrition*, 7th ed.; American Academy of Pediatrics: Elk Grove Village, IL, USA, 2014.
12. Georgieff, M.K.; Brunette, K.E.; Tran, P.V. Early life nutrition and neural plasticity. *Dev. Psychopathol.* **2015**, *27*, 411–423. [CrossRef]
13. Mun, J.G.; Legette, L.L.; Ikonte, C.J.; Mitmesser, S.H. Choline and DHA in Maternal and Infant Nutrition: Synergistic Implications in Brain and Eye Health. *Nutrients* **2019**, *11*, 1125. [CrossRef] [PubMed]
14. Dietary Guidelines Advisory Committee. *Scientific Report of the 2020 Dietary Guidelines Advisory Committee: Advisory Report to the Secretary of Agriculture and the Secretary of Health and Human Services*; U.S. Department of Agriculture, Agricultural Research Service: Washington, DC, USA, 2020. [CrossRef]
15. Eldridge, A.L.; Catellier, D.J.; Hampton, J.C.; Dwyer, J.T.; Bailey, R.L. Trends in Mean Nutrient Intakes of US Infants, Toddlers, and Young Children from 3 Feeding Infants and Toddlers Studies (FITS). *J. Nutr.* **2019**, *149*, 1230–1237. [CrossRef] [PubMed]
16. Krebs, N.F.; Miller, L.V.; Hambidge, K.M. Zinc deficiency in infants and children: A review of its complex and synergistic interactions. *Paediatr. Int. Child Health* **2014**, *34*, 279–288. [CrossRef]
17. World Health Organization. Infant and Young Child Feeding. Nutrition Landscape Information System (NLiS) 2022. Available online: https://www.who.int/data/nutrition/nlis/info/infant-and-young-child-feeding (accessed on 23 September 2022).
18. Domellöf, M.; Braegger, C.; Campoy, C.; Colomb, V.; Decsi, T.; Fewtrell, M.; Hojsak, I.; Mihatsch, W.; Molgaard, C.; Shamir, R.; et al. Iron requirements of infants and toddlers. *J. Pediatr. Gastroenterol. Nutr.* **2014**, *58*, 119–129. [CrossRef] [PubMed]
19. International Zinc Nutrition Consultative Group; Brown, K.H.; Rivera, J.A.; Bhutta, Z.; Gibson, R.S.; King, J.C.; Lonnerdal, B.; Ruel, M.T.; Sandtrom, B.; Wasantwisut, E.; et al. International zinc nutrition consultative group (IZiNCG) technical document #1. Assessment of the risk of zinc deficiency in populations and options for its control. *Food Nutr. Bull.* **2004**, *25*, S99–S203.
20. Hambidge, K.M.; Sheng, X.; Mazariegos, M.; Jiang, T.; Garces, A.; Li, D.; Westcott, J.; Tshefu, A.; Sami, N.; Pasha, O.; et al. Evaluation of meat as a first complementary food for breastfed infants: Impact on iron intake. *Nutr. Rev.* **2011**, *69*, S57–S63. [CrossRef]
21. Krebs, N.F.; Westcott, J.E.; Butler, N.; Robinson, C.; Bell, M.; Hambidge, K.M. Meat as a First Complementary Food for Breastfed Infants: Feasibility and Impact on Zinc Intake and Status. *J. Pediatr. Gastroenterol. Nutr.* **2006**, *42*, 207–214. [CrossRef]
22. Georgieff, M.K.; Ramel, S.E.; Cusick, S.E. Nutritional influences on brain development. *Acta Paediatr.* **2018**, *107*, 1310–1321. [CrossRef]
23. An, R.; Nickols-Richardson, S.M.; Khan, N.; Liu, J.; Liu, R.; Clarke, C. Impact of Beef and Beef Product Intake on Cognition in Children and Young Adults: A Systematic Review. *Nutrients* **2019**, *11*, 1797. [CrossRef]
24. Blanton, C. Improvements in Iron Status and Cognitive Function in Young Women Consuming Beef or Non-Beef Lunches. *Nutrients* **2013**, *6*, 90–110. [CrossRef]
25. Kim, J.; Peterson, K.E. Association of Infant Child Care With Infant Feeding Practices and Weight Gain Among US Infants. *Arch. Pediatr. Adolesc. Med.* **2008**, *162*, 627–633. [CrossRef] [PubMed]
26. Harrison, M.; Brodribb, W.; Hepworth, J. A qualitative systematic review of maternal infant feeding practices in transitioning from milk feeds to family foods. *Matern. Child Nutr.* **2016**, *13*, e12360. [CrossRef] [PubMed]
27. National Cattlemen's Beef Association. Fact Sheet: What Parents Think about Introducing Beef as a First Food. 2020. Available online: https://www.beefresearch.org/resources/market-research-planning/fact-sheets/what-parents-think-about-introducing-beef-as-a-first-food (accessed on 7 May 2021).
28. U.S. Department of Agriculture National Agricultural Statistics Service. *2017 Census of Agriculture*; 2017. Available online: www.nass.usda.gov/AgCensus (accessed on 7 May 2021).
29. Setia, M.S. Methodology series module 5: Sampling strategies. *Indian J. Dermatol.* **2016**, *61*, 505–509. [CrossRef]
30. Jirout, J.; LoCasale-Crouch, J.; Turnbull, K.; Gu, Y.; Cubides, M.; Garzione, S.; Evans, T.M.; Weltman, A.L.; Kranz, S. How Lifestyle Factors Affect Cognitive and Executive Function and the Ability to Learn in Children. *Nutrients* **2019**, *11*, 1953. [CrossRef] [PubMed]
31. Bayley, N.; Aylward, G. *Bayley Scales of Infant and Toddler Development*, 4th ed.; NCS Pearson, Inc.: Bloomington, MN, USA, 2019.
32. Alfonso, V.C.; Engler, J.R.; Turner, A.D. *Essentials of Bayley-4 Assessment*; John Wiley & Sons, Inc.: Hoboken, NJ, USA, 2022.
33. Weintraub, S.; Dikmen, S.S.; Heaton, R.K.; Tulsky, D.S.; Zelazo, P.D.; Bauer, P.J.; Carlozzi, N.E.; Slotkin, J.; Blitz, D.; Wallner-Allen, K.; et al. Cognition assessment using the NIH Toolbox. *Neurology* **2013**, *80*, S54–S64. [CrossRef] [PubMed]
34. Mejía-Rodríguez, F.; Neufeld, L.M.; García-Guerra, A.; Quezada-Sanchez, A.D.; Orjuela, M.A. Validation of a food frequency questionnaire for retrospective estimation of diet during the first 2 years of life. *Matern. Child Health J.* **2014**, *18*, 268–285. [CrossRef] [PubMed]
35. Roess, A.A.; Jacquier, E.F.; Catellier, D.J.; Carvalho, R.; Lutes, A.C.; Anater, A.S.; Dietz, W.H. Food Consumption Patterns of Infants and Toddlers: Findings from the Feeding Infants and Toddlers Study (FITS) 2016. *J. Nutr.* **2018**, *148*, 1525S–1535S. [CrossRef]

6. Sharma, S.; Kolahdooz, F.; Butler, L.; Budd, N.; Rushovich, B.; Mukhina, G.L.; Gittelsohn, J.; Caballero, B. Assessing dietary intake among infants and toddlers 0-24 months of age in Baltimore, Maryland, USA. *Nutr. J.* **2013**, *12*, 52. [CrossRef]
7. ESHA Research, Food Processor SQL. *Food Processor Nutrition and Fitness Software*; Processor SQL Inc.: Salem, OR, USA, 2022.
8. Kohn, M.; Senyak, J. Sample Size Calculators. 2022. Available online: http://sample-size.net/ (accessed on 19 September 2022).
9. Institute of Medicine. *Dietary Reference Intakes for Thiamin, Riboflavin, Niacin, Vitamin B6, Folate, Vitamin B12, Pantothenic Acid, Biotin, and Choline*; The National Academies Press: Washington, DC, USA, 1998.
10. Institute of Medicine. *Dietary Reference Intakes for Vitamin A, Vitamin K, Arsenic, Boron, Chromium, Copper, Iodine, Iron, Manganese, Molybdenum, Nickel, Silicon, Vanadium, and Zinc*; The National Academies Press: Washington, DC, USA, 2001.
11. Institute of Medicine. *Dietary Reference Intakes for Energy, Carbohydrate, Fiber, Fat, Fatty Acids, Cholesterol, Protein, and Amino Acids*; The National Academies Press: Washington, DC, USA, 2005.
12. Fisher, J.O.; Butte, N.F.; Mendoza, P.M.; Wilson, T.A.; Hodges, E.A.; Reidy, K.C.; Deming, D. Overestimation of infant and toddler energy intake by 24-h recall compared with weighed food records. *Am. J. Clin. Nutr.* **2008**, *88*, 407–415. [CrossRef]
13. Bailey, R.L.; Catellier, D.J.; Jun, S.; Dwyer, J.T.; Jacquier, E.F.; Anater, A.S.; Eldridge, A. Total Usual Nutrient Intakes of US Children (Under 48 Months): Findings from the Feeding Infants and Toddlers Study (FITS) 2016. *J. Nutr.* **2018**, *148* (Suppl. 3), 1557S–1566S. [CrossRef]
14. Krebs, N.F. Dietary zinc and iron sources, physical growth and cognitive development of breastfed infants. *J. Nutr.* **2000**, *130*, 358S–360S. [CrossRef] [PubMed]
15. Venkatramanan, S.; Armata, I.E.; Strupp, B.J.; Finkelstein, J.L. Vitamin B-12 and Cognition in Children. *Adv. Nutr. Int. Rev. J.* **2016**, *7*, 879–888. [CrossRef] [PubMed]
16. Deoni, S.; Dean, D.; Joelson, S.; O'Regan, J.; Schneider, N. Early nutrition influences developmental myelination and cognition in infants and young children. *NeuroImage* **2018**, *178*, 649–659. [CrossRef] [PubMed]

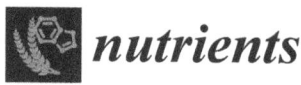 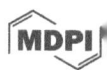

Article

Indexing of Fatty Acids in Poultry Meat for Its Characterization in Healthy Human Nutrition: A Comprehensive Application of the Scientific Literature and New Proposals

Alessandro Dal Bosco [1], Alice Cartoni Mancinelli [1,*], Gaetano Vaudo [2], Massimiliano Cavallo [2], Cesare Castellini [1] and Simona Mattioli [1]

[1] Department of Agricultural, Environmental and Food Science, University of Perugia, Borgo XX Giugno 74, 06124 Perugia, Italy; alessandro.dalbosco@unipg.it (A.D.B.); cesare.castellini@unipg.it (C.C.); simona.mattioli@unipg.it (S.M.)

[2] Department of Medicine and Surgery, University of Perugia, Piazzale Gambuli 1, 06132 Perugia, Italy; gaetano.vaudo@unipg.it (G.V.); massimilianocavallotr@gmail.com (M.C.)

* Correspondence: acartonimancinelli@gmail.com; Tel.: +39-075-585-7123

Abstract: Chicken meat is becoming the most consumed in the world for both economic and nutritional reasons; regarding the latter, the lipid profile may play positive or negative roles in the prevention and treatment of diseases. In this study, we define the state of the art of lipid-based nutritional indexes and used the lipid content and fatty acid profile (both qualitative and quantitative) of breast meat of two poultry genotypes with different growth rates and meat traits. Further, we summarize and review the definitions, implications, and applications of nutritional indexes used in recent years and others of our own design to provide a useful tool to researchers working in the field of meat quality (not only in poultry) to select the most appropriate index for their own scientific purposes. All indexes show advantages and disadvantages; hence, a rational choice should be applied to consider the nutritional effect of meat on human health and for a possible assessment of the most suitable rearing systems (genotype, feeding, farming system or postmortem handling).

Keywords: fatty acids; chicken; meat quality; metabolism; human nutrition; index

Citation: Dal Bosco, A.; Cartoni Mancinelli, A.; Vaudo, G.; Cavallo, M.; Castellini, C.; Mattioli, S. Indexing of Fatty Acids in Poultry Meat for Its Characterization in Healthy Human Nutrition: A Comprehensive Application of the Scientific Literature and New Proposals. *Nutrients* 2022, *14*, 3110. https://doi.org/10.3390/nu14153110

Academic Editor: Joanna Stadnik

Received: 28 June 2022
Accepted: 26 July 2022
Published: 28 July 2022

Publisher's Note: MDPI stays neutral with regard to jurisdictional claims in published maps and institutional affiliations.

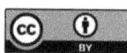

Copyright: © 2022 by the authors. Licensee MDPI, Basel, Switzerland. This article is an open access article distributed under the terms and conditions of the Creative Commons Attribution (CC BY) license (https://creativecommons.org/licenses/by/4.0/).

1. Introduction

For many years, meat has been considered not only a source of nutritional elements such as proteins, lipids and minerals, but also a food capable of providing fundamental bioactive compounds for a whole series of metabolic functions that are at the basis of an optimal state of human health [1].

Many reviews have been published on the importance of the fatty acid composition of various meats and on the technologies used to improve their nutritional profile, mainly concerning the polyunsaturated fractions [2–5].

In these and other scientific studies, plentiful evidence has been given for all the metabolic functions that different fatty acids possess and in particular on the positive or negative roles in the prevention or onset of different chronic diseases, depending on their nature (i.e., presence or absence of double bonds and the number and/or position of them). Indeed, saturated fatty acids (SFAs) can increase the development of coronary heart diseases, multiple sclerosis and other metabolic dysfunctions [6], while polyunsaturated fatty acids (PUFAs) may have positive effects and beneficial actions on cardiovascular diseases, neurological diseases, allergic diseases, and so on [7].

These fatty acids are mainly obtained from various dietary sources, which have very different compositions and consequently have different effects on health outcomes. For this reason, the precise assessment of the fatty acid profile must be determined to rank foods based on their nutritional/functional properties, especially in fatty-acid-rich foods, food supplements and herb-based medicines.

It is well known that Long-Chain n-3 PUFAs (LC-PUFAs) are found predominantly in oily fish, but their consumption is declining [8], as well as that of all meats, with the exception of poultry, which has increased in consumption by 73% in the last 30 years [9]. From a nutritional point of view, comparing the n-3 PUFA content of poultry meat with that of mammal livestock, it seemingly has lower levels of n-3 and higher levels of n-6 [5], but it is also true that the fatty acid composition of poultry could easily be modified through feeding or management strategies [3,10,11]. In this scenario, organic or extensive rearing systems of poultry improve in the consideration of consumers, such as respect for animal welfare, environmental sustainability and food quality, due to the richness of some bioactive compounds, including n-3 PUFAs [9,12,13].

Based on the belief that the determination of the fatty acid profile, especially if expressed as a percentage, is not sufficient to explain the nutritional properties of a food and, taking a cue from a recent review on the nutritional indexes of meat and fish [14], we aimed to trace the state of the art of nutritional indexing, with indexes taken from the bibliography and other new ones of our conception. Therefore, the aim of the present study was to update the situation of lipid nutritional indexing in poultry meat and, on this basis, conceive other indexes that more effectively explore potential uses in the determination of nutritional properties by comparing two poultry genotypes with extremely different growth rates and fat contents. This study could help researchers working in the field of meat fatty acid composition to select the most appropriate index for their purposes. Indeed, after a reasonable evaluation of the best index, a more systematic research process has been used:

- to come to valid considerations about the nutritional effects of different meats on human health; and
- to provide a useful evaluation of the most suitable genotype and/or management practices (choice of the most appropriate feeding strategies, farming systems or post-mortem handling).

2. Materials and Methods

2.1. Animals and Diets

To obtain a complete dataset on lipid content and the profile to be indexed, an experimental trial was carried out at the poultry farm of the University of Perugia (Italy), using 100 subjects for each of two very different genotypes (50/50 sex ratio). In particular, the genotypes were extremely different in growth rate: slow-growing (SG, growth rhythm <20 g/d), originating from a conservation flock at the Department of Agricultural, Environmental and Food Science in the 1960s, and fast-growing (FG, growth rhythm >40 g/d), furnished by a commercial poultry farm (Avicola Berlanda, Italy). We chose these two divergent genotypes to differentiate the carcass and meat characteristics, particularly for lipid content and fatty acid composition (% of total fatty acids and mg/100 g) of meat (as reviewed by Dal Bosco et al. [15]), to verify the indexes considered in the present study.

All animals were reared according to EU regulation 834/07 on animal welfare for experimental and other scientific purposes. Furthermore, the experimental protocol was positively evaluated by an internal university committee (prot. 112606 of 12 January 2021). Chickens were kept separate after hatching until 20 d of age in an environmentally controlled poultry house with temperatures ranging from 20 to 32 °C and with relative humidity ranging from 65 to 75%. Incandescent light (30 lux) placed at the bird level was used for heating and illumination. Chicks were vaccinated against Marek and Newcastle diseases. At 21 days of age, the chicks were transferred to straw-bedded indoor pens (0.10 m^2/bird), each equipped with feeders and drinkers and with free access to a forage paddock (4 m^2/bird). Each genotype was represented in four replicates containing 25 chicks each. Birds were confined to indoor pens during the night. Chickens were fed ad libitum with the same starter (1–21 d) and grower–finisher (22 d to slaughter) diets (Table 1).

Table 1. Ingredient composition and calculated analysis of diets.

	Starter	Finisher
Ingredients		
Maize	52.0	46.0
Full-fat soybean	30.5	12.5
Wheat	-	20.0
Soybean meal	9.00	14.0
Alfalfa meal	2.80	2.80
Corn gluten feed	3.00	2.00
Vitamin-mineral premix [1]	1.00	1.00
Dicalcium phosphate	1.00	1.00
Sodium bicarbonate	0.50	0.50
NaCl	0.20	0.20
Chemical composition		
Dry matter	90.9	90.8
Crude protein (%)	22.3	18.0
Ether extract (%)	7.95	4.98
Crude fiber (%)	4.67	4.01
Ash (%)	5.76	5.59
NDF—Neutral Detergent Fiber	10.7	10.1
ADF—Acid Detergent Fiber	5.58	5.06
Cellulose (%)	4.22	3.56
ADL—Acid Detergent Liquid	1.03	1.11
Hemicellulose (%)	5.16	5.05
Metabolizable Energy (Mj/kg DM)	12.5	12.9

[1] Amounts per kg: Vit. A 11.000 IU; Vit. D3 2.000 IU; Vit. B1 2.5 mg; Vit. B2 4 mg; Vit. B6 1.25 mg; Vit. B12 0.01 mg; α-tocopheryl acetate 30 mg; biotin 0.06 mg; Vit. K 2.5 mg; niacin 15 mg; folic acid 0.30 mg; pantothenic acid 10 mg; choline chloride 600 mg; Mn 60 mg; Fe 50 mg; Zn 15 mg; I 0.5 mg; Co 0.5 mg.

Access to feed and water was freely available, and all diets were formulated to contain adequate nutrient levels as defined by the NRC [16] and several authors [17]. Considering the very different growth rates of the birds, slaughter was carried out when 70% of the adult weight was reached, at approximately 110 days for SG and 45 days for FG.

2.2. Sampling and Analysis

A sample of 20 birds per strain, each weighing between ±10% of the population mean, was slaughtered in a slaughterhouse approved by the EU, 12 h after feed withdrawal. Chickens were electrically stunned (110 V; 350 Hz) before killing. After killing, the carcasses were placed in hot water (56.5 °C for 1 min) and then plucked, eviscerated (nonedible viscera: intestines, proventriculus, gall bladder, spleen, esophagus and full crop), and stored for 24 h at 4 °C. From the carcass, the pectoralis major muscle was excised for analysis. Samples were transported in refrigerated conditions to the department's laboratory and immediately analyzed in duplicate to determine the lipid amounts. Total lipids were extracted in duplicate from 5 g of each homogenized sample and calculated gravimetrically [18]. Fatty acids were quantified as methyl esters (FAMEs) with a gas chromatography system (CP 3800 VARIAN, Varian Medical Systems Italia S.P.A., Milan, Italy) equipped with an FID detector and a capillary column of 100 m length × 0.25 mm × 0.2 μm film (Supelco, Bellefonte, PA, USA). To calculate the amount of each FA, heneicosanoic acid was used as the internal standard (C21:0, Sigma—Aldrich analytical standard, Steinfeld, Germany), and data were expressed as mg/100 g of meat (quantitative evaluation) and % of total FA (qualitative evaluation). The average amount of each fatty acid was used to calculate the sum of the SFAs, monounsaturated fatty acids (MUFAs) and PUFAs.

2.3. Indexes

All the indexes considered in this review were categorized into subgroups based on the aim for which they were conceived, and in particular into qualitative, nutritional, metabolic and lipid- or energy-related content indexes, as summarized in Table 2.

Table 2. Summary of the studied indexes and their significance regarding health effects (D = direct; I = indirect).

Sub-Categories	Indexes	Unit	Sign.	References
Qualitative	• PUFA/SFA	%	D	Many Authors
	• n-6/n-3 ratio	%	I	Simopoulus, 2008 [1];
	• LA/ALA	%	I	Undurti, 2006 [2];
	• EPA + DHA%	%	D	Holub, 2009 [3], Crupi and Cuzzocreas, 2022 [4];
	• Unsaturation Index (UI)	%	I	Shahidi and Zhong, 2010 [5].
Nutritional	• Nutrition Value Index	%	D	Chen et al., 2016 [6];
	• Index of Atherogenicity (IA)	%	I	Ulbricht and Southgate, 1991 [7];
	• Index of Thrombogenicity (IT)	%	I	Ulbricht and Southgate, 1991 [7];
	• Hypocholesterolemic/Hypercholesterolemic (HH)	%	D	Santos-Silva et al., 2002 [8];
	• Health-Promoting Index (HPI)	%	D	Chen et al., 2004 [9];
	• Fish Lipid Quality/Flesh Lipid Quality (FLQ)	%	D	Xie et al., 2022 [10].
Metabolic	• Elongase	%	-	Zhang et al., 2007 [12];
	• Thioesterase	%	-	Zhang et al., 2007 [12];
	• Δ 9-desaturase (18.0)	%	-	Vessby et al., 2002 [13];
	• Δ 9-desaturase (16.0 + 18.0)	%	-	Vessby et al., 2002 [13];
	• Δ5-desaturase + Δ6-desaturase	%	-	Sirri et al., 2011 [14];
	• Activity index	%	-	Failla et al., 2021 [19].
Lipid- or energy-related content indexes	• EPA + DHA quantity	mg/100 g	D	Godbe, 1994 [20];
	• Index of nutritional quality	mg/100 g	D	Sorenson et al., 1976 [21];
	• QuantiN-3 index	mg/100 g	D	Present paper;
	• Healthy fatty index 1	mg/100 g	D	Present paper;
	• Healthy fatty index 2	mg/100 g	D	Present paper.

PUFA: polyunsaturated fatty acid; SFA: saturated fatty acid; LA: linoleic acid; ALA: α-linolenic acid; EPA: eicosapentaenoic acid; DHA: docosahexaenoic acid.

2.3.1. Qualitative Indexes

Polyunsaturated Fatty Acid/Saturated Fatty Acid (PUFA/SFA)

$$\text{PUFA/SFA} = (\Sigma \text{ Polyunsaturated Fatty Acids})/(\Sigma \text{ Saturated Fatty Acids}) \quad (1)$$

The index reported in (1) is the most-used index for evaluating the impact of a particular food on cardiovascular health, assuming that all PUFAs are able to reduce low-density lipoprotein cholesterol and serum cholesterol, whereas all SFAs can contribute to increasing serum cholesterol. Thus, this is a direct index: higher values indicate a better (positive) effect (or the contrary), given by a certain meat or meat product intake.

n-6/n-3 Ratio

$$\text{n-6/n-3} = (C18:2n\text{-}6 + C20:2n\text{-}6 + C20:3n\text{-}6 + C20:4n\text{-}6)/ \\ (C18:3n\text{-}3 + C20:3n\text{-}3 + C20:5n\text{-}3 + C22:5n\text{-}3 + C22:6n3) \quad (2)$$

As a complement to the aforementioned index, it could be coupled with the n-6/n-3 ratio (2) defined by Simopoulus [1,22], which has now become a way of evaluating the nutritional quality of foods used by thousands of researchers. A lower ratio of n-6/n-3 fatty acids is more desirable for reducing the risk of many of the chronic diseases of high prevalence in Western societies, as well as in developing countries [23].

Linoleic Acid/α-Linolenic Acid (LA/ALA) Ratio

$$\text{LA/ALA} = (C18:2n\text{-}6)/(C18:3n\text{-}3) \quad (3)$$

This ratio (3) was developed as an evaluation tool for dietary infant formula. These two fatty acids cannot be synthesized in the mammalian body hence, they must be obtained by diet.

Moreover, they compete for the same desaturase and elongase enzymes, which permit the synthesis of LC-PUFAs. Due to the low conversion rate of ALA, the LA/ALA ratio reduction only provides a modest improvement in the levels of some n-3 LC-PUFAs (i.e., EPA, DPA and DHA; [2]); thus, the index can be considered a first step for LC-PUFA estimation.

Sum of Eicosapentaenoic Acid and Docosahexaenoic Acid (EPA + DHA%)

$$EPA + DHA\% = \%C20{:}5n{-}3 + \%C22{:}6n{-}3 \qquad (4)$$

The two fatty acids of this index (4) are n-3 LC-PUFAs involved and positively correlated with human health, mainly in the reduction of the risk of cardiovascular diseases, hypertension, inflammation [3] and reproductive functions [24,25].

Unsaturation Index (UI)

$$UI = (\%\ monoenoic) + (2 \times \%\ dienoic) + (3 \times \%\ trienoic) + (4 \times \%\ tetraenoic) + (5 \times \%\ pentaenoic) + (6 \times \%\ hesaenoic) \qquad (5)$$

This index (5) adds information on the degree of unsaturation of fatty acids rather than dwelling only on the sum of them. Indeed, UI indicates the degree of unsaturation of each fatty acid and is calculated as the sum of each unsaturated fatty acid (%) multiplied by the number of its double bonds, thus giving different weights to the different unsaturated classes. This index does not distinguish the two different series of fatty acids (n-3 and n-6); hence, it is not very specific for nutritional aspects, while it is of great importance for establishing the oxidative stability of livestock feed or human food and defining some oxidative protection strategies [5].

2.3.2. Nutritional Indexes
Nutrition Value Index

$$\text{Nutrition Value Index} = (C18{:}0 + C18{:}1n9)/(C16{:}0) \qquad (6)$$

This index (6) was developed by Chen and coworkers [6]; it considers only the dominant fatty acids in a food of animal origin: palmitic (C16:0), stearic (C18:0) and oleic (C18:1n-9) acids, due to their higher concentrations.

Index of Atherogenicity (IA)

$$IA = [C12{:}0 + (4 \times C14{:}0) + C16{:}0]/(\Sigma\ UFA) \qquad (7)$$

This index (7) was developed by Ulbricht and Southgate in 1991 [7], who published an article in *The Lancet* aimed to characterize the atherogenic potential of fatty acids of foods. The two researchers wanted to define a more specific index compared to PUFA/SFA, considered too general and weak an indicator to assess the atherogenicity of food. In particular, the IA indicates the relationship between the sum of SFAs, with the exception of stearic acid (C18:0), not considered pro-atherogenic by the authors because of the capacity of humans to desaturate it to oleic acid (C18:1n-9). In contrast, lauric (C12:0), myristic (C14:0) and palmitic (C16:0) acids favor the adhesion of lipids to cells of the circulatory and immunological systems and the accumulation of atherogenic plaques, and they reduce the levels of phospholipids and esterified fatty acids [26]. The IA has been used widely for evaluating seaweeds, crops, meat, fish and dairy products. Contrary to the previous index, a lower value indicates better nutritional characteristics of the food.

Index of Thrombogenicity (IT)

$$IT = (C14{:}0 + C16{:}0 + C18{:}0)/[(0.5 \times MUFA) + (0.5 \times \Sigma n{-}6\ PUFA) + (3 \times \Sigma n{-}3\ PUFA) + (\Sigma n{-}3\ PUFA/\Sigma n{-}6\ PUFA)] \qquad (8)$$

This index (8) was also developed by Ulbricht and Southgate [7], together with IA, to further characterize the thrombogenic potential of fatty acids, separating them on the basis of the effects triggered by some derivatives (eicosanoids) in pro-thrombogenic (C12:0, C14:0, and C16:0) and anti-thrombogenic FAs, such as MUFAs, n-3 and n-6 PUFAs, although current studies have demonstrated the negative implication of n-6 PUFAs on thrombogenesis [27]. Therefore, the consumption of foods or products with a lower IT is beneficial for human health (indirect index).

Hypocholesterolemic/Hypercholesterolemic (HH) Ratio

$$HH\ ratio = (C18:1 + \Sigma\ PUFA)/(C12:0 + C14:0 + C16:0) \tag{9}$$

In 2002, Santos-Silva et al. [8] proposed this index (9) following their studies on lamb meat to better assess the nutritional properties of this meat. The authors developed the HH with the intention of focusing on the relationships between dietary fatty acids and plasma low-density lipoproteins relating the hypocholesterolemic fatty acids (C18:1n-9 and PUFA) and hypercholesterolemic fatty acids (C12:0, C14:0, C16:0).

Health-Promoting Index (HPI)

$$HPI = (\Sigma\ UFA)/[C12:0 + (4 \times C14:0) + C16:0] \tag{10}$$

In 2004, Chen and coworkers [9] proposed this index (10) to assess the nutritional value of fat, with particular emphasis on the effects of fatty acids on cardiovascular diseases. It is immediately evident that this index is exactly the inverse of the IA and thus has become a direct index mainly used in research on dairy products.

Fish Lipid Quality/Flesh Lipid Quality (FLQ)

$$FLQ = 100 \times (C20:5n-3 + C22:6n-3)/(\Sigma\ Saturated\ Fatty\ Acids) \tag{11}$$

This index (11) was originally used for assessing the lipid quality of fish or flesh [28,29]. Its aim is similar to that of the sum EPA + DHA, but the sum of EPA and DHA is calculated as a percentage of fatty acids. It can be used as an ancillary to EPA + DHA since the absolute quantity for EPA and DHA is more important.

2.3.3. Metabolic Indexes

Several indexes were used to estimate the activities of desaturases and elongases of muscle tissue through the enzyme approach "products/substrate ratio" [30].

The elongase index (12) was calculated as the ratio of C18:0 to C16:0, whereas the thioesterase index (13) was calculated as the ratio of C16:0 to myristic acid (C14:0) [12].

$$Elongase = ((C18:0)/(C16:0)) \times 100 \tag{12}$$

$$Thioesterase = ((C16:0)/(C14:0)) \times 100 \tag{13}$$

Estimated desaturase activities (14–15) are often used, and among many authors, Vessby et al. [13] reported that the calculated activities of $\Delta 9$-, $\Delta 5$- and $\Delta 6$-desaturase can be used as surrogates of the measure of true desaturase activity in the laboratory [31].

$$\Delta 9\text{-desaturase}\ (C:18:1) = ((C18:1n-9)/(C18:0 + C18:1n-9)) \times 100 \tag{14}$$

$$\Delta 9\text{-desaturase}\ (C16:1 + C:18:1) = ((C16:1n-7 + C18:1n-9)/(C16:0 + C18:0 + C16:1n-7 + C18:1n-9)) \times 100 \tag{15}$$

To evaluate the activities of both Δ5- and Δ6-desaturase (16), the enzymes catalyzing the formation of long-chain n-6 and n-3 polyunsaturated fatty acids (PUFAs) starting from the precursors C18:2n-6 and C18:3n-3, the following equation was used [14]:

$$\Delta 5\text{-desaturase} + \Delta 6\text{-desaturase} = (C20:2n\text{-}6 + C20:4n\text{-}6 + C20:5n\text{-}3 + C22:5n\text{-}3 + C22:6n\text{-}3)/(C18:2n\text{-}6 + C18:3n\text{-}3 + C20:2n\text{-}6 + C20:4n\text{-}6 + C20:5n\text{-}3 + C22:5n\text{-}3 + C22:6n\text{-}3) \quad (16)$$

In this view, the rate of n-3 β-oxidation in the muscle (e.g., n-3 LC-PUFA/ALA) can adequately describe n-3 LC-PUFA mobilization used for energy production (i.e., movement; [32]) and the resulting oxidative status. The ratio between n-3 LC-PUFA and ALA could be taken as an indicator of energy consumption (β-oxidation; (17)). This should be higher in oxidative than in glycolytic muscles [19] and therefore in animals with higher kinetic activity [33].

$$\text{Activity Index} = (\Sigma \text{ n-3 PUFA})/(C18:3n\text{-}3) \quad (17)$$

2.3.4. Lipid- or Energy-Related Content Indexes

Sum of Eicosapentaenoic Acid and Docosahexaenoic Acid (EPA + DHA Quantity)

$$\text{EPA + DHA quantity} = \text{mg}/100 \text{ g } C20:5n\text{-}3 + \text{mg}/100 \text{ g } C22:6n\text{-}3 \quad (18)$$

In 1994, Godbe [20] developed the first (18) of these last groups of indexes, while the other three have been conceived by us. These indexes differ from the others because they consider the quantity of fat or energy that is related to the quantity/quality of fatty acids in the food. We also calculated the percentage with respect to the daily requirements of various lipid classes, especially PUFAs, in a 150 g standard portion of chicken meat. This standard meal contains approximately 30 g of proteins, which is 35% of the 1800 kcal diet, based on 55:35:20% contents of carbohydrates, lipids and proteins [34]. To better understand the nutritional value of chicken meat lipid content in a real-life setting, we propose to examine the implication (in %) with respect to an ideal healthy meal in the context of a balanced Mediterranean Diet.

Index of Nutritional Quality

The index of nutritional quality (INQ; (19)) was calculated based on the eicosapentaenoic (EPA) + docosahexaenoic (DHA) acid content, considering the energy content of the meat (expressed as Kcal of every nutrient) and the EPA and DHA daily requirements.

$$\text{INQ} = (((\Sigma \text{ mg}/100 \text{ g EPA + DHA}))/(\text{Energy content Kcal } 100 \text{ g}))/(\text{EPA + DHA daily requirement}) \quad (19)$$

Proposed New Indexes

In the following indexes, our intention was to relate the fatty-acid profile with the total lipid content, in the belief that these nutritional properties cannot be evaluated separately. We propose a deeper lipid study through the development of three progressive indexes.

QuantiN-3 Index

In particular, the quantiN-3 index (20) relates the polyunsaturated fatty acids of the n-3 series expressed in quantity (mg/100 g) of meat with the quantity (g/100 g) of fat.

$$\text{QuantiN-3 index} = (\text{mg}/100 \text{ g of n-3 PUFA})/(\text{g}/100 \text{ g of Total Lipids}) \quad (20)$$

Healthy Fatty Indexes 1 and 2

In the two latter indexes, we wanted to further deepen the previous quantiN-3 index through the careful differentiation of the various classes of fatty acids (by unsaturation and by the position of the double bonds), partly following the indications of Ulbricht and

Southgate [7] but always relating everything to the quantity of lipids (Healthy Fatty Index 1—HFI1, (21)). Furthermore, in Healthy Fatty Index 2 (22), the contents of the different classes of fatty acids and their properties were considered. The rationale of this last index is to consider the dietary lipid input not only from a nutritional viewpoint but also with a health approach. In particular, the idea is to consider the various classes of fatty acids by increasing or decreasing (using some empirically unknown constants: MUFA = 2; n-6 PUFA = 4; n-3 PUFA = 8, partly derived from Ulbricht and Southgate [7]) their relative content expressed in weight according to their health impact, deduced from the consolidated scientific literature.

The resulting value is divided by the fat, weighted on the quantity of various classes (SFAs, MUFAs, n-3 PUFAs and n-6 PUFAs). This decreases the values because of their negative effects on human health through specific constants (reciprocal of the constants in the numerator, i.e., SFA = 1, MUFA = 1/2 = 0.5, n-6 PUFA = 1/4 = 0.25, n-3 PUFA = 1/8 = 0.125). From this perspective, more weight is given to the n-3/n-6 ratio (or reversed): specifically, the numerator reports variables that accentuate the positive value of n-3 fatty acids (i.e., MUFA, n-6 PUFA, n-3 PUFA and n-3/n-6), and in the denominator, we amplify the lower health effect by introducing the weight of fatty acid classes. In particular, we enhance the n-6 PUFA effects by reversing the ratio (n-6/n-3).

$$\text{HFI1} = ((\text{mg}/100 \text{ g of MUFA} \times 2) + (\text{mg}/100 \text{ g of n-6} \times 4) + (\text{mg}/100 \text{ g of n-3} \times 8) + (\text{mg}/100 \text{ g n-3}/\text{mg}/100 \text{ g n-6}))/(\text{mg}/100 \text{ g of Total Lipids}) \qquad (21)$$

$$\text{HFI2} = ((\text{mg}/100 \text{ g of MUFA} \times 2) + (\text{mg}/100 \text{ g of n-6} \times 4) + (\text{mg}/100 \text{ g of n-3} \times 8) + (\text{mg}/100 \text{ g n-3}/\text{mg}/100 \text{ g n-6}))/((\text{mg}/100 \text{ g of SFA}) + (\text{mg}/100 \text{ g of MUFA} \times 0.5) + (\text{mg}/100 \text{ g of n-6} \times 0.25) + (\text{mg}/100 \text{ g of n-3} \times 0.125) + (\text{mg}/100 \text{ g n-6}/\text{mg}/100 \text{ g n-3})) \qquad (22)$$

2.4. Statistical Analyses

The data were analyzed with a linear model (STATA, 2015, College Station, TX, USA; [35]) to evaluate the effect of strain; the significance of differences ($p < 0.05$; $p < 0.0001$) was evaluated by Bonferroni multiple *t*-tests.

3. Results and Discussion

3.1. Fatty Acid Composition (The Dataset)

The lipid contents and the fatty acid profiles of the breast meat are shown in Table 3, expressed as % or in quantitative form (mg/100 g f.m.). The analysis of these results shows that the initial objective of the experiment was largely achieved; indeed, the choice of two divergent genotypes resulted in different lipid contents and fatty acid profiles.

As reported in our review [15], the genotype interacts with movement, intake of antioxidants, antioxidant capacity of the body, plasma, and fatty acid profile of meat. In particular, the SG chickens had a high kinetic behavior that may be matched with a more exploratory attitude, improving their meat's nutritional characteristics. In contrast, FG chickens showed some kinetic problems, especially in the last phase of the cycle. The strain effect reported herein also implicates a different behavior of birds in terms of the amount of feed/forage intake. These genotypes, which were selected for high precocity and ability to reach high live weight at an early age, are not compatible with longer periods of raising [36]. The combination of age, low kinetic activity and high feed intake resulted in higher fat accumulation in muscles.

Table 3. Lipid contents (g/100 g meat) and fatty acid compositions (g/100 g fatty acids and mg/100 g meat) of breast meat from different genotypes.

	SG	FG	SEM	SG	FG	SEM
Lipids (g/100 g meat)	0.25 B	1.45 A	0.13			
	% of total FA			mg/100 g meat		
C12:0	0.20 B	0.62 A	0.09	0.43 B	7.41 A	1.03
C14:0	0.71 B	1.04 A	0.21	1.54 B	12.42 A	2.21
C16:0	27.98 b	30.01 a	2.03	60.53 B	358.45 A	125.14
C18:0	12.02 a	11.00 b	1.61	30.33 B	131.39 A	20.14
Others	2.49	2.07	0.20	7.55 B	24.72 A	3.56
Total SFA	43.40 a	44.74 b	2.11	100.38 B	534.39 A	156.48
C14:1n-6	0.15	0.11	0.04	0.32 B	1.31 A	0.24
C16:1n-7	0.61 A	1.39 B	0.19	1.32 B	16.60 A	3.14
C18:1n-9	19.50 A	23.04 B	2.31	40.02 B	275.20 A	10.41
Others	0.26	0.17	0.91	0.56 a	2.03 b	0.48
Total MUFA	20.52 A	23.94 B	1.75	42.23 B	293.95 A	23.47
C18:2n-6	18.09 B	20.70 A	2.18	39.14 B	247.25 A	25.36
C20:2n-6	0.68 a	0.20 b	0.16	1.47 b	2.39 a	0.23
C20:3n-6	0.17	0.16	0.03	0.37 B	1.91 A	0.47
C20:4n-6	10.60 a	8.03 b	1.36	22.93 B	95.91 A	15.98
Total n-6	29.54	29.09	2.47	63.91 B	347.46 A	36.98
C18:3n-3	2.03 a	0.98 b	0.74	2.23 B	11.71 A	4.12
C20:3n-3	0.04	0.03	0.01	0.09 B	0.36 A	0.13
C20:5n-3	0.68 A	0.09 B	0.27	0.39 B	1.07 A	0.32
C21:5n-3	0.87 A	0.03 B	0.47	1.88 A	0.36 B	0.24
C22:5n-3	1.37 A	0.92 B	0.25	2.96 B	10.99 A	1.79
C22:6n-3	1.05 A	0.18 B	0.29	2.26	2.15	0.14
Total n-3	4.54 A	2.23 B	1.75	9.81 B	26.64 A	3.49
Total PUFA	35.58 A	31.32 B	3.04	73.72 B	374.10 A	98.85

SG: Slow-growing; FG: Fast-growing; SEM: standard error mean; SFA: saturated fatty acids; MUFA: monounsaturated fatty acids; PUFA: polyunsaturated fatty acids; Number: 20 samples per group; A,B: $p < 0.0001$; a,b: $p < 0.05$.

Breeds were also a source of variation for the main fatty acids. Differences in the fatty acid profiles were observed in the content of SFAs, where a higher value was observed in SG chickens and a lower value was observed in commercial lines. Additionally, SG chickens exhibited higher amounts of stearic acid (C18:0). In general, these strains produce very lean meats; despite the anatomical cut (breast) and the absence of skin, the difference between the genotypes was very significant ($p < 0.0001$), with an obvious modification of fatty acid amount. As an example, the sum of the n-3 PUFAs, which was double in the breast meat of SG subjects, was three times higher in the FG subjects from a quantitative point of view.

The MUFAs, which in chickens are related either to endogenous synthesis or to gut absorption from the diet, showed the highest levels in FG genotypes. These MUFAs were mainly represented by oleic and palmitoleic acids. The low MUFA level observed in SG genotypes can be attributed to the higher intake of pasture (average MUFA value 227 mg/100 g) with respect to the feed (average MUFA value 1134 mg/100 g) and to the different intramuscular fat content of birds [14]. Meat of slow-growing genotypes compared with fast-growing ones was characterized by a high percentage of PUFAs (both n-3 and n-6). Despite the increased consumption of fresh forage, lower levels of ALA in the meat of slow-growing strains could be explained by the higher conversion of this fatty acid in the long-chain derivatives [37].

3.2. Indexes

The different indexes are shown in Table 4 and are discussed following complexity and dealing with general and specific considerations for the meat of the two chicken genotypes.

As already stated, all indexes were grouped into subcategories based on their underlying qualitative, nutritional and metabolic principles and considering the relationships between fatty acids and lipid- or energy content-related indexes of meat. The large difference in values obtained with the different indexes strongly underlines their different meanings and thus the use of each index in different conditions.

Table 4. Indexes of breast muscle of different chicken genotypes.

Indexes	SG	FG	SEM
Qualitative			
Polyunsaturated/Saturated Fatty Acids	0.81 a	0.70 b	0.06
n-6/n-3 Fatty Acids Ratio	4.89 B	13.04 A	1.89
Linoleic Acid/α-Linolenic Acid	8.91 B	21.12 A	2.15
Sum of EPA and DHA	1.73 A	0.27 B	0.23
Unsaturation Index	128.05 A	107.75 B	5.36
Nutritional			
Nutritional Value Index	1.11	1.14	0.14
Index of Atherogenicity	0.55 b	0.63 a	0.07
Index of Thrombogenicity	0.94 b	1.24 a	0.10
Hypocholesterolemic/Hypercholesterolemic	1.91 A	1.21 B	0.12
Health-Promoting Index	1.81 a	1.59 b	0.17
Fish Lipid Quality/Flesh Lipid Quality	1.73 A	0.27 B	0.12
Metabolic			
Elongase Index	0.47 a	b	0.09
Thioesterase Index	42.7 A	30.9 B	4.23
Δ9-Desaturase (18)	58.0 B	68.7 A	3.65
Δ9-Desaturase (16 + 18)	31.40 b	37.51 a	6.32
Δ5/Δ6-Desaturase	52.48 A	23.55 B	4.92
Activity index	1.97 A	1.28 B	0.12
Lipid- or energy-related content indexes			
Sum of EPA and DHA (mg/100 g meat)	3.72 a	3.22 b	0.15
Index of Nutritional Quality	9.42 A	7.29 B	0.74
Quanti n-3 Index	53.23 A	18.37 B	4.05
Healthy Fatty Index 1	1.80 a	1.49 b	0.08
Healthy Fatty Index 2	3.22 A	2.80 B	0.12

Calculated on 20 samples per group; A,B on the same line: $p < 0.0001$; a,b: $p < 0.05$.

3.3. Qualitative Indexes

Concerning the PUFA/SFA index, it is evident that the two groups showed different values ($p < 0.05$), demonstrating the higher unsaturation levels of the SG meat, as reported above. It is also evident that in this index, the effect of monounsaturated fatty acids (MUFAs) was neglected (i.e., possible regulation of plasma LDL concentrations). Indeed, oleic acid (C18:1 n-9), the most representative MUFA in poultry meat, increases the activity of low-density lipoprotein receptors and decreases the cholesterol concentration in serum [38]. In addition, not all SFAs contribute equally to increasing the serum cholesterol concentration.

Even the generalization of the SFA is very explanatory of the negative action of these FAs in increasing the cholesterol concentration in serum by inhibiting the activity of the aforementioned receptors. Indeed, some short chain SFAs are rapidly oxidized by acetyl-CoA in the liver, and they have a very feeble action on LDL receptors; in contrast, C12:0, C14:0, and C16:0 fatty acids show a greater effect on the increase in serum cholesterol. In addition, not all PUFA classes can have the same positive effectiveness toward the prevention of CVD [39]. In general, a value of this index greater than 0.45 is recommended in human diets to prevent CVD and other chronic diseases [40]. Therefore, it is possible to state that the poultry meats analyzed here can be considered of high quality on the basis of this index (especially that produced by SG chickens). In contrast, the same thing cannot be said for the quality of the indexes, which appears outdated due to its scarce specificity toward the single fatty acids and classes. Even the discriminatory capacity, although significant, is low considering the great diversity of the two chicken strains.

Concerning the n-6/n-3 ratio, it should be emphasized that, with an increased specificity of the index, the two experimental groups showed much more evident differences (4.89 vs. 13.04, respectively, for SG and FG birds; $p < 0.0001$). Simoupolus [1] suggests that the human diet in Western countries is unbalanced in terms of the n-6/n-3 ratio (15–16/1 vs. 4/1 recommended), basically because Western diets are deficient in n-3 fatty acids, contrary to what was found in the diets of our ancestors [41]. This situation could promote the pathogenesis of many diseases, including CVD, cancer, and inflammatory and autoimmune diseases, while increased levels of n-3 PUFAs can exert suppressive effects. In the prevention of cardiovascular diseases, a 4/1 ratio was associated with a 70% decrease in total mortality [39]. A ratio of 2.5/1 reduced rectal cell proliferation in colorectal cancer patients, while a ratio of 4/1 with the same amount of n-3 PUFA had no effect [42]. This is consistent with the fact that chronic diseases are multigenic and multifactorial.

Thus, food with a lower n-6/n-3 ratio is more desirable for reducing the risk of many chronic diseases of high prevalence in Western societies. This index shows that SG meat has an equilibrated ratio of PUFAs, whereas FG meat has a much higher ratio. This index is more specific than PUFA/SFA, although it still has some gaps that does not make it suitable for food from animal origins. From a nutritional point of view, the exact content of the various classes of lipids could not completely explain the nutritional value of chicken meat. Even if SG presents a useful lipid profile with an n-6/n-3 ratio of 4.8, closer to the abovementioned desirable 4, the total content of lipids and PUFAs is approximately six times less than that of FG (0.25 vs. 1.45 g/100 g, respectively). These considerations further corroborate the need for developing indexes more specifically dedicated to nutritional quality.

Following this line of evaluation and analyzing the linoleic acid/α-linolenic acid index, it can be seen how strong the effect of the chicken breed is. This index highlights that SG meat is even more interesting, always remaining in a strictly qualitative context. It is common knowledge that the essential PUFAs (LA and ALA) have a different effect on human health, and for this reason, the suggested intake is not equal. LA and ALA compete for the same metabolic pathway in elongase and desaturase reactions to generate active LC-PUFAs. However, the n-3 pathway has a higher metabolic energy expenditure than the n-6 pathway; thus, the latter is the preferential route in the mammalian body, with few exceptions [43,44]. Furthermore, the LA/ALA indexes also showed a first picture of the conversion efficiency of ALA and LA into their longer chain homologs. Harnack et al. [45] suggested that a dietary ALA/LA ratio of 1:1 would lead to the highest formation of n-3 LC-PUFAs, given that the conversion of precursors depends on the n-6/n-3 ratio of the diet. In the above context, even the sum of EPA and DHA (%) gives higher values for SG meat, richer in PUFA, as also demonstrated by the UI and by the most recent references [11,46,47].

The UI represents the relationship between the FA profile and its susceptibility to oxidation, providing useful information on the shelf life of meat. The index highlights the relationship between antioxidant protections and PUFA content and the development of undesirable effects of oxidative stress associated with the formation of lipid peroxides. These processes in turn have been suggested to contribute to the processes of aging and many diseases, such as atherosclerosis [40,48–50]. In the present study, meat from FG chickens showed a lower ($p < 0.0001$) value of UI with respect to that of SG, indicating a lower risk of fatty acid autooxidation, but also a lower healthy value of fat obtained from the meat of these lines.

3.4. Nutritional Indexes

As already stated, the AI index points out the relationship between the main saturated fatty acids and the main classes of unsaturated fatty acids, considering the former as proatherogenic and as promoters of the activation of immunological cells; thus, they adhere to the vessel wall, whereas the others are antiatherogenic (inhibiting the aggregation of plaque and diminishing the levels of esterified fatty acids, cholesterol and phospholipids, thereby preventing the appearance of micro- and macro-coronary diseases [51]).

The TI indicates the predisposition to form clots in blood vessels. This is defined as the relationship between pro-thrombogenic (saturated) and anti-thrombogenic fatty acids (MUFAs, n-6 PUFAs and n-3 PUFAs). Both AI and TI indicate a potential for stimulating platelet aggregation [52]. Thus, smaller AI and TI values suggest a protective potential for coronary artery health. In terms of human health, an AI and TI in the diet of less than 1.0 and 0.5, respectively, are recommended [53]. However, one critical point of the TI index is the consideration of n-6 PUFAs as anti-thrombogenic agents, whereas in recent years, the relative pro-aggregation properties of n-6 derivatives have been clearly established [38].

Regardless, the obtained values for the meat of the two poultry genotypes can be considered to have high nutritional value, but between them, the SG breast showed the most desirable values. The ratio between hypocholesterolemic and hypercholesterolemic fatty acids indicated the different effects on cholesterol metabolism: higher values are considered more beneficial for human health. In this study, we obtained values for SG and FG chickens of 1.91 and 1.21, respectively ($p < 0.0001$). The health-promoting index, as already reported, represented the inverse of the IA, thus showing inverse values compared with IA (1.81 vs. 1.59, respectively, in SG and FG).

Finally, flesh lipid quality is similar to that of EPA + DHA, calculated as a percentage of total fatty acids. Because it is not affected by lipid content, SG meat showed an almost six-fold higher value than FG meat, underscoring the higher content of n-3 LC-PUFA of the first strain.

3.5. Metabolic Indexes

The relevance of these indexes is also connected with their ability to be considered substitutes for expensive laboratory activities [31]. It should be noted that these indexes were developed for identifying the metabolism of animals and have low relevance for discriminating meat quality. Indeed, these indexes are of low nutritional importance because they are not able to discriminate metabolic changes due to dietary effects. All these indexes showed that the SG genotype strongly diverged from the FG genotype. In particular, slow-growing strains had higher levels of elongase, thioesterase and $\Delta 5/\Delta 6$ desaturase, accompanied by a lower $\Delta 9$ index, confirming our previous results obtained by comparing native poultry breeds with commercial strains [37].

In fatty acid synthesis, thioesterase is responsible for terminating the reaction and releasing the newly synthesized fatty acid. The ratio of C16:0 to C14:0 could be useful in understanding the selective division of thioesterase on C14-acyl-acyl carrier protein or C16-acyl-acyl carrier protein; in this experiment, the significantly higher thioesterase index observed in SG birds is probably related to less cleavage of C14-acyl-acyl carrier protein. Conversely, the $\Delta 9$-desaturase that catalyzes the conversion of C16:0 and C18:0 to C16:1 and C18:1 [54] was lower in SG chickens, suggesting that the lower concentrations of C16:1 in SG chickens (1.32 vs. 16.60 mg/100 g muscle, respectively, for SG and FG) could be attributed to higher $\Delta 9$-desaturase activity [55]. An interesting inference comes from the findings of Kouba et al. [56] in pigs, who related the dietary intake of ALA to $\Delta 9$-desaturase activity. The same authors observed a negative correlation of this index with the intake of ALA. Our results agree with this assumption, and it could be argued that the higher intake of ALA through forage SG chickens could partly contribute to such $\Delta 9$-desaturase lowering. These assumptions are also confirmed by Poureslami et al. [57], who analyzed the interactive effect of diet and age on SFA and MUFA metabolism in poultry, concluding that both factors affected deposition, elongation and $\Delta 9$ desaturation activities as well as the oxidation process of fatty acids.

The most evident differences, however, were observed in the $\Delta 5/\Delta 6$-desaturase complex, which represents the most valid tool to verify the capacity of animals to synthesize LC-PUFAs from precursors. The higher $\Delta 5/\Delta 6$-desaturase index (more than double) of the

SG genotype demonstrates once again the higher efficiency in LC-PUFA synthesis of the native breeds with respect to commercial hybrids [14,58].

Another interesting finding is related to the competition between n-6 and n-3 fatty acids. A previous investigation [44,58] demonstrated that the n-3 precursor is the preferred substrate in the desaturation and elongation pathway of local breeds with respect to high-performance strains, and that the rate-limiting step in the enzymatic pathways of PUFA biosynthesis could be Δ6-desaturase activity [36,59]. Cherian and Sim [60], investigating the effects of dietary ALA of laying hens on the fatty acid composition of liver microsomes and the activity of Δ6-desaturase in hatched chicks, observed increases in long-chain 20- and 22-carbon fatty acids, which may be attributed to the use of ALA as the preferred substrate over LA. Concordantly, our previous in vitro results revealed that a significant inhibition of Δ-6 desaturase activity occurs with high amounts of ALA in rabbit liver [44].

We can therefore conclude that this category of indexes is efficient in both the discrimination between poultry genotypes characterized by very different lipid metabolism and the replacement of complex and expensive laboratory analyses for the determination of enzymatic activity in microsomes.

The activity index is based on the indirect evaluation of β-oxidation activity in red and white chicken muscles to estimate their energy expenditure. In our case, the two genotypes showed differences (1.97 vs. 1.28, $p < 0.0001$, respectively, for SG and FG), magnified by the extensive rearing system, where the birds were allowed to walk in an outdoor run. The activity index is therefore an attempt to measure the energy expenditure due to the movement developed throughout the entire life of the chicken, with all the qualitative and nutritional consequences that this entails in its meat. This index can only be measured by evaluating the FA profile of the muscle after slaughter, and is surely a valid and objective tool for measuring the adaptability of a genetic line to extensive rearing systems, because it accounts for all the activity exerted during the life of the animal and can be used for an ex post welfare assessment.

3.6. Lipid- or Energy Content-Related Indexes

The analysis of all the indexes considered thus far have highlighted some strengths, such as the discriminatory capacity between different poultry genotypes and the effectiveness in replacing complex and expensive analytical practices. However, many gaps have been highlighted, mainly from the nutritional viewpoint. To fill these gaps, our idea was to relate the content of fatty acids with high nutritional value with that of total lipids, in the belief that the two parameters have to be considered together. Establishing precise relationships between these components can provide interesting and definitive information on the nutritional value of a food.

The sum of EPA and DHA (in mg/100 g f.m.; previously discussed as a percentage of the total fatty acids) is very important, as it is well known that the roles of n-3 LC-PUFAs in human metabolism [27] provide information on their absolute presence, which is inextricably linked to the quantities of meat lipids. This index is recognized worldwide, and recommendations for these two fatty acids and their precursors have been made by the Food and Agriculture Organization of the United Nations. In particular, 0.5–0.6% ALA per day is useful to prevent deficiency symptoms, whereas the n-3 LC-PUFA recommendation is approximately 250–2000 mg per day. For adult males and nonpregnant/nonlactating females, 250 mg/day EPA plus DHA is recommended, with insufficient evidence to set a specific minimum intake of either EPA or DHA. For adult pregnant and lactating females, the minimum intake for optimal adult health and fetal and infant development is 300 mg/d EPA + DHA, of which at least 200 mg/d should be DHA [39].

As the last index, we wanted to simulate a portion of 150 g of chicken meat containing approximately 33 g of proteins, which represents a correct amount to cover the protein requirement of a balanced meal (20% of total energy in a 1800 kcal balanced Mediterranean diet). In this context, investigating the lipid contribution of a standard portion of chicken in a balanced Mediterranean diet could allow us to establish a dietary plan with other sources of lipids (i.e., olive oil) to both reach the right amount of lipid-derived energy per meal (approximately 35% of energy expressed in calories) and counterbalance levels of different PUFA classes (n-6/n-3 ratio).

Chicken meat obviously cannot represent the only source of lipids in a balanced diet, but knowing its exact lipid composition and the dietary implications could help in the elaboration of a high-quality dietary plan. This analysis could also allow meat scientists, clinicians, and experts in nutrition to engage in better dialog for improving the lipid content of chicken meat by intervening in farming techniques, nutrition and additives for livestock. Undoubtedly, this manuscript allows nutrition experts to gain in-depth knowledge of lipid quality in terms of health promotion and preservation and to elaborate balanced dietary plans.

With a portion of SG or FG breast meat in a standard meal, we can reach EPA plus DHA intake levels of 5.58 and 4.83 mg, respectively. These quantities are low considering the differences between terrestrial plants and animals with respect to seafood [61], particularly fish, but surely interesting considering the low lipid contents of these meats. Indeed, it should be considered that deskinned breast meat has a very low-fat content: the same portions obtained from other body parts (i.e., drumstick, thigh) have quite the same fatty acid profile, but with approximately 10 times more fat, with up to 20–25% of the daily recommendation. A further increase in n-3 LC-PUFAs of meat could also be attained with dietary supranutritional administration of LNA [56].

The large difference between the two genotypes lies in the fact that in the SG meat, the content depends on the high unsaturation, while in the FG meat, it depends on the high content of lipids (relative to SG, of course), which in any case provides good quantities of EPA and DHA.

The amount of 150 grams of chicken contains approximately 100 mg of n-6 in SG meat vs. 500 mg in FG meat and 15 mg of n-3 in SG vs. 40 in FG. Considering 1 g of n-3 as an adequate dose for a meal, we see that the percentages of both SG and FG are very low, demonstrating that chicken breast meat cannot represent a primary source of lipids, but at the same time, these data give us information on how to build a balanced diet by using meat containing good lipids that at the same time bring the n-6/n-3 ratio more toward 4/1 and provide the right amount of lipids. At this point of the discussion, a relevant question arose: are the high quantities of n-3 LC-PUFA contained in foods rich in lipids advisable in a healthy human diet? Is it, perhaps, necessary to deepen the relationship between these components?

INQ, which relates the quantities of EPA and DHA to the energy content of the food (weighted for the daily requirements of these two fatty acids), offers more precise nutritional information, emphasizing the goodness of the SG meat (high PUFA and low-fat content), but as previously mentioned, a simultaneous relationship between fat and the fatty acid profile is needed. In particular, the QuantiN-3 index relates the polyunsaturated fatty acids of the n-3 series expressed in mg/100 g meat with the quantity of fat (g/100 g). Because the concentration of fatty acids with respect to the total lipids varies from 0.83 to 0.91 on the basis of animal species [56], we also considered going into more detail with regard to the total amount of fat added.

Based on the critical analysis of the indexes previously reported, we constructed two indexes (healthy fatty indexes 1 and 2). The concept of HFI1, which then evolved into HFI2, is to give different weights to the various categories of fatty acids, relying on their healthy properties. In particular, in the first-mentioned index, all fatty acids with more or less pronounced positive action on human health are reported in the numerator. All classes were multiplied by empirical constants partly derived from Ulbricht and Southgate [7], two for MUFAs, four for n-6, and eight for n-3, to consider the nutritional and health implications of the various classes.

As in the Quanti n-3 index, the denominator shows the total lipids. Fatty meat lowers the index and the relative nutritional quality; however, not all lipids have the same nutritional effect, which must be represented in the index. Hence, in building a new index (HFI2), nothing changes in the numerator, but the lipids in the denominator are given different weights, obviously in the opposite manner to that described above. SFAs are considered fully, whereas MUFAs, n-6 PUFAs and n-3 PUFAs are reduced by half, a quarter and an eighth, respectively, using the math fraction of the constants in the numerator to consider their less negative effect. Furthermore, the n-3/n-6 ratio (with the ratio in a positive sense, i.e., reversed ratio) was introduced to consider the healthy importance of their balance.

In our opinion, this careful categorization of the different classes of fatty acids can allow a comprehensive lipid indexing of food, taking into consideration their quality and nutritional characteristics, with an evaluation of the quantities of lipids that carry these bioactive compounds. In other words, is it better to eat fatty meat that still brings many n-3 PUFAs even if not very rich in percentages, or is a lean meat with a high percentage of unsaturation preferred?

From the analysis of the HFI2 in Table 3, there is no doubt, as the lean meat of SG chickens showed significantly ($p < 0.0001$) higher values than that of FG chickens (3.22 vs. 2.80, respectively); however, increasing the quantity of lipids should not be demonized if the meat presents healthy FA classes, especially in a monogastric species such as chicken. In our case, hypothetically bringing the levels of n-3 in FG meat to the levels observed in SG meat, the HFI2 index would rise to 3.22, a value even higher than that of the very lean SG meat.

4. Conclusions

This study clearly demonstrates how complex it is to index fatty acids in order to assess the nutritional or health potential of chicken meat. Our conclusion is related to the concept that an overall and final evaluation must consider the many factors that regulate the nutritional properties of food. In particular, the level of fats, the FA profiles and the relationships between them is of fundamental importance for the design and adoption of an index. We believe that Healthy Fatty Index 2 collects all this information. It is tentative and will certainly require adjustment in light of further evidence, especially in the assessment of the constant values.

Further investigations are necessary to better define the weights of the different classes of fatty acids (or of the single fatty acid), the discriminatory capacity of this index (within different foods) and its parameterization with a standard dose of meat for consumption. Moreover, when Healthy Fatty Index 2 will be validated, it is our intention to broaden our horizon to other meats and foods (both of animal and vegetable origin) in order to create a new-generation nutritional quality database.

Author Contributions: Conceptualization, A.D.B., C.C. and G.V.; methodology, A.D.B.; software, A.D.B. and C.C.; formal analysis, S.M.; investigation, A.D.B., A.C.M., C.C. and S.M.; resources, A.D.B. and C.C.; data curation, A.D.B., G.V., M.C., C.C. and S.M.; writing—original draft preparation, A.D.B. and S.M.; writing—review and editing, A.C.M., G.V., M.C. and C.C.; funding acquisition, C.C. All authors have read and agreed to the published version of the manuscript.

Funding: This research was partially funded by PRIN2017 grant number 2017S229WC.

Institutional Review Board Statement: The study was conducted in accordance with EU regulation 834/07 on animal welfare for experimental and other scientific purposes. Furthermore, the experimental protocol was positively evaluated by the internal university committee (protocol code 112606 of 12 January 2021).

Data Availability Statement: The data are available upon justified request.

Acknowledgments: The authors wish to thank Giovanni Migni, Osvaldo Mandoloni and Cinzia Boldrini for their contributions in animal handling.

Conflicts of Interest: The authors declare no conflict of interest.

References

1. Simopoulos, A.P. The importance of the omega-6/omega-3 fatty acid ratio in cardiovascular disease and other chronic diseases. *Exp. Biol. Med.* **2008**, *233*, 674–688. [CrossRef] [PubMed]

1. Das, U.N. Essential fatty acids: Biochemistry, physiology and pathology. *Biotechnol. J.* **2006**, *1*, 420–439. [CrossRef] [PubMed]
2. Holub, B.J. Docosahexaenoic acid (DHA) and cardiovascular disease risk factors. *Prostaglandins Leukot. Essent. Fat. Acids* **2009**, *81*, 199–204. [CrossRef] [PubMed]
3. Crupi, R.; Cuzzocrea, S. Role of EPA in Inflammation: Mechanisms, Effects, and Clinical Relevance. *Biomolecules* **2022**, *12*, 242. [CrossRef] [PubMed]
4. Fereidoon, S.; Ying, Z. Lipid oxidation and improving the oxidative stability. *Chem. Soc. Rev.* **2010**, *39*, 4067–4079. [CrossRef]
5. Chen, Y.; Qiao, Y.; Xiao, Y.; Chen, H.; Zhao, L.; Huang, M.; Zhou, G. Differences in physicochemical and nutritional properties of breast and thigh meat from crossbred chickens, commercial broilers, and spent hens. *Asian-Australas. J. Anim. Sci.* **2016**, *29*, 855–864. [CrossRef]
6. Ulbricht, T.L.V.; Southgate, D.A.T. Coronary heart disease: Seven dietary factors. *Lancet* **1991**, *338*, 985–992. [CrossRef]
7. Santos-Silva, J.; Bessa, R.J.B.; Santos-Silva, F. Effect of genotype, feeding system and slaughter weight on the quality of light lambs. II. Fatty acid composition of meat. *Livest. Prod. Sci.* **2002**, *77*, 187–194. [CrossRef]
8. Chen, S.; Bobe, G.; Zimmerman, S.; Hammond, E.G.; Luhman, C.M.; Boylston, T.D.; Freeman, A.E.; Beitz, D.C. Physical and sensory properties of dairy products from cows with various milk fatty acid compositions. *J. Agric. Food Chem.* **2004**, *52*, 3422–3428. [CrossRef]
9. Xie, D.; Guan, J.; Huang, X.; Xu, C.; Pan, Q.; Li, Y. Tilapia can be a Beneficial n-3 LC-PUFA Source due to Its High Biosynthetic Capacity in the Liver and Intestine. *J. Agric. Food Chem.* **2022**, *70*, 2701–2711. [CrossRef]
10. Cartoni Mancinelli, A.; Mattioli, S.; Twining, C.; Dal Bosco, A.; Donoghue, A.M.; Arsi, K.; Angelucci, E.; Chiattelli, D.; Castellini, C. Poultry meat and eggs as an alternative source of n-3 long-chain polyunsaturated fatty acids for human nutrition. *Nutrients* **2022**, *14*, 1969. [CrossRef]
11. Zhang, S.; Knight, T.J.; Stalder, K.J.; Goodwin, R.N.; Lonergan, S.M.; Beitz, D.C. Effects of breed, sex, and halothane genotype on fatty acid composition of pork longissimus muscle. *J. Anim. Sci.* **2007**, *85*, 583–591. [CrossRef]
12. Vessby, B.; Gustafsson, I.; Tengblad, S.; Boberg, M.; Andersson, A. Desaturation and elongation of fatty acids and insulin action. *Ann. N. Y. Acad. Sci.* **2002**, *967*, 183–195. [CrossRef]
13. Sirri, F.; Castellini, C.; Bianchi, M.; Petracci, M.; Meluzzi, A.; Franchini, A. Effect of fast-, medium- and slow-growing strains on meat quality of chickens reared under the organic farming method. *Animals* **2011**, *5*, 312–319. [CrossRef]
14. Dal Bosco, A.; Mattioli, S.; Cartoni Mancinelli, A.; Cotozzolo, E.; Castellini, C. Extensive rearing systems in poultry production: The right chicken for the right farming system. A review of twenty years of scientific research in Perugia University, Italy. *Animals* **2021**, *11*, 1281. [CrossRef]
15. Hosie, R.C. National Research Council. *For. Regen. Ont.* **2019**, 91–93.
16. Leeson, S.; Summers, J.D. *Commercial Poultry Nutrition*; Nottingham University Press: Nottingham, UK, 2009; Volume 3, ISBN 9781904761785.
17. Folch, J.; Lees, M.; Sloane Stanley, G.H. A simple method for the isolation and purification of total lipides from animal tissues. *J. Biol. Chem.* **1957**, *226*, 497–509. [CrossRef]
18. Failla, S.; Buttazzoni, L.; Zilio, D.M.; Contò, M.; Renzi, G.; Castellini, C.; Amato, M.G. An index to measure the activity attitude of broilers in extensive system. *Poult. Sci.* **2021**, *100*, 101279. [CrossRef]
19. Godbe, J.S. Nutritional value of muscle foods. In *Muscle Foods: Meat, Poultry and Seafood Technology*; Kinsman, D.M., Kotula, A.W., Breidenstein, B.C., Eds.; Chapman & Hall: London, UK; New York, NY, USA, 1994; p. 430.
20. Sorenson, A.W.; Wyse, B.W.; Wittwer, A.J.; Hansen, R.G. An Index of Nutritional Quality for a balanced diet. New help for an old problem. *J. Am. Diet. Assoc.* **1976**, *68*, 236–242. [CrossRef]
21. Simopoulos, A.P. The omega-6/omega-3 fatty acid ratio: Health implications. *Oléagineux Corps Gras Lipides* **2010**, *17*, 267–275. [CrossRef]
22. Timmis, A.; Vardas, P.; Townsend, N.; Torbica, A.; Katus, H.; De Smedt, D.; Gale, C.P.; Maggioni, A.P.; Petersen, S.E.; Huculeci, R.; et al. European Society of Cardiology: Cardiovascular disease statistics 2021. *Eur. Heart J.* **2022**, *43*, 716–799. [CrossRef]
23. Castellini, C.; Mattioli, S.; Signorini, C.; Cotozzolo, E.; Noto, D.; Moretti, E.; Brecchia, G.; Dal Bosco, A.; Belmonte, G.; Durand, T.; et al. Effect of Dietary n-3 Source on Rabbit Male Reproduction. *Oxid. Med. Cell. Longev.* **2019**, *2019*, 3279670. [CrossRef]
24. Rodríguez, M.; Rebollar, P.G.; Mattioli, S.; Castellini, C. n-3 PUFA sources (precursor/products): A review of current knowledge on rabbit. *Animals* **2019**, *9*, 806. [CrossRef]
25. Omri, B.; Chalghoumi, R.; Izzo, L.; Ritieni, A.; Lucarini, M.; Durazzo, A.; Abdouli, H.; Santini, A. Effect of dietary incorporation of linseed alone or together with tomato-red pepper mix on laying hens' egg yolk fatty acids profile and health lipid indexes. *Nutrients* **2019**, *11*, 813. [CrossRef]
26. Calder, P.C. Polyunsaturated fatty acids and inflammation. *Prostaglandins Leukot. Essent. Fat. Acids* **2006**, *75*, 197–202. [CrossRef]
27. Abrami, G.; Natiello, F.; Bronzi, P.; McKenzie, D.; Bolis, L.; Agradi, E. A comparison of highly unsaturated fatty acid levels in wild and farmed eels (*Anguilla anguilla*). *Comp. Biochem. Physiol.* **1992**, *101*, 79–81. [CrossRef]
28. Krajnovi'c-Ozretic, M.; Najdek, M.; Ozreti'c, B. Fatty acids in liver and muscle of farmed and wild sea bass (*Dicentrarchus labrax* L.). *Comp. Biochem. Physiol.* **1994**, *109*, 611–617. [CrossRef]
29. Okada, T.; Furuhashi, N.; Kuromori, Y.; Miyashita, M.; Iwata, F.; Harada, K. Plasma palmitoleic acid content and obesity in children. *Am. J. Clin. Nutr.* **2005**, *82*, 747–750. [CrossRef]

31. Mattioli, S.; Cartoni Mancinelli, A.; Cotozzolo, E.; Mancini, S.; Castellini, C.; Dal Bosco, A. Comparison of an estimated index of fatty acid metabolism and liver delta6-desaturase activity in rabbit. In Proceeding of 12th World Rabbit Congress, Nantes, France, 3–5 November 2021.
32. Kriketos, A.D.; Pan, D.A.; Sutton, J.R.; Hoh, J.F.; Baur, L.A.; Cooney, G.J.; Storlien, L.H. Relationships between muscle membrane lipids, fiber type, and enzyme activities in sedentary and exercised rats. *Am. J. Physiol.* **1995**, *269*, 1154–1162. [CrossRef]
33. Dal Bosco, A.; Mugnai, C.; Ruggeri, S.; Mattioli, S.; Castellini, C. Fatty acid composition of meat and estimated indices of lipid metabolism in different poultry genotypes reared under organic system. *Poult. Sci.* **2012**, *91*, 2039–2045. [CrossRef] [PubMed]
34. Simopoulos, A.P. Genetic variation and dietary response: Nutrigenetics/nutrigenomics. *Asia Pac. J. Clin. Nutr.* **2002**, *11*, S117–S128. [CrossRef]
35. StataCorp. *Stata Statistical Software: Release 14*; StataCorp LP.: College Station, TX, USA, 2015.
36. Mancinelli, A.C.; Di Veroli, A.; Mattioli, S.; Cruciani, G.; Dal Bosco, A.; Castellini, C. Lipid metabolism analysis in liver of different chicken genotypes and impact on nutritionally relevant polyunsaturated fatty acids of meat. *Sci. Rep.* **2022**, *12*, 1888. [CrossRef] [PubMed]
37. Dal Bosco, A.; Mugnai, C.; Mattioli, S.; Rosati, A.; Ruggeri, S.; Ranucci, D.; Castellini, C. Transfer of bioactive compounds from pasture to meat in organic free-range chickens. *Poult. Sci.* **2016**, *95*, 2464–2471. [CrossRef]
38. Wood, J.D.; Richardson, R.I.; Nute, G.R.; Fisher, A.V.; Campo, M.M.; Kasapidou, E.; Sheard, P.R.; Enser, M. Effects of fatty acids on meat quality: A review. *Meat Sci.* **2004**, *66*, 21–32. [CrossRef]
39. FAO. *Fats and Fatty Acids in Human Nutrition*; Report of an Expert Consultation; FAO: Rome, Italy, 2010; Volume 91, pp. 1–189.
40. Kang, M.J.; Shin, M.S.; Park, J.N.; Lee, S.S. The effects of polyunsaturated:saturated fatty acids ratios and peroxidisability index values of dietary fats on serum lipid profiles and hepatic enzyme activities in rats. *Br. J. Nutr.* **2005**, *94*, 526–532. [CrossRef]
41. Simopoulos, A.P. Human requirement for N-3 polyunsaturated fatty acids. *Poult. Sci.* **2000**, *79*, 961–970. [CrossRef]
42. Harris, W.S.; Von Schacky, C. The Omega-3 Index: A new risk factor for death from coronary heart disease? *Prev. Med.* **2004**, *39*, 212–220. [CrossRef]
43. Mohrhauer, H.; Christiansen, K.; Gan, M.V.; Deubig, M.; Holman, R.T. Chain elongation of linoleic acid and its inhibition by other fatty acids in vitro. *J. Biol. Chem.* **1967**, *242*, 4507–4514. [CrossRef]
44. Castellini, C.; Dal Bosco, A.; Mattioli, S.; Davidescu, M.; Corazzi, L.; MacChioni, L.; Rimoldi, S.; Terova, G. Activity, Expression, and Substrate Preference of the δ6-Desaturase in Slow- or Fast-Growing Rabbit Genotypes. *J. Agric. Food Chem.* **2016**, *64*, 792–800. [CrossRef]
45. Harnack, K.; Andersen, G.; Somoza, V. Quantitation of alpha-linolenic acid elongation to eicosapentaenoic and docosahexaenoic acid as affected by the ratio of n6/n3 fatty acids. *Nutr. Metab.* **2009**, *6*, 8. [CrossRef]
46. Mancinelli, A.C.; Silletti, E.; Mattioli, S.; Bosco, A.D.; Sebastiani, B.; Menchetti, L.; Koot, A.; van Ruth, S.; Castellini, C. Fatty acid profile, oxidative status, and content of volatile organic compounds in raw and cooked meat of different chicken strains. *Poult. Sci.* **2020**, *100*, 1273–1282. [CrossRef] [PubMed]
47. Mattioli, S.; Cartoni Mancinelli, A.; Menchetti, L.; Dal Bosco, A.; Madeo, L.; Guarino Amato, M.; Moscati, L.; Cotozzolo, E.; Ciarelli, C.; Angelucci, E.; et al. How the kinetic behavior of organic chickens affects productive performance and blood and meat oxidative status: A study of six poultry genotypes. *Poult. Sci.* **2021**, *100*, 101297. [CrossRef] [PubMed]
48. Sinanoglou, V.J.; Strati, I.F.; Bratakos, S.M.; Proestos, C.; Zoumpoulakis, P.; Miniadis-Meimaroglou, S. On the Combined Application of Iatroscan TLC-FID and GC-FID to Identify Total, Neutral, and Polar Lipids and Their Fatty Acids Extracted from Foods. *ISRN Chromatogr.* **2013**, *2013*, 859024. [CrossRef]
49. Mattioli, S.; Collodel, G.; Signorini, C.; Cotozzolo, E.; Noto, D.; Cerretani, D.; Micheli, L.; Fiaschi, A.I.; Brecchia, G.; Menchetti, L.; et al. Tissue antioxidant status and lipid peroxidation are related to dietary intake of n-3 polyunsaturated acids: A rabbit model. *Antioxidants* **2021**, *10*, 681. [CrossRef]
50. Castellini, C.; Mattioli, S.; Moretti, E.; Cotozzolo, E.; Perini, F.; Dal Bosco, A.; Signorini, C.; Noto, D.; Belmonte, G.; Lasagna, E.; et al. Expression of genes and localization of enzymes involved in polyunsaturated fatty acid synthesis in rabbit testis and epididymis. *Sci. Rep.* **2022**, *12*, 2637. [CrossRef]
51. Wołoszyn, J.; Haraf, G.; Okruszek, A.; Wereńska, M.; Goluch, Z.; Teleszko, M. Fatty acid profiles and health lipid indices in the breast muscles of local Polish goose varieties. *Poult. Sci.* **2020**, *99*, 1216–1224. [CrossRef]
52. Ghaeni, M.; Ghahfarokhi, K.N.; Zaheri, L. Fatty acids profile, atherogenic (IA) and thrombogenic (IT) health lipid indices in Leiognathusbindus and Upeneussulphureus. Journal of Marine Science. *Res. Dev.* **2013**, *3*, 1.
53. Fernandes, A.P.; Gandin, V. Selenium compounds as therapeutic agents in cancer. *Biochim. Biophys. Acta (BBA)—Gen. Subj.* **2015**, *1850*, 1642–1660. [CrossRef]
54. Wood, J.D.; Enser, M.; Fisher, A.V.; Nute, G.R.; Sheard, P.R.; Richardson, R.I.; Hughes, S.I.; Whittington, F.M. Fat deposition, fatty acid composition and meat quality: A review. *Meat Sci.* **2008**, *78*, 343–358. [CrossRef]
55. Laborde, F.L.; Mandell, I.B.; Tosh, J.J.; Wilton, J.W.; Buchanan-Smith, J.G. Breed effects on growth performance, carcass characteristics, fatty acid composition, and palatability attributes in finishing steers. *J. Anim. Sci.* **2001**, *79*, 355–365. [CrossRef]
56. Kouba, M.; Mourot, J. A review of nutritional effects on fat composition of animal products with special emphasis on n-3 polyunsaturated fatty acids. *Biochimie* **2011**, *93*, 13–17. [CrossRef] [PubMed]
57. Poureslami, R.; Raes, K.; Turchini, G.M.; Huyghebaert, G.; De Smet, S. Effect of diet, sex and age on fatty acid metabolism in broiler chickens: N-3 and n-6 PUFA. *Br. J. Nutr.* **2010**, *104*, 189–197. [CrossRef] [PubMed]

58. Boschetti, E.; Bordoni, A.; Meluzzi, A.; Castellini, C.; Dal Bosco, A.; Sirri, F. Fatty acid composition of chicken breast meat is dependent on genotype-related variation of FADS1 and FADS2 gene expression and desaturating activity. *Animal* **2016**, *10*, 700–708. [CrossRef] [PubMed]
59. Twining, C.W.; Brenna, J.T.; Hairston, N.G.; Flecker, A.S. Highly unsaturated fatty acids in nature: What we know and what we need to learn. *Oikos* **2016**, *125*, 749–760. [CrossRef]
60. Cherian, G.; Sim, J.S. Maternal dietary α-linolenic acid (18:3n-3) alters n-3 polyunsaturated fatty acid metabolism and liver enzyme activity in hatched chicks. *Poult. Sci.* **2001**, *80*, 901–905. [CrossRef]
61. Twining, C.W.; Brenna, J.T.; Lawrence, P.; Winkler, D.W.; Flecker, A.S.; Hairston, N.G. Aquatic and terrestrial resources are not nutritionally reciprocal for consumers. *Funct. Ecol.* **2019**, *33*, 2042–2052. [CrossRef]

MDPI AG
Grosspeteranlage 5
4052 Basel
Switzerland
Tel.: +41 61 683 77 34

Nutrients Editorial Office
E-mail: nutrients@mdpi.com
www.mdpi.com/journal/nutrients

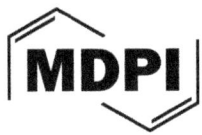

Disclaimer/Publisher's Note: The statements, opinions and data contained in all publications are solely those of the individual author(s) and contributor(s) and not of MDPI and/or the editor(s). MDPI and/or the editor(s) disclaim responsibility for any injury to people or property resulting from any ideas, methods, instructions or products referred to in the content.

www.ingramcontent.com/pod-product-compliance
Lightning Source LLC
LaVergne TN
LVHW070704100526
838202LV00013B/1030